Physical Activity for Public Health

Physical Activity for Public Health

Guest Editor

Ukadike Chris Ugbolue

MDPI

Basel • Beijing • Wuhan • Barcelona • Belgrade • Novi Sad • Cluj • Manchester

Guest Editor
Ukadike Chris Ugbolue
School of Health and Life Sciences
University of the West of Scotland
Glasgow
UK

Editorial Office
MDPI AG
Grosspeteranlage 5
4052 Basel, Switzerland

This is a reprint of the Special Issue, published open access by the journal *International Journal of Environmental Research and Public Health* (ISSN 1660-4601), freely accessible at: https://www.mdpi.com/journal/ijerph/special_issues/Phys_Act_Pub_Health.

For citation purposes, cite each article independently as indicated on the article page online and as indicated below:

Lastname, A.A.; Lastname, B.B. Article Title. *Journal Name* **Year**, *Volume Number*, Page Range.

ISBN 978-3-7258-7727-0 (Hbk)
ISBN 978-3-7258-7728-7 (PDF)
https://doi.org/10.3390/books978-3-7258-7728-7

Contents

About the Editor

Ukadike Chris Ugbolue

Ukadike Chris Ugbolue is a Lecturer in Applied Biomechanics at the University of the West of Scotland (UWS) and a member of the Sport Performance and Active Living research community. He also holds an honorary position as Associate Professor at Ningbo University, China. His research focuses on human movement analysis, sports biomechanics, and the application of emerging technologies to enhance athletic performance, rehabilitation, and health. His expertise includes motion capture, electromyography, wearable sensing technologies, and biomechanical modelling to examine movement patterns in sport, clinical, and functional settings. Dr. Ugbolue's work spans interdisciplinary areas including sports performance analysis, injury prevention, neuromuscular function, and rehabilitation technologies. A key aspect of his research involves translating biomechanical insights into practical applications that support athletes, clinicians, and rehabilitation specialists. His research has contributed to understanding movement mechanics in sports such as golf, boxing, and running, alongside broader investigations into fatigue, neuromuscular control, and musculoskeletal health. In addition to his academic research, Dr. Ugbolue is actively engaged in innovation and translational research. He is currently developing assistive technologies, including a rehabilitation glove designed to support stroke recovery and improve upper-limb function. This work integrates biomechanics, wearable technology, and clinical rehabilitation principles to develop practical solutions for patient care. Dr. Ugbolue has authored and co-authored numerous peer-reviewed publications in biomechanics, sports science, and bioengineering, and collaborates with international researchers and industry partners. Through his research, teaching, and editorial activities, he contributes to advancing the understanding of human movement and technology-driven approaches to sport performance and rehabilitation.

Preface

Physical activity remains one of the most powerful yet underutilized tools for protecting and enhancing public health. Recent global disruptions, particularly the COVID 19 pandemic, have exposed the profound physical, psychological, and social consequences of prolonged inactivity across all age groups. These challenges have reinforced the need for evidence based strategies that promote active lifestyles, equitable access to movement opportunities, and accurate methods for assessing physical activity and health.

This Special Issue brings together interdisciplinary research that advances our understanding of physical activity from behavioural, physiological, biomechanical, and socioecological perspectives. By bridging scientific insight with real world application, the contributions collectively aim to inform policy, guide practice, and support sustainable public health interventions across diverse populations and settings.

Ukadike Chris Ugbolue
Guest Editor

International Journal of
Environmental Research and Public Health

MDPI

Article

Comparing the activPAL CREA and GHLA Algorithms for the Classification of Postures and Activity in Free-Living Children

Duncan S. Buchan * and Ukadike C. Ugbolue

Division of Sport and Exercise, School of Health and Life Sciences, University of the West of Scotland, Lanarkshire Campus, Scotland G72 0LH, UK
* Correspondence: duncan.buchan@uws.ac.uk

Abstract: The activPAL accelerometer has been used extensively in research to assess sedentary behaviour (SB) and physical activity (PA) outcomes. The aim of this study was to assess the comparability of PA and SB outcomes from two automated algorithms (CREA and GHLA) applied to the activPAL accelerometer. One hundred and twenty participants aged 8–12 years wore an activPAL accelerometer on their right thigh continuously for seven days on two occasions, providing valid data from 1058 days. The PALbatch software downloaded the data after applying the CREA and GHLA (latest) algorithms. The comparability of the algorithms were assessed using the mean absolute percent error (MAPE), intra-class correlation coefficients (ICC), and equivalence testing. Comparisons for daily wear time, primary lying, sitting and standing time, sedentary and stepping time, upright time, total number of steps, sit–stand transitions and stepping time $\leq$ 1 min revealed mainly small MAPE ($\leq$2%), excellent ICCs (lower bound 95% CI $\geq$ 0.97), and equivalent outcomes. Time spent in sitting bouts > 60 min and stepping bouts > 5 min were not equivalent with the absolute zone needed to reach equivalence ($\geq$7%). Comparable outcomes were provided for wear time and postural outcomes using the CREA or GHLA algorithms, but not for time spent in sitting bouts > 60 min and stepping bouts > 5 min.

Keywords: agreement; equivalence; free-living; sedentary behaviour; accelerometry

1. Introduction

Leading a physically active lifestyle provides several health-related benefits in physical and mental health, cognitive function, and academic outcomes [1]. Yet in adolescents aged between 11–17 years, recent estimates suggest that 81% of adolescents are insufficiently active, with significant differences in prevalence estimates evident between genders and countries [2]. Alongside physical activity (PA), it is important to consider the role of sedentary behaviour in the health of children and adolescents. Sedentary behaviour (SB) can be defined "as any waking behaviour characterized by an energy expenditure $\leq$ 1.5 metabolic equivalents, while in a sitting, reclining, or lying position" [3]. In adults, excessive SB is associated with morbidity and all-cause mortality [4,5]. Although there is currently insufficient evidence available to establish whether there is a dose–response relationship between time spent sedentary and adverse health outcomes in children and adolescents, current understanding suggests that less time spent sedentary will be better for health outcomes [6]. This is reflected in current recommendations for children and adolescents offered by the World Health Organisation to limit the amount of time spent sedentary [1] and, internationally, through public health guidelines [7–9]. Given the importance given to reducing SB, accurate monitoring of this behaviour is essential.

The gold standard device for the objective measurement of SB is the thigh-worn activPAL (PAL Technologies Ltd., Glasgow, UK) [10]. Wearing the activPAL on the thigh enables users to differentiate between seated and upright postures as well as stationary and non-stationary activity, which can then be used to estimate time spent in sedentary and non-sedentary activities [11]. The validity of the activPAL device is well established, demonstrating a sensitivity of 96% to 98% for correctly identifying steps and posture against direct observation in laboratory settings [12,13]. Precise estimates of steps and posture from the activPAL has also been observed in free-living settings and has shown a sensitivity to reductions in sitting time [14]. Prior to late 2018, users only had the option of using activPAL's proprietary VANE (standard) classification algorithm, which calculates time spent sitting, standing, and stepping as well as posture transitions. As the activPAL is often encouraged to be worn continuously throughout the monitoring period, the inability of the VANE algorithm to identify periods of non-wear time or time in bed can be problematic. Indeed, errors in the estimates of sedentary time can occur when time in bed is classified as sedentary time and when true sedentary time (i.e., lying down during the day) is misclassified as time in bed [15]. Equally, inflated estimates of sedentary time could occur when true non-wear time is not identified and misclassified as awake wear time. To overcome the limitations of the VANE algorithm, participants are requested to complete a log of non-wear times and in-out of bed times [11]. With this increased participant burden, however, logs are often incomplete, which raises the questions of how missing data are dealt with (if not described) and/or the inability to compare study findings if different methods are used.

With the full release of an enhanced "CREA" algorithm by the manufacturers of activPAL (PAL Technologies Ltd.) in mid 2019, users now have the ability to report on additional metrics to those provided by the VANE algorithm including non-wear time, time in bed, lying, cycling, and seated transport. The appeal for researchers being able to document time spent in different behaviours (i.e., sleep, PA, and SB) and explore their relationships with indicators of health is obvious [1,7]. Despite the appeal of activPAL's CREA algorithm, limited studies have examined the equivalence of this algorithm against sleep logs or other available algorithms. In adults, Courtney et al. [16] reported that the CREA algorithm was equivalent to self-reported logs for time going to bed, but not for wake time, whereas Leister et al. [17] reported a lack of equivalence between self-reported logs and the CREA algorithm for sleep time (i.e., difference between bedtime and wake time). While these two studies focused on the accuracy of the time in and out of bed estimates of the CREA algorithm, others have compared the comparability of activity and posture outcomes provided by the VANE and CREA algorithms for adults [18]. In this study, the authors found equivalent estimates between the two activPAL algorithms for steps, activity score, stepping time, bouts of stepping, and upright time, but non-equivalent estimates for posture transitions and bouts of sitting.

Although these recent studies have extended our understanding of the comparability of the CREA algorithm with self-reported logs and other algorithms [16–18], they all involved adults. To the best of our knowledge, only one study has explored the agreement between self-reported diary and the CREA algorithm in children and adolescents [15]. Here, the authors reported the agreement between participant diaries and the CREA algorithm in a small sample of youths (n = 20) and found an overall accuracy of 90% for accurately classifying time out of bed. Despite also reporting non-significant differences between the CREA algorithm and participant diaries for several additional outcomes including out-of-bed time, total sedentary time, mean bout duration, number of breaks, etc., these findings included both adults and youth. Moreover, only a limited number of outcomes were reported in this study [15]. Given the recently proposed standardized Core Research Outcomes for Sedentary Behaviour research [19], it is important that future SB research begins to report these outcomes in order to enhance the accumulation of pooled evidence and opportunities for meta-analyses.

Continued advances in the assessment of SB and PA mean that software updates and new algorithms are routinely developed by manufacturers and are available for the user. In May 2022, a new updated "GHLA" algorithm was added to the activPAL software [20]. Other than stating that the GHLA algorithm is an updated version of the CREA algorithm with sensor calibration, no other information is provided. It is unclear therefore whether comparable outcomes are provided from the CREA and GHLA algorithms. To the best of our knowledge, no study has compared outputs from activPAL's CREA and GHLA algorithms. Therefore, the purpose of this study is to compare activity and posture outcomes from the CREA and GHLA algorithms in free-living children and to establish which outcomes are equivalent.

2. Materials and Methods

The data used for the current study came from a previous study that explored the feasibility and acceptability of a classroom-based Active Breaks intervention [21]. Ethical approval for the study was received from the University of the West of Scotland with baseline measures undertaken in October 2018. Briefly, 146 child participants aged 8–12 years attending eight primary schools in North Lanarkshire, Scotland, volunteered to participate and provided baseline measures. Following the end of the intervention 6 weeks later, 117 participants completed the same baseline measures as described below.

Participants' stature and mass were measured using a calibrated scale (Seca Digital Scales, Seca Ltd., Birmingham, UK) and stadiometer (Seca Stadiometer, Seca Ltd., Birmingham, UK), respectively, without shoes and in light clothing. Participants were asked to wear the activPAL Micro4 (PAL Technologies Ltd., Glasgow, UK; herein activPAL) accelerometer. The activPAL was placed into a nitril sleeve fitted to each participant on the anterior midline of their right thigh using hypoallergenic Hypafix (BSN Medical, Hull, UK) dressings. All participants were encouraged to wear the device at all times for 7 days. Prior to dissemination, each device was synchronized with Greenwich Mean Time and initialized using the manufacturers proprietary software (activPAL Professional, v7.2.28) to start data collection at 06:30 a.m. on the following day at 20 Hz. A valid day of wear time included $\geq$20 h of wear time, no data errors identified by the software, and 1440 min of recording time.

2.1. Data Processing

Upon the return of the activPAL devices, time- and date-stamped activPAL data files were immediately downloaded using the manufacturer proprietary software (activPAL Professional, v7.2.28) for later processing. Using the manufacturers proprietary software (PALbatch v8.11.1.36), the participant data were averaged across valid days using activPAL's CREA algorithm (version 1.3) to provide the following outcomes, including wear time, valid wear time days, sedentary time, sitting time, stepping time, standing time, upright time, total number of steps, the number of sit–stand transitions, and primary lying. Primary lying is used by the CREA and GHLA (version 2.2) algorithms to estimate time spent sleeping. Alongside these measures, several additional outcomes were provided including time spent in sitting bouts longer than 30 and 60 min, and stepping time for the following durations of $\leq$1 min, >1 min to $\leq$5 min, >5 min to $\leq$10 min, >10 min to $\leq$20 min, and >20 min. The following outcomes were also provided from PALbatch when using the GHLA algorithm. To ensure consistency, the default of 10 s was used to classify the minimum non-upright and upright periods for both algorithms. Finally, outcomes provided by both algorithms were aligned for each participant.

2.2. Statistical Analysis

Participant data were averaged across valid days and separately at each data collection point. Once valid days were identified from the algorithms, the daily validation and daily summary outcome spreadsheets were downloaded to confirm the same valid days were identified by both algorithms. In addition, these spreadsheets were used to confirm no data errors were evident and that 1440 min of recording time was captured. Agreement between algorithms for each outcome was examined using mean percent error (MPE), mean absolute percent error (MAPE), intraclass correlation coefficients (ICC, two-way mixed effects, single measures, absolute agreement) with 95% confidence intervals (CI), equivalence tests and Bland–Altman plots as recommended [22]. MPE was provided to indicate the direction and magnitude of error at a group-level, whereas the MAPE provided an indicator of individual agreement by accounting for each participant's error. To aid interpretations, a threshold of <5% for MPE was used to consider the practical relevance of the agreement between outcomes from each algorithm [23], whereas an MAPE of <3% denoted excellent agreement, as used elsewhere [18]. Values < 0.5, 0.5–0.75, 0.75–0.9, and >0.90 were indicative of poor, moderate, good, and excellent agreement, respectively, based on the lower bound 95%CI of the ICC estimate [24]. Finally, Bland–Altman plots were used to assess the agreement in outcomes between algorithms and to visualize the magnitude of differences [25].

The pairwise 95% equivalence tests were used to explore whether the 95% CI of the outcome mean from one algorithm fell within the proposed equivalence zone for each outcome [26]. Although applying a 10% equivalence zone is common in similar studies [27,28], such an approach can be problematic. For instance, the use of a 10% zone can be strict when values are highly variable and smaller but lax when values are very high and across a narrow range of values [29]. Therefore, the absolute equivalence zone needed to reach equivalence is provided alongside the relative equivalence zone presented as a proportion of the SD [30]. To aid interpretations, a strict threshold of 3%, indicative of excellent agreement between algorithms, was used to aid interpretations of the absolute equivalence zone [26]. All equivalence testing was undertaken twice. In the first instance, outcomes from the CREA algorithm were used as the reference method followed by outcomes provided by the GHLA algorithm. Statistical analyses were undertaken using IBM SPSS statistical software for Windows version 25 (IBM, Armonk, NY, USA), whereas equivalence testing was undertaken in Minitab (v17) with alpha set at 0.05.

3. Results

Of the 263 accelerometer data files that could have been provided, eight participants withdrew consent and four were removed by their teacher (n = 24), five participants failed to return their activPAL device, and one activPAL device suffered a battery malfunction shortly after distribution (n = 30). This left 233 accelerometer files from participants (n = 143) available for the subsequent analysis. Fifteen accelerometer files were further removed as they failed to provide $\geq$20 h of wear time for $\geq$1 day. This left 218 accelerometer files from 120 participants (68 girls; mean age: 10.4 $\pm$ 0.8 years) providing 1058 valid days, with an average of 4.9 valid days, to be processed in the subsequent analysis. The findings of the MPE, MAPE, and ICCs are provided in Table 1.

The findings from the MPE revealed that the group level differences for outcomes processed using the CREA and GHLA algorithms were all less than <5%. Findings from the MAPE revealed that individual level differences were mostly <3%, denoting excellent agreement in these outcomes between algorithms. Nonetheless, large MAPE values were evident for sitting bouts and stepping time > 5 to 10 min. Agreement from the ICCs were found to be excellent for all outcomes apart from stepping time > 5 to 10 min which demonstrated good agreement between the algorithms.

The findings from the equivalency analysis are displayed in Figure 1. The relative zone needed to reach equivalence for almost all outcomes was $\leq$0.1 SDs. Although the relative zone for total daily wear-time was 0.5 SDs, this was likely a consequence of the very small SD for this outcome. The absolute zone needed to reach equivalence was in the main $\leq$ 3%, apart from time spent in sitting bouts > 60 min, stepping time > 5 to 10 min, and stepping time > 10 to 20 min, which demonstrated absolute equivalence zones ranging from 7% to 9%.

To examine the differences in these outcomes in more detail, Bland–Altman plots were undertaken with the findings displayed in Figure 2. The mean bias between the CREA and GHLA algorithms for time spent in sitting bouts > 60 min was 1.3 min with limits of agreement (LoA) of −31 to 33 min. The mean bias for stepping time > 5 to 10 min was 0.1 min with LoA of −9.4 to 9.5 min, whereas the mean bias for stepping time > 10 to 20 min was 0.2 min with LoA of −1.6 to 2.0 min.

Table 1. Comparison of outcomes provided from the CREA and GHLA algorithms.

Domain & Reporting Statistic	Outcome	CREA Algorithm	GHLA Algorithm	MPE ± SD	MAPE ± SD	ICC (95% CI)
Device Wear Time	Daily wear time (h/d)	23.9 ± 0.5	23.9 ± 0.5	−0.01 ± 0.37	0.02 ± 0.20	0.99 (0.99, 0.99)
	Valid wear time days	4.9 ± 1.5	4.9 ± 1.5	−0.09 ± 0.33	0.40 ± 3.45	0.99 (0.99, 0.99)
Posture Outcomes	Primary lying (min/d)	606.6 ± 56.1	605.6 ± 57.1	0.16 ± 1.86	0.19 ± 1.50	0.99 (0.99, 0.99)
	Sedentary time (min/d)	515.6 ± 73.1	514.9 ± 77.7	0.13 ± 5.97	1.35 ± 2.57	0.99 (0.99, 0.99)
	Sitting time (min/d)	347.3 ± 77.6	351.3 ± 78.8	−1.13 ± 1.50	3.76 ± 6.14	0.98 (0.97, 0.98)
	Stepping time (min/d)	132.7 ± 33.1	131.4 ± 33.1	1.00 ± 0.16	1.28 ± 1.87	0.99 (0.99, 0.99)
	Standing time (min/d)	175.6 ± 50.1	179.8 ± 51.2	−2.22 ± 4.24	3.43 ± 2.94	0.98 (0.97, 0.99)
	Upright time (min/d)	308.3 ± 69.8	311.1 ± 71.9	−0.86 ± 2.94	1.96 ± 2.02	0.99 (0.98, 0.99)
	Total number of steps	10,587.2 ± 2780.7	10,481.6 ± 2784.9	1.01 ± 0.17	1.25 ± 2.00	0.99 (0.99, 0.99)
Sitting bouts	Sit–stand transitions (number/d)	92 ± 22	92 ± 22	−0.22 ± 0.07	1.67 ± 2.01	0.99 (0.99, 0.99)
	Time (min) spent in sitting bouts > 30 min	92.9 ± 66.3	92.8 ± 66.3	−0.70 ± 3.22	7.92 ± 16.92	0.94 (0.93, 0.96)
	Time (min) spent in sitting bouts > 60 min	26.1 ± 44.3	25.7 ± 45.4	3.21 ± 0.96 *	10.32 ± 29.37	0.96 (0.95, 0.97)
Stepping bouts	Stepping time (min) ≤ 1 min	82.6 ± 19.6	82.2 ± 19.6	0.41 ± 0.63	1.23 ± 1.85	0.99 (0.99, 0.99)
	Stepping time (min) > 1 to 5 min	39.1 ± 14.8	38.3 ± 15.1	1.61 ± 1.22	3.46 ± 4.57	0.99 (0.99, 0.99)
	Stepping time (min) > 5 to 10 min	7.8 ± 7.3	7.8 ± 6.9	2.18 ± 8.76 †	142.3 ± 287.1	0.78 (0.72, 0.83)
	Stepping time (min) > 10 to 20 min	3.0 ± 4.6	2.8 ± 4.5	1.98 ± 4.50 ‡	2.58 ± 9.92	0.98 (0.97, 0.98)
	Stepping time (min) > 20 min	0.3 ± 1.4	0.3 ± 1.4	0.26 ± 0.16	0.02 ± 0.31	0.97 (0.96, 0.98)

MPE = mean percent error; MAPE = mean absolute percent error; ICC = interclass correlation coefficient. * n = 201 as 17 files were removed as one algorithm provided data (CREA = 12; GHLA = 5) and the other did not. † n = 173 as 45 files were removed as one algorithm provided data (CREA = 24; GHLA = 21) and the other did not. ‡ n = 213 as 5 files were removed as one algorithm provided data (CREA = 4; GHLA = 1) and the other did not.

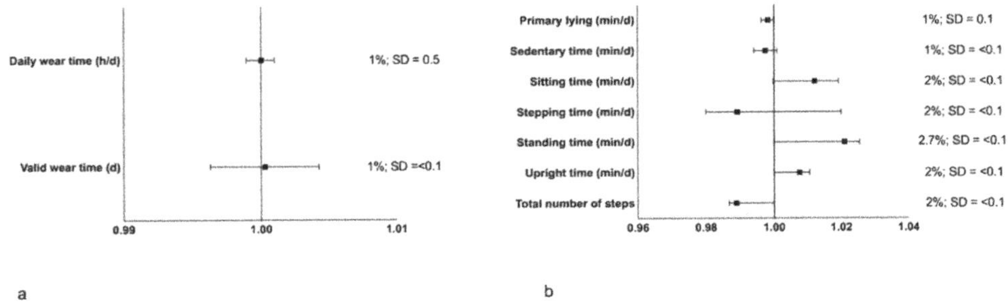

Figure 1. *Cont.*

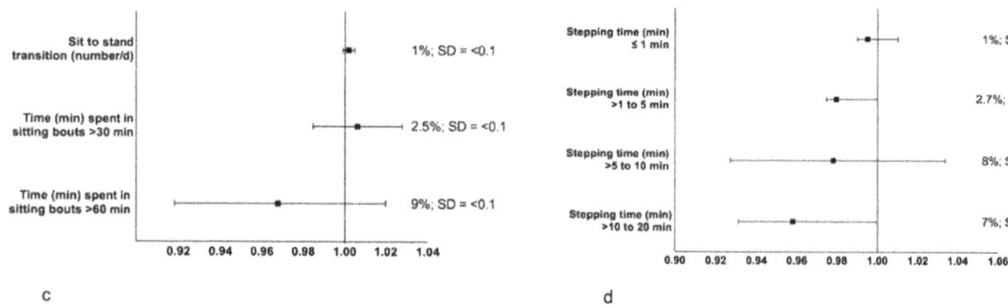

Figure 1. Equivalence of outcomes provided from the CREA and GHLA algorithms for (**a**) device wear time, (**b**) posture outcomes, (**c**) sitting bouts, and (**d**) stepping bouts. The solid squares represent the mean difference, whereas the horizontal lines show the 95% CI. To the right of each figure, the absolute zone needed to reach equivalence is provided as a %, alongside the zone necessary to achieve equivalence as a proportion of the SD. Outcomes from the CREA algorithm were used as the reference in all analyses and are presented here. All equivalence testing was repeated using the GHLA algorithm outcomes as the reference and provided identical results (not presented). An equivalence test not undertaken for stepping time > 20 min as only 13 cases provided values with the remaining comparisons all being zeros.

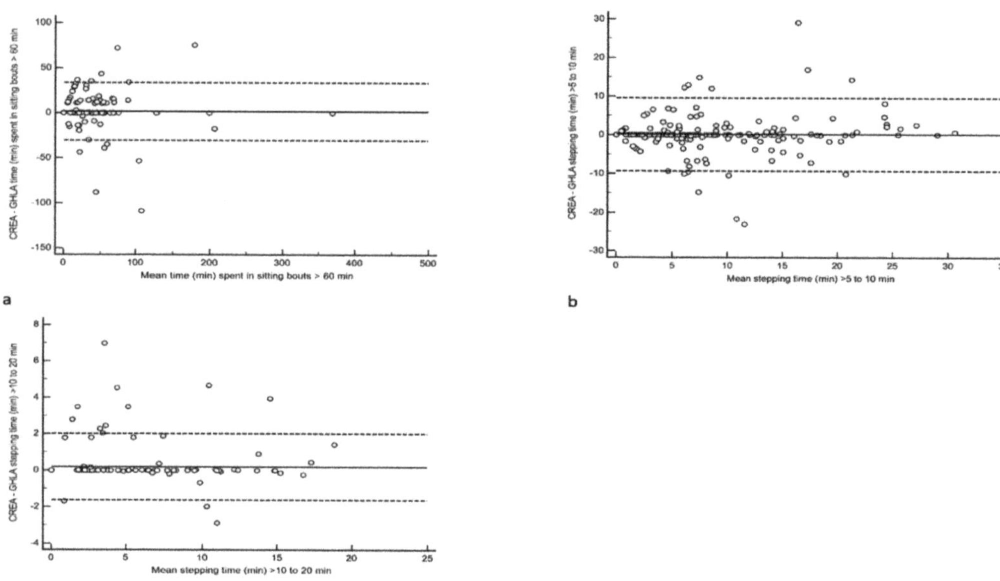

Figure 2. Bland–Altman plots comparing the outcomes provided from the CREA and GHLA algorithms for (**a**) time (min) spent in sitting bouts > 60 min, (**b**) stepping time (min) > 5 to 10 min, and (**c**) stepping time (min) > 10 to 20 min.

4. Discussion

The aim of this study was to compare the comparability of outcomes collected from activPAL devices using PAL Technologies CREA and GHLA algorithms. Excellent agreement and equivalence of outcomes were evident for measures of daily wear time and posture outcomes. At a group level, the differences for daily wear time, valid days, and most postural outcomes (primary lying, sedentary time, sitting time, stepping time, upright time, and total number of steps) were ≤1%. These findings suggest that near identical values are provided for these outcomes when calculated by the CREA and GHLA algorithms at the group level. For the number of sit–stand transitions, time spent in sitting bouts > 30 min, stepping time $\leq$ 1 min, >1 to 5 min, and >20 min, near identical values were provided by the CREA and GHLA algorithms, demonstrating excellent comparability. Yet, the high absolute zone needed to reach equivalence for time spent in sitting bouts > 60 min and stepping time > 5 to 10 min and 10 to 20 min suggest caution is warranted if looking to compare these outcomes when processed using different algorithms. These findings suggest that device wear time and postural outcomes calculated using the CREA and GHLA algorithms are comparable and may facilitate study comparisons. Conversely, caution is advised when comparing time spent in sitting bouts > 60 min and bouts of stepping time > 5 min across studies if calculated using different algorithms.

To the best of our knowledge, this is the first study to compare outcomes from the CREA and GHLA algorithms. As such, it is difficult to draw comparisons between our findings and those previously published. In this study, poor agreement and a lack of equivalence was evident between algorithms for time spent in sitting bouts > 60 min. This is similar to a previous study, albeit involving older adults, that compared outcomes from the VANE and CREA algorithms [18]. Here Montoye et al., (2022) reported an MPE of 531% and a MAPE of 141% for time spent in sitting bouts > 60 min with the VANE algorithm providing the larger values. Similar MPE and MAPE values were also observed when comparing overall sitting time. The lack of comparability noted by the authors for overall sitting time is unsurprising given that the VANE algorithm combines sitting, lying down, and non-wear time into a single metric, whereas the CREA algorithm provides these as separate outcomes. In an attempt to prove a fairer comparison for sitting time, an adjusted sitting time outcome was calculated for the CREA algorithm by summing the overall sitting + primary lying + secondary lying + non-wear. The adjusted sitting time outcome subsequently demonstrated good agreement and equivalence between algorithms. Unfortunately, similar adjustments were not reported for time spent in sitting bouts > 60 min. In our study, overall sitting time demonstrated good comparability between the CREA and GHLA algorithms, which suggests that both algorithms calculate this outcome in a similar way.

An outcome that can affect time sitting is the number of transitions from a sedentary to upright posture, and vice versa. In the study by Montoye et al. (2022), poor comparability was evident between the number of sedentary to upright transitions (and vice versa) between the VANE and CREA algorithms. With the cause of differences in nearly all participant files being a result of the VANE algorithm identifying more transitions than the GHLA algorithm. In this study, excellent comparability was evident in the number of sit–stand transitions identified by the algorithms, with near identical values provided. Similar findings were also evident for the number of stand–sit transitions (data not reported). Therefore, our findings suggest that the poor comparability of time spent in sitting bouts > 60 min was not a consequence of how the algorithms calculated posture transitions or overall sitting time. When exploring the data in more detail, 17 files had to be removed from the MPE and MAPE analysis as one algorithm provided data (CREA = 12; GHLA = 5) when the other algorithm did not. From the outliers identified within the B&A plot (Figure 2a), most of the outliers were a result of the GHLA algorithm providing a higher value than the CREA algorithm, with differences ranging from 109%–202%.

When using the batch processing software PALbatch, both the CREA and GHLA algorithms provided details of accelerometer alignment with a value of 100%, indicative of the device being 100% aligned, whereas 50% alignment is indicative of a 45-degree angle offset [31]. None of the outlier files were perfectly aligned with differences ranging from 0% to 6%, and in all cases the alignment from CREA was greater than that from GHLA. For the three outliers that had the greatest differences in alignment (4%, 5%, and 6%), differences in time spent in sitting bouts > 60 min were 202%, 109%, and 158%, respectively. It is worth noting, nonetheless, that other outliers that had differences in alignment of 0% and 2% had differences of 113% and 177%, respectively. In the absence of an agreed consensus on how to deal with files that are not perfectly aligned, we examined the effect of excluding those files (n = 24) that displayed ≥3% differences in alignment. We found that MPE reduced slightly to <3%, whereas MAPE was reduced to 8.2%. Similar positive effects were also seen on the absolute zone needed to reach equivalence. Future work should therefore consider the impact of device alignment on outcomes, and whether there is a need to establish a consensus on the degree of alignment needed to warrant the inclusion of files in subsequent analyses. Finally, the alignment of all files from CREA was slightly greater than that from GHLA (95.8% vs. 94.6%, respectively) with both MPE and MAPE below 1.5%.

We also observed poor comparability for stepping time in bouts that were longer than 5 min. Despite excellent agreement at the group level for stepping time in bouts > 5 to 10 min, the MAPE was high at 142%. This is likely a consequence of the occasional outlier as seen from the B&A plot in Figure 2b, which resulted in wide SDs. Furthermore, time spent stepping in bouts > 5 to 10 min was generally low and on average less than 8 min, regardless of the algorithm, with no participant spending more than 31 min in stepping bouts > 5 to 10 min. There were also a considerable number of files that had to be removed from the analysis for this outcome (n = 45), as on occasion, one algorithm provided data (CREA = 24; GHLA = 21) and the other did not. Absolute differences between algorithms can thus appear substantial, when in fact the differences are only a matter of minutes. When examining those files that demonstrated a MAPE difference greater than 100% (n = 31, range 104% to 2738%), GHLA provided higher values than CREA for all comparisons. With the difference in alignment between these 31 files being less than 0.5%, these findings suggest that there are differences in how these two algorithms calculate stepping time longer than 5 min. Although we found excellent agreement for the number of sit–stand transitions (and vice versa) and overall stepping time, our findings do appear to suggest that algorithms calculate stepping bouts differently.

The importance of breaking up prolonged bouts of SB for health are reflected in current recommendations for children and adolescents that recognize the benefits of reducing the quantity of SB [1,7–9]. As our understanding of the most effective means of breaking up SB to induce health benefits evolves [32,33], it is important that valid measures of this behaviour are available. As this study used previously collected data however, we were unable to establish which algorithm is more accurate for measuring time spent in sitting and stepping bouts. Further work should therefore explore the validity of CREA and GHLA and establish which is more accurate for identifying time spent in sitting and stepping bouts across different durations.

The strengths of this study include the large sample of children that provided, on average, five free-living days of valid wear time to be analysed. The use of several standardized approaches to explore the comparability of outcomes provided detailed comparisons, allowing future studies to compare their findings to ours. Furthermore, being able to download data from one device removed the need for additional devices and concerns over different device placements when comparing outcomes. There were some limitations to the study, including the lack of criterion measure to establish which algorithm was the most accurate for measuring outcomes where poor agreement was evident. Finally, the sample was recruited from one geographical area and comprised of children of a narrow age range, which may limit the generalizability of our findings to younger children and adolescents.

5. Conclusions

In conclusion, our findings suggest that comparable findings were evident for outcomes reporting daily wear time, posture, transitions between sedentary and upright postures, as well as time spent in sitting bouts > 30 min and stepping time in bouts lasting less than 5 min when calculated using PAL Technologies CREA and GHLA algorithms. These findings suggest that these outcomes may be compared across studies that have used either of these algorithms. Caution is advised if looking to compare time spent in sitting bouts > 60 min and stepping time > 5 to 10 min and 10 to 20 min if calculated using the

CREA and GHLA algorithms. Future work should thus provide details of the algorithm used to calculate the outcomes from the activPAL device to facilitate study comparisons.

Author Contributions: D.S.B.: Conceptualization, design, formal analysis, and writing—original draft. U.C.U.: Writing—review and editing. All authors have read and agreed to the published version of the manuscript.

Funding: This research received no external funding.

Institutional Review Board Statement: The study was conducted according to institutional ethical requirements, and approval for data security and handling was obtained from the University of the West of Scotland (application 5147-3767) and in accordance with the latest revision of the Declaration of Helsinki.

Informed Consent Statement: Informed consent was obtained from all subjects and guardians involved in the study.

Data Availability Statement: The data presented in this study are available upon reasonable request from the corresponding author.

Conflicts of Interest: The authors declare no conflict of interest.

References

1. World Health Organization. *Guidelines on Physical Activity and Sedentary Behaviour*; World Health Organization: Geneva, Switzerland, 2020.
2. Guthold, R.; Stevens, G.A.; Riley, L.M.; Bull, F.C. Global Trends in Insufficient Physical Activity among Adolescents: A Pooled Analysis of 298 Population-Based Surveys with 1.6 Million Participants. *Lancet Child Adolesc. Health* **2020**, *4*, 23–35. [CrossRef] [PubMed]
3. Tremblay, M.S.; Aubert, S.; Barnes, J.D.; Saunders, T.J.; Carson, V.; Latimer-Cheung, A.E.; Chastin, S.F.M.; Altenburg, T.M.; Chinapaw, M.J.M. Sedentary Behavior Research Network (SBRN)–Terminology Consensus Project Process and Outcome. *Int. J. Behav. Nutr. Phys. Act.* **2017**, *14*, 75. [CrossRef] [PubMed]
4. Biswas, A.; Oh, P.I.; Faulkner, G.E.; Bajaj, R.R.; Silver, M.A.; Mitchell, M.S.; Alter, D.A. Sedentary Time and Its Association with Risk for Disease Incidence, Mortality, and Hospitalization in Adults: A Systematic Review and Meta-Analysis. *Ann. Intern. Med.* **2015**, *162*, 123–132. [CrossRef] [PubMed]
5. Patterson, R.; McNamara, E.; Tainio, M.; de Sá, T.H.; Smith, A.D.; Sharp, S.J.; Edwards, P.; Woodcock, J.; Brage, S.; Wijndaele, K. Sedentary Behaviour and Risk of All-Cause, Cardiovascular and Cancer Mortality, and Incident Type 2 Diabetes: A Systematic Review and Dose Response Meta-Analysis. *Eur. J. Epidemiol.* **2018**, *33*, 811–829. [CrossRef] [PubMed]
6. Chaput, J.-P.; Willumsen, J.; Bull, F.; Chou, R.; Ekelund, U.; Firth, J.; Jago, R.; Ortega, F.B.; Katzmarzyk, P.T. 2020 WHO Guidelines on Physical Activity and Sedentary Behaviour for Children and Adolescents Aged 5–17 Years: Summary of the Evidence. *Int. J. Behav. Nutr. Phys. Act.* **2020**, *17*, 141. [CrossRef] [PubMed]
7. Tremblay, M.S.; Carson, V.; Chaput, J.-P.; Connor Gorber, S.; Dinh, T.; Duggan, M.; Faulkner, G.; Gray, C.E.; Gruber, R.; Janson, K.; et al. Canadian 24-Hour Movement Guidelines for Children and Youth: An Integration of Physical Activity, Sedentary Behaviour, and Sleep. *Appl. Physiol. Nutr. Metab.* **2016**, *41*, S311–S327. [CrossRef]
8. Department of Health and Social Care. UK Chief Medical Officers' Physical Activity Guidelines. 2019, 66p. Available online: https://assets.publishing.service.gov.uk/government/uploads/system/uploads/attachment_data/file/832868/ukchief-medical-officers-physical-activity-guidelines.pdf (accessed on 10 September 2022).
9. Australian Government. Physical Activity and Exercise Guidelines for All Australians. Available online: https://www.health.gov.au/health-topics/physical-activity-and-exercise/physical-activity-and-exercise-guidelines-for-all-australians (accessed on 1 September 2022).
10. Chastin, S.F.M.; Dontje, M.L.; Skelton, D.A.; Čukić, I.; Shaw, R.J.; Gill, J.M.R.; Greig, C.A.; Gale, C.R.; Deary, I.J.; Der, G.; et al. Systematic Comparative Validation of Self-Report Measures of Sedentary Time against an Objective Measure of Postural Sitting (ActivPAL). *Int. J. Behav. Nutr. Phys. Act.* **2018**, *15*, 21. [CrossRef]
11. Edwardson, C.L.; Winkler, E.A.H.; Bodicoat, D.H.; Yates, T.; Davies, M.J.; Dunstan, D.W.; Healy, G.N. Considerations When Using the ActivPAL Monitor in Field-Based Research with Adult Populations. *J. Sport Health Sci.* **2017**, *6*, 162–178. [CrossRef]
12. Grant, P.M.; Ryan, C.G.; Tigbe, W.W.; Granat, M.H. The Validation of a Novel Activity Monitor in the Measurement of Posture and Motion during Everyday Activities. *Br. J. Sports Med.* **2006**, *40*, 992–997. [CrossRef]
13. Sellers, C.; Dall, P.; Grant, M.; Stansfield, B. Validity and Reliability of the ActivPAL3 for Measuring Posture and Stepping in Adults and Young People. *Gait Posture* **2016**, *43*, 42–47. [CrossRef]
14. Kozey-Keadle, S.; Libertine, A.; Lyden, K.; Staudenmayer, J.; Freedson, P.S. Validation of Wearable Monitors for Assessing Sedentary Behavior. *Med. Sci. Sports Exerc.* **2011**, *43*, 1561–1567. [CrossRef]

15. Carlson, J.A.; Tuz-Zahra, F.; Bellettiere, J.; Ridgers, N.D.; Steel, C.; Bejarano, C.; LaCroix, A.Z.; Rosenberg, D.E.; Greenwood-Hickman, M.A.; Jankowska, M.M.; et al. Validity of Two Awake Wear-Time Classification Algorithms for ActivPAL in Youth, Adults, and Older Adults. *J. Meas. Phys. Behav.* **2021**, *4*, 151–162. [CrossRef] [PubMed]
16. Courtney, J.B.; Nuss, K.; Lyden, K.; Harrall, K.K.; Glueck, D.H.; Villalobos, A.; Hamman, R.F.; Hebert, J.R.; Hurley, T.G.; Leiferman, J.; et al. Comparing the ActivPAL Software's Primary Time in Bed Algorithm against Self-Report and van Der Berg's Algorithm. *Meas. Phys. Educ. Exerc. Sci.* **2021**, *25*, 212–226. [CrossRef]
17. Leister, K.R.; Garay, J.; Barreira, T. Validity of a Novel Algorithm to Detect Bedtime, Wake Time, and Sleep Time in Adults. *J. Meas. Phys. Behav.* **2022**, *5*, 76–84. Available online: https://journals.humankinetics.com/view/journals/jmpb/5/2/article-p76.xml (accessed on 5 September 2022). [CrossRef]
18. Montoye, A.H.K.; Vondrasek, J.D.; Neph, S.E.; Basu, N.; Paul, L.; Bachmair, E.-M.; Stefanov, K.; Gray, S.R. Comparison of the ActivPAL CREA and VANE Algorithms for Characterization of Posture and Activity in Free-Living Adults. *J. Meas. Phys. Behav.* **2022**, *5*, 49–57. [CrossRef]
19. Curran, F.; Dowd, K.P.; Peiris, C.L.; van der Ploeg, H.P.; Tremblay, M.S.; O'Donoghue, G. A Standardised Core Outcome Set for Measurement and Reporting Sedentary Behaviour Interventional Research: The CROSBI Consensus Study. *Int. J. Environ. Res. Public. Health* **2022**, *19*, 9666. [CrossRef] [PubMed]
20. PAL Technologies Version History–PAL Knowledge Base. Available online: https://kb.palt.com/articles/palanalysis-version-history/ (accessed on 6 September 2022).
21. McLellan, G.; Arthur, R.; Donnelly, S.; Bakshi, A.; Fairclough, S.J.; Taylor, S.L.; Buchan, D.S. Feasibility and Acceptability of a Classroom-Based Active Breaks Intervention for 8–12-Year Old Children. *Res. Q. Exerc. Sport* **2021**, *93*, 813–824. [CrossRef]
22. DeShaw, K.J.; Ellingson, L.; Bai, Y.; Lansing, J.; Perez, M.; Welk, G. Methods for Activity Monitor Validation Studies: An Example with the Fitbit Charge. *J. Meas. Phys. Behav.* **2018**, *1*, 130–135. [CrossRef]
23. Feito, Y.; Garner, H.; Bassett, D. Evaluation of ActiGraph's Low-Frequency Filter in Laboratory and Free-Living Environments. *Med. Sci. Sports Exerc.* **2014**, *47*, 211–217. [CrossRef]
24. Koo, T.K.; Li, M.Y. A Guideline of Selecting and Reporting Intraclass Correlation Coefficients for Reliability Research. *J. Chiropr. Med.* **2016**, *15*, 155–163. [CrossRef]
25. Bland, J.M.; Altman, D.G. Statistical Methods for Assessing Agreement between Two Methods of Clinical Measurement. *Lancet Lond. Engl.* **1986**, *1*, 307–310. [CrossRef]
26. Dixon, P.M.; Saint-Maurice, P.F.; Kim, Y.; Hibbing, P.; Bai, Y.; Welk, G.J. A Primer on the Use of Equivalence Testing for Evaluating Measurement Agreement. *Med. Sci. Sports Exerc.* **2018**, *50*, 837–845. [CrossRef]
27. Buchan, D.S.; Boddy, L.M.; McLellan, G. Comparison of Free-Living and Laboratory Activity Outcomes from ActiGraph Accelerometers Worn on the Dominant and Non-Dominant Wrists. *Meas. Phys. Educ. Exerc. Sci.* **2020**, *24*, 247–257. [CrossRef]
28. Buchan, D.S. Equivalence of Activity Outcomes Derived from Three Research Grade Accelerometers Worn Simultaneously on Each Wrist. *J. Sports Sci.* **2022**, *40*, 797–807. [CrossRef] [PubMed]
29. Rowlands, A.V.; Plekhanova, T.; Yates, T.; Mirkes, E.M.; Davies, M.; Khunti, K.; Edwardson, C.L. Providing a Basis for Harmonization of Accelerometer-Assessed Physical Activity Outcomes Across Epidemiological Datasets. *J. Meas. Phys. Behav.* **2019**, *2*, 131–142. [CrossRef]
30. O'Brien, M.W. Implications and Recommendations for Equivalence Testing in Measures of Movement Behaviors: A Scoping Review. *J. Meas. Phys. Behav.* **2021**, *4*, 353–362. [CrossRef]
31. PAL Technologies Average Valid Day Summaries–PAL Knowledge Base. Available online: https://kb.palt.com/articles/average-valid-day-summaries/ (accessed on 25 October 2022).
32. Dunstan, D.W.; Kingwell, B.A.; Larsen, R.; Healy, G.N.; Cerin, E.; Hamilton, M.T.; Shaw, J.E.; Bertovic, D.A.; Zimmet, P.Z.; Salmon, J.; et al. Breaking Up Prolonged Sitting Reduces Postprandial Glucose and Insulin Responses. *Diabetes Care* **2012**, *35*, 976–983. [CrossRef]
33. Hadgraft, N.T.; Winkler, E.; Climie, R.E.; Grace, M.S.; Romero, L.; Owen, N.; Dunstan, D.; Healy, G.; Dempsey, P.C. Effects of Sedentary Behaviour Interventions on Biomarkers of Cardiometabolic Risk in Adults: Systematic Review with Meta-Analyses. *Br. J. Sports Med.* **2021**, *55*, 144–154. [CrossRef]

International Journal of
Environmental Research and Public Health

MDPI

Article

Perceived Constraints on Active Recreational Sport Participation among Residents in Urban China

Lan Lin [1], Qun Liu [1,*], Xiao Xiao [2] and Qin Luo [1]

1 School of Geographical Sciences, Institute of Tourism, Fujian Normal University, Fuzhou 350117, China
2 School of Community Resources and Development, Arizona State University, Phoenix, AZ 85004, USA
* Correspondence: liuqun@fjnu.edu.cn

Abstract: Recreational sport participation is an important pathway to improving the quality of life. While facilities for recreational sports are provided in many urban areas in China, how urban residents might be aware of or use these facilities for recreational sport participation is still a vague notion in the literature. This study explored the linkages between perceived leisure constraints and active participation in recreational sports among urban residents. We collected data samples from 2901 urban residents in China to identify their perceived constraints and the effects of the perceived constraints on active recreational sport participation by structural equation models. Five perceived constraints of active recreational sport participation were identified: intrapersonal, interpersonal, environmental condition, facility-service management, and leisure opportunity constraints. More specifically, leisure opportunity, intrapersonal, facility-service management, and interpersonal constraints were the four most important constraints limiting active recreational sport participation of urban residents. Theoretical and practical implications to facilitate the active recreational sport participation of Chinese urban residents were discussed.

Keywords: perceived constraints; leisure opportunities; active recreational sport participation; urban residents; China

1. Introduction

Over the past two decades, the inactive and inadequate participation in recreational sports have been a challenging issue for the urban residents' quality of life. Urban areas should provide a dwelling, work, transportation, and recreation functions to satisfy the urban residents' diverse needs [1]. Meanwhile, the fundamental role of people-oriented functions of a city rather than the material-based or political power-based functions is highlighted in the modern urban development agenda. Therefore, the concept of "leisure cities" and "healthy cities" has been widely promoted and implemented in many urban areas in China [2–4]. Through these initiatives, the diverse culture and lifestyles of urban residents are valued, which empowers urban residents to freely choose health-friendly leisure behaviors, and guarantees the physical fitness and leisure rights of urban residents through various urban development and revitalization processes.

Inspired by the national strategy "Healthy China" initiated in 2017, a large number of recreational facilities for physical exercise, leisure space, and service management were developed to encourage mass sports and fitness at the national level. Nowadays, many cities in urban areas have built varying levels of physical exercise facilities and leisure resources. Based on the statistics of the Sixth National Stadium Census Data Bulletin (2013), there are 82 types of sports complexes in total in China, with 1,694,600 sports venues; the number of sports venues in urban areas is 96,270 with an area of 1.337 billion square meters. Consequently, participating in physical activities during one's leisure time has become one of the primary leisure activities for urban residents. Among all types of leisure activities, recreational sport is one of the most popular leisure activities in China.

Recreational sporting activities are leisure activities that combine both sport and recreation. These activities fall under the umbrella of play [5], and do not have to be competitive or require particular equipment or rules [1,6,7]. A number of studies have examined the positive outcomes of the physical activity component of recreational sports and reported that recreational sport activity enhances circulatory health, provides mental clarity, promotes successful aging, and promotes social interaction [8–12]. However, the benefits of recreational sport participation vary between rural and urban areas [13].

While urban areas have provided the resources for recreational sport, urban residents might encounter constraints when participating in recreational sports. Inadequate facilities, lack of leisure time, and lack of knowledge are common constraints for urban residents to engage in urban recreational sport [14]. In China, the leisure activities of urban residents are highly constrained by socio-economic resources and time [15]. Crawford and Godbey's [16] framework of leisure constraints has discussed the link between perceived constraints and non or less leisure participation, and the framework has been widely applied to different types of recreation settings. Moreover, leisure activity participation might be different among social groups, as racial/ethnic minority groups, women, adolescents [17,18], and people with disabilities were traditionally disadvantaged groups in leisure participation. However, most leisure constraint studies have focused on specific group/populations in North America [19,20], Europe, and Australia, and the content are constraint determinants for the level of participation in leisure time physical activity (LTPA) in general [21–24]. The application and extension of this framework research to recreational sport participation are limited [25,26]. From the theoretical perspective, very few studies have examined the perceived constraints of urban residents for active recreational sporting participation in China. The urban population is growing rapidly in China, accounting for nearly two-thirds of the population, and more and more residents actively participate in recreational sports activities. Active recreational sport participants have been the main users of urban leisure sports venues and facilities. Whether the recreational facilities and leisure resources could meet the urban residents' recreational sport activity needs is an emerging question for park managers and urban designers. To better explore recreational sport, academics and professionals must understand and appreciate the perceived constraints facing urban active recreational sport participants. Specifically, the study aimed to (a) identify the perceived constraints affecting active recreational sport participation; (b) test the relationships between perceived constraints and active recreational sport participation, and (c) examine the differences in the perceived constraints and active recreational sport participation by gender. We tried to test and extend the leisure constraints model [16] in non-Western contexts, which not only seek to understand the choice determinants of the active participant, but also to comprehend the range of perceived constraints preventing active sport participants from becoming inactive or non-sport participants in urban China.

2. Literature Review

2.1. Recreational Sport Participation in Urban Area

Recreational sport activities are typically conducted during leisure time and are an unstructured means of entertainment [27–29], which is valued as a way to improve an individual's quality of life [25]. Recreational sport participation can bring benefits to individuals from both physiological and psychological perspectives. Physiologically, regular participation in recreational sports might promote health including reducing the risks of cardiovascular disease [30], diabetes [31], and extending the length of life [30]. Psychologically, the social interactions of recreational sport participation can enhance the individuals' self-esteem and facilitate positive emotions [32]. These benefits were manifested in studies among different regions and across time, for example, a longitudinal study found that regular recreation sport participation could improve fitness, develop healthy lifestyles, enhance mood, and strengthen attitudes toward fitness [33]. A few pilot studies have examined the scales of recreational sport participation and found that the participation was a multi-facet process that involves: (1) challenge, (2) victory, (3) sensory, (4) workout, and

(5) social [34]. In addition, recreational sport participation levels might be different among socio-demographic groups. Gender has been one of the most important socio-demographic factors that lead to disparities in recreational sport participation levels, and females are more likely to encounter constraints in participating in recreational sports than males in general [25,35]. Perceived constraints are not only barriers that might influence motivation, but also as potential motivators for participation [36,37].

Recreational sport participation also varies greatly between urban and rural areas. For instance, a recent study found that rural residents were less interested in recreational sports than urban residents. Similarly, a study examined factors associated with youth sport participation and found that children in rural communities experienced more constraints of sport participation than those living in urban communities [38]. Chick et al. [39] found that older people listed constraints related to age and health more frequently than younger people while younger informants were more concerned with resources such as money in the urban Taiwanese.

Recreational sports, as an important pathway to facilitate mass sports and healthy cities in China, have been highlighted in the recent National Agenda. Providing sports facilities, organizing public sports activities, and enhancing the awareness of physical exercises can facilitate engagement of recreational sport participation for the general public [40]. The participation of Chinese urban residents in sports activities is spatially clustered in recreation areas and facilities such as parks, neighborhood gardens, and urban squares [41]. Although recreational sports participation is encouraged at the local, regional, and national levels, research on the participation of Chinese urban residents in recreation sport is still in a notably nascent stage, and more research is needed to examine the perceived constraints for the active participation of urban residents in recreational sports in China.

2.2. Leisure Constraints among Urban Residents

Leisure research in Western countries is one of the oldest domains of social science research, which has a long history of more than 130 years. Since Crawford and Godbey put forward the concept of leisure constraint in 1987, which has been widely assumed in the constraints literature, that the constraints people perceive lead either to nonparticipation or to reduced leisure participation. Constraints have been defined as "the factors that are assumed by researchers and perceived by individuals to inhibit or prohibit participation and enjoyment in leisure" [42] with additional possibilities to enable leisure [36]. Scholars generally agree that the process of people striving for leisure rights is also a process of overcoming various leisure constraints.

Constraints occur at the intrapersonal, interpersonal, and structural levels that operate in a hierarchy [16,36], which was subsequently expanded by Crawford et al. [43]. Since that time, many researchers have debated the scholarship on leisure constraints and noted possible interactions between intrapersonal, interpersonal, and structural constraints [44–46]. Intrapersonal constraints are the individuals' characters, values, and personalities that prohibit the participation in recreational sports [16] such as a lack of skills and interests, stress, and health concerns [47,48]. Interpersonal constraints, however, stem from interactions and relationships with social groups such as a lack of companions, family support, or encountering discrimination from other leisure participants [32]. Structural constraints are external factors intervening in recreational sport participation such as socio-economic resources, weather, and work schedule. Findings on the impacts of the three types of constraints on recreational sport participation are mixed in earlier studies [32], while a few studies have suggested that intrapersonal constraints seemed to be the most powerful predictors of commitment to recreational sport participation [25,37,49].

Although considerable research efforts have been focused on examining leisure constraints in the Western context, research on the leisure constraints in the non-Western context is at a notably nascent stage, in particular, recreational sport constraints in urban China. Dong and Chick [15] examined leisure constraints for urban residents in six cities in China and found that a lack of time and money were the primary constraints for leisure participation of Chinese urban residents. Chick et al. [39,50,51] found that cultural consonance can be a moderator between leisure constraints and leisure satisfaction for urban residents in China. Liu and Walker [52] examined the effects of urbanization, motivation, and constraint on the participation of Chinese people in leisure time physical activity and found that structural constraint was the most important constraint, followed by interpersonal barrier. On the other hand, perseverance was the most motivation positively influenced LTPA, followed by enjoyment. Moreover, Chen [53] and Lin et al. [54] noted that spatial, social, and structural constraints (e.g., distance to facilities/venues and lacks of time) were key factors influencing Chinese people's LTPA.

2.3. Extended Three Dimensions of Leisure Constraints

Although the three types of leisure constraints have been applied and tested widely in earlier studies, a few studies have highlighted the concern that constraints may not easily be delineated into a categorization of intrapersonal, interpersonal, and structural constraints [46,55–59]. Other researchers have also noted possible interactions between intrapersonal, interpersonal, and structural constraints [44,59,60]. Some researchers have investigated how combinations of personal characteristics (e.g., motivation, gender, age, socio-economic status, and race/ethnicity) affected the individuals' constraints to outdoor recreation [45,61–63]. Alexandris et al. [37] provided evidence that motivation acts as an intervening variable between constraints and recreational sport participation. A few recent studies have identified additional factors impacting leisure participation rather than the traditional three-dimension approach. Leisure-related facilities and service management, leisure opportunities, and cultural consonance are important factors associated with leisure participation. For example, Perry et al. [64] found that the lack of transportation facilities was an important constraint for racial/ethnic minority groups to participate in leisure activities in national parks. Leisure opportunities or initiatives such as more efficient and accessible transportation facilities and programs can facilitate leisure participation for marginalized groups [63,64]. However, the coherent impacts of these factors with the three dimensions of constraints on recreational sport participation have not been fully documented in earlier studies, particularly in the context of urban areas in China. There is still limited understanding of cultural variation in leisure constraints [15,50,65–67]. Perceived constraints on recreational sport participation requires more cross-cultural and comparative research.

3. Materials and Methods

3.1. Hypotheses and Theoretical Model

Drawing on leisure constraints theory [16,43,47] and previous leisure constraint research, a hierarchy model of leisure constraints proposes that intrapersonal, interpersonal, and structural constraints influence the individual's preferences for leisure activities and participation coherently. Building on the hierarchy model of leisure constraints and additional factors associated with leisure participation identified in earlier studies, we propose a five-category hierarchical model of recreational sport perceived constraints. Two categories were referred to as intrapersonal and interpersonal perceived constraints [27,28]. Structural perceived constraints were divided into three sub-dimensions: environmental, leisure opportunity, and facility-service management [59]. We first proposed an initial theoretical model and posited that all five perceived constraints would influence the individuals' preferences and frequency of active recreational sport participation. In order to test the multi-variate relationship between the five perceived constraints and active recreational sport participation in leisure time, five hypotheses were stated in the following and are presented in Figure 1.

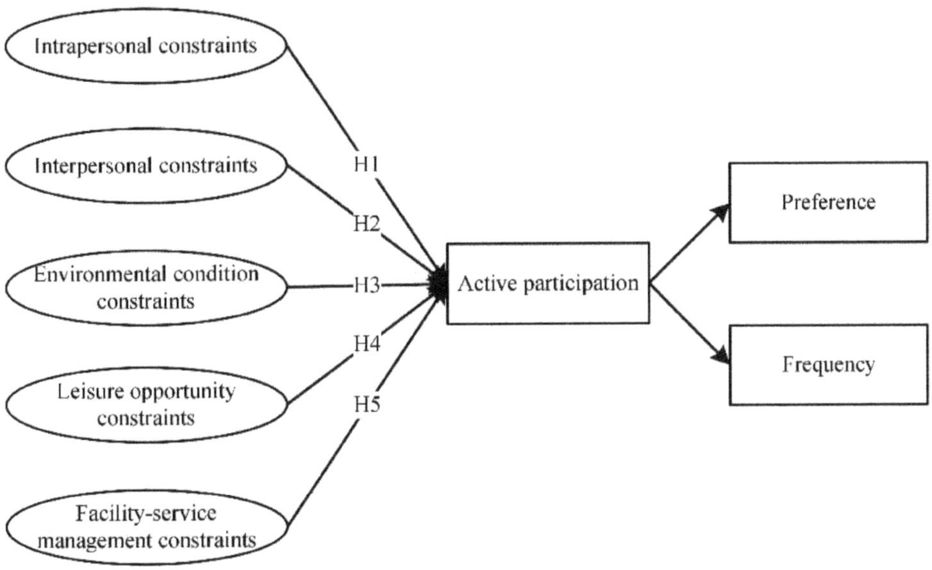

Figure 1. Hypothesized perceived constraints and the active recreational sport participation model.

H1: *The intrapersonal constraints would have a negative relationship with active recreational spor participation.*

H2: *The interpersonal constraints would have a negative relationship with active recreational sport participation.*

H3: *The environmental condition constraints would have a negative relationship with active recreational sport participation.*

H4: *The leisure opportunity constraints would have a negative relationship with active recreational sport participation.*

H5: *The facility-service management constraints would have a negative relationship with active recreational sport participation.*

3.2. Perceived Constraints

Constraints were measured by modified variables from Hubbard and Mannell [27], White [28], and Zhu et al. [59] to make the content aligned to the recreational sport activities in the study locations. Participants were asked to report on the degree of agreement with 23 items of perceived constraints for active recreation sport participation. The 23 items included physical problems, psychological problems, negative attitudes toward fitness, lack of interests, not skilled enough, lack of partners, negative attitudes of family and friends, lack of coaches' guidance, bad weather, fear of safety, poor hygiene, limited opening hours, lack of time, lack of fitness fees, fitness activities are limited, fitness fees are too high, inaccessibility, unattractive programs, lack of personalized services, lack of professional management, inadequate programs and facilities, lack of information, and environment-unfriendly. A five-point scale (1 = "strongly disagree", 2 = "disagree", 3 = "neither agree or disagree", 4 = "agree", 5 = "strongly agree") was used to measure the respondents' agreement with the perceived constraints. A principal components analysis was conducted to identify the dimensions of the perceived constraints.

3.3. Recreational Sport Participation

Recreational sport participation was measured by 10 activities based on the Sixth National Stadium Census Data Bulletin (2013). The Sixth National Stadium Census Data Bulletin is a nationwide survey on sport participation for Chinese residents, which was commissioned from 2011 to 2014. The ten activities included team sports (e.g., football, badminton, and basketball); fitness-related activities (e.g., aerobics, dancing); and individual activities (e.g., swimming, yoga, walking, and jogging). Respondents were asked as to which recreational sport activities they always participated in during their leisure-time, then answered the preferences and frequency for the activity that influenced the desire to active participate. In this study, all of the respondents were asked to rate two statements by preference for (e.g., 1 = "not like at all", 2 = "like it slightly", 3 = "like it moderately", 4 = "like it a lot", 5 = "like it extremely") and the frequency of participation (e.g., 1 = "once to twice times per month", 2 = "one time per week", 3 = " twice to three times per week", 4 = "four to five times per week", 5 = "more than 6 times per week").

3.4. Data Collection

The survey was conducted by members of our research team. Our research object was to investigate the perceived constraints of active participation. The samples recruited in the study consisted of citizens who had actively participated in recreational sport activities. A self-administered, on-site questionnaire survey was distributed randomly in both public physical exercise places and private physical fitness clubs in three Chinese cities (i.e., Nanjing, Fuzhou, and Xiamen). Nanjing, Fuzhou, and Xiamen are important pilot cities for national sports promotion, and residents in these three cities have relatively higher levels of awareness about recreational sport participation, making them rational and representative for a recreational sport constraints study. The survey was administered across both weekends and weekdays from July 2014 to August 2016.

The questionnaire included three main parts: the behavioral characteristics of active recreational sport participation (i.e., degree of preference and participation frequency), perception of the constraints in recreational sport participation, and demographic information (e.g., gender, age, lifestyle, occupational status, income, and education). Overall, 2927 citizens participated in the study, and 99.11% of them completed the questionnaire (N = 2901). The sample sizes from Nanjing, Fuzhou, and Xiamen were 926, 1049, and 926, respectively.

4. Results

4.1. Demographic Characteristics of the Sample

Of the 2901 sample, 35.3% were females and 67.7% were males. As shown in Table 1, the age profile was mixed among various age groups including people aged 46 to 65 (14.8%), 36 to 45 (21.4%), 26 to 35 (36.7%), 19 to 25 (20.2%), and less than 18 (6%). For the education background, 45.5% of the respondents had an undergraduate degree and 23.9% had junior college qualifications, respectively. Personal monthly income primarily fell into the classifications of lower than 3000 yuan (20.8%) and from 3001 to 5000 yuan (33.6%). In terms of occupation, 30.1% of the respondents were working at state-owned enterprises, and 27% were working at government-sponsored institutions. Students and public functionaries were 13.4% and 12.1%, respectively.

Table 1. The demographic characteristics of the sample.

Variables	Category	Number	Percentage
Gender	Man	1878	64.7
	female	1023	35.3
Age	≤18	173	6.0
	19–25	586	20.2
	26–35	1064	36.7
	36–45	620	21.4
	46–55	323	11.1
	56–65	108	3.7
	>65	27	0.9
Education	Junior high school or lower	176	6.0
	High school/Technical secondary school	405	14.0
	Junior college	693	23.9
	Undergraduate	1320	45.5
	Postgraduate	307	10.6
Personal monthly income (RMB)	≤3000	603	20.8
	3001–5000	976	33.6
	5001–7000	505	17.4
	7001–10,000	440	15.2
	≥10,001	377	13.0
Occupation	Public functionary	352	12.1
	State-owned enterprise	873	30.1
	Private enterprise	260	9.0
	Government-sponsored institution	782	27.0
	Student	390	13.4
	Liberal professions	85	2.9
	Retirement	84	2.9
	Other	75	2.6

4.2. Principal-Component Analysis

A principal component analysis was conducted to categorize the 23 items related to the recreational sport participation scale. Cronbach's alpha was used to test the reliability and internal consistency, and the values of KMO and Bartlett's spherical were used to test for sampling adequacy. Results showed that the Cronbach's α of the whole scale was 0.95. The value of KMO was 0.96, which was greater than 0.7. Bartlett's spherical test value was 43,573.25, which reached a significant level under the condition of 253 degrees of freedom and $p < 0.001$. The data were suitable for principal component analysis (PCA).

The PCA was conducted by the SPSS 17.0 Factor program and AMOS 22.0. Only those components with an eigenvalue greater than 1.0 were retained and rotated, and both orthogonal and oblique rotations were used. After 66 times of factor-analysis, it indicated that the six initial constraint items with factor loadings were less than 0.7 and deleted. The PCA was employed again for the remaining 17 items, and five factors emerged to account for 74.87% of the variance (Table 2). The Cronbach's α of the whole scale was 0.91. The value of KMO was 0.93, which was greater than 0.7. Bartlett's spherical test value was 30,631.49, which reached a significant level under the condition of 171 degrees of freedom and $p < 0.001$. The internal consistency reliability of the whole scale was 0.83. All items proved to have acceptable internal consistency reliability and validity. The five extracted factors were defined as follows: intrapersonal constraints, interpersonal constraints, environmental condition constraints, leisure opportunity constraints, and facility-service management constraints.

Table 2. The principal component analysis results for 17 items (n = 2901).

Perceived Constraints Factors	Sub-Constraints Factors	Factor Loadings	Eigen Value	Contribution Rate (%)	Cumulative (%)
Intrapersonal constraints	Physical problems	0.80	1.20	7.07	64.56
	Psychological problems	0.78			
	Negative attitudes toward fitness	0.76			
	Lack of interests	0.71			
Interpersonal constraints	Lack of partners	0.81	0.82	4.84	74.87
	Negative attitudes of family and friends	0.79			
Environmental condition constraints	Bad weather	0.73	0.93	5.48	70.04
	Fear of safety	0.75			
	Poor hygiene	0.71			
Leisure opportunity constraints	Lack of fitness fees	0.82	1.77	10.40	57.49
	Lack of time	0.80			
	Fitness activities are limited	0.77			
	Fitness fees are too high	0.73			
Facility-service management constraints	Lack of personalized services	0.81	8.01	47.09	47.09
	Lack of professional management	0.81			
	Inadequate programs and facilities	0.75			
	Lack of information	0.74			

4.3. *Confirmatory Factor Analysis*

The validity of the hypothesized measurement model was tested in the AMOS 22.0 using confirmatory factor analysis (CFA), followed by a test of the hypothesized structural relationships. Results of the CFA demonstrated that the measurement model was an acceptable fit to the data (χ^2 = 939.83, df = 109, $\rho < 0.01$; RMSEA = 0.05, 90% lower = 0.05, 90% upper = 0.05; CFI = 0.97; NNFI = 0.97). A full summary of the CFA results including the means, standard deviation, standardized factor loading, bootstrapped standard error, critical ratio, average variance explained, and composite reliability were shown for each of the variables in Table 3. The mean score for all perceived constraints indicated that urban residents rated the intrapersonal constraints as the most important perceived constraint (M = 4.02) that limits the active recreational sport participation. Interpersonal constraints were rated as the second important perceived constraint (M = 3.75), followed by environmental condition constraints (M = 3.75) and facility-service management constraints (M = 3.70). The leisure opportunity constraints had the lowest mean of 3.67 among the five perceived constraints. The variables in the intrapersonal constraints dimension ranged from 3.83 to 4.23, and the lack of interests and physical problems were the most important factors in this dimension. Poor hygiene and negative attitudes toward fitness of the two constraint subscale scores were also higher, which were rated as important reasons for active participation. For the preferences for active participation, respondents were generally likely to participate in recreational sport activities a lot (M = 4.19). The average frequency of active participation was 3.57, which indicated that urban residents wished to participate in recreational sport activities twice to three times to four to five times per week.

Table 3. Results of the confirmatory factor analysis.

Variables (α)	M (SD)	Λ (Boot. SE)	z-Value	AVE	ρ
Intrapersonal constraints (α = 0.83)	4.02 (0.78)	0.53 (0.02)	23.30 ***	0.56	0.84
Physical problems	4.05 (0.94)	0.78 (0.01)	28.59 ***		
Psychological problems	3.83 (1.01)	0.79 (0.01)	27.64 ***		
Negative attitudes toward fitness	3.95 (3.95)	0.77 (0.01)	28.78 ***		
Lack of interests	4.23 (4.23)	0.66 (0.01)	33.33 ***		
Interpersonal constraints (α = 0.74)	3.75 (0.96)	0.68 (0.03)	19.82 ***	0.58	0.74
Lack of partners	3.82 (1.11)	0.75 (0.02)	23.04 ***		
Negative attitudes of family and friends	3.69 (1.06)	0.78 (0.02)	20.01 ***		
Environmental condition constraints (α = 0.79)	3.75 (0.92)	0.42 (0.03)	15.56 ***	0.61	0.82
Bad weather	3.49 (1.16)	0.56 (0.03)	35.87 ***		
Fear of safety	3.80 (1.09)	0.88 (0.01)	19.31 ***		
Poor hygiene	3.95 (1.04)	0.86 (0.01)	22.25 ***		
Leisure opportunity constraints (α = 0.90)	3.67 (0.93)	0.83(0.03)	26.55 ***	0.70	0.90
Lack of fitness fees	3.58 (1.10)	0.83 (0.01)	30.10 ***		
Lack of time	3.80 (1.07)	0.86 (0.01)	27.95 ***		
Fitness activities are limited	3.68 (1.04)	0.86 (0.01)	27.55 ***		
Fitness fees are too high	3.62 (1.03)	0.79 (0.01)	31.85 ***		
Facility-service management constraints (α = 0.91)	3.70 (0.88)	0.75 (0.03)	29.31 ***	0.72	0.91
Lack of personalized services	3.68 (0.99)	0.88 (0.01)	27.50 ***		
Lack of professional management	3.75 (0.98)	0.88 (0.01)	27.60 ***		
Inadequate programs and facilities	3.74 (1.01)	0.82 (0.01)	31.72 ***		
Lack of information	3.63 (1.01)	0.82 (0.01)	31.55 ***		
Active participation	3.88 (0.61)	—	—	—	—
Preference	4.19 (0.71)				
Frequency	3.57 (1.03)				

Note. C.R. = critical ratio; AVE = average variance explained; ρ = composite reliability; *** p-value < 0.001.

Measurement model constructs indicated acceptable reliability with values of the Cronbach's alpha (e.g., $\alpha \geq 0.7$) calculated for each item, and ranged from 0.74 to 0.91. Campbell and Fiske (1959) stressed a successful evaluation of discriminant validity that showed that a test of a concept is not highly correlated with other tests designed to measure theoretically different concepts. Test statistics and composite reliability were also acceptable ($\rho \geq 0.7$), and the average variance explained was validity (AVE ≥ 0.5). In Table 4, the discriminant validity was acceptable for all of the latent constructs (less than 0.85).

Table 4. Test for the convergent and discriminant validity of the latent constructs.

Construct	Correlation Coefficients				
Intrapersonal constraints	1				
Interpersonal constraints	0.67	1			
Environmental condition constraints	0.483	0.444	1		
Leisure opportunity constraints	0.569	0.573	0.627	1	
Facility-service management constraints	0.561	0.512	0.752	0.709	**1**

4.4. Structural Equation Models

In this study, we followed a two-step modeling procedure for structural equation modeling (SEM) to test the hypothesized measurement model. The 17 measuring perceived constraint scales obtained from PCA were the observed variables in the SEM. Intrapersonal constraints, interpersonal constraints, environmental condition constraints, leisure opportunity constraints, and facility-service management constraints were the latent variables of cause in the SEM. The preference and frequency of active participation were treated as latent variables of SEM. Figure 1 shows the five hypothesized paths between the perceived constraint latent factors and active participation latent factors, followed by a test of the hypothesized measurement structural relationships for latent variable modeling.

The SEM model fit was judged by using multiple fit indices, and widely-used indices including the chi-square (χ^2)/degree of freedom ratio, normed fit index (NFI), comparative fit index (CFI), non-normed fit index (NNFI), and root mean square error of approximation (RMSEA). The chi-squared test is biased against sample size and model complexity. While a non-significant value of chi-square/degree of freedom ratio suggests a good fit to the data, the statistics are known to be highly sensitive to sample size. When the sample size is greater than 200, the chi-square/degree of freedom ratio is often not used as an insightful index to test the goodness-of-fit for the SEM model. The indices of NFI, CFI, and NNFI should be greater than 0.9, and the RMSEA value of less than 0.08 also indicates an acceptable model fit. These criteria were used in assessing the fit of our models. Considering the relatively large sample size of our SEM model (N = 2901), we used NFI, CFI, NNFI, and RMSEA as the goodness-of-fit indices for the SEM model.

We first tested the fit indicators of the initial measurement model. In Table 5, the results of the initial measurement model indicated a poor goodness-of-fit (GFI = 0.76, RMSEA = 0.12, AGFI = 0.69, NFI = 0.78, CFI = 0.79, IFI = 0.79), which meant the initial measurement model needed to be modified by correlating a new structural relationship among the error variables and using the modification indices. All indices showed a high goodness-of-fit of the revised SEM model (GFI = 0.96, RMSEA = 0.05, AGFI = 0.95, NFI = 0.97, CFI = 0.97, IFI = 0.97). A summary of the overall fit indices for the initial measurement model and the final structural model is presented in Table 5.

Table 5. Summary of the overall fit indices for the initial measurement model and final SEM model.

Overall	Absolute Fit Indices		Incremental Fit Indices		Parsimonious Fit Indices			
Fit Indices	GFI	RMSEA	AGFI	NFI	CFI	IFI	AIC	ECVI
Ideal indices	>0.9	<0.08	>0.9	>0.9	>0.9	>0.9	N/A	N/A
Initial measurement model	0.76	0.12	0.69	0.78	0.79	0.79	6683.48	0.35
Final structural model	0.96	0.05	0.95	0.97	0.97	0.97	1027.83	0.11

The test of the final structural model also revealed that the standardized parameter coefficients were significant and the data supported all of the hypotheses except for Hypotheses 3 (Table 6). The leisure opportunity constraints had a direct negative effect on active participation (S.E = 0.01, $p < 0.001$) and was the strongest factor impacting active participation in the SEM. Intrapersonal constraints also had a direct negative relationship with active recreational sport participation (S.E = 0.02, $p < 0.001$) (Figure 2). The facility-service management constraints had a negative impact on active participation (S.E = 0.02, $p < 0.001$). and the interpersonal constraints had a negative impact on active recreation sport participation, while the impact was weaker compared to the other three factors. However, we did not find support for the hypothesized relationship between the environmental condition constraints and active participation.

Table 6. Summary of the hypothesized SEM model (n = 2901).

The Hypothesized Paths	The Standardized Parameter Coefficients	Standard Errors	z-Value	Test Results
H1: Intrapersonal constraints→participation	−0.24	0.02	−4.40 ***	Acceptable
H2: Interpersonal constraints→participation	−0.22	0.02	−2.58 **	Acceptable
H3: Environmental condition constraints→participation	−0.004	0.02	−0.08	Not accepted
H4: Leisure opportunity constraints→participation	−0.28	0.01	−5.33 ***	Acceptable
H5: Facility-service management constraints→participation	−0.17	0.02	−3.31 ***	Acceptable

Note: *** p-value < 0.001, ** p-value < 0.01; For all analyses, n = 2901.

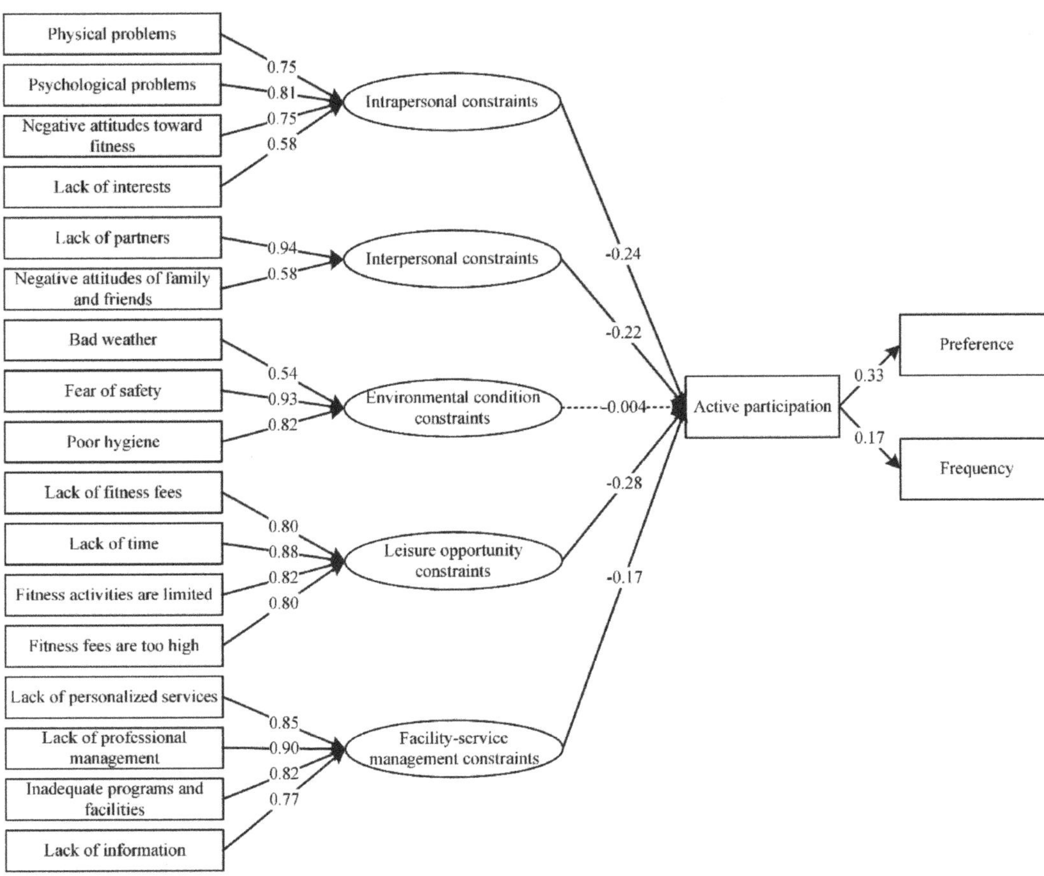

Figure 2. Graphical summary of the structural model results. Dotted line indicates the non-significant results.

4.5. Multi-Group Comparisons

To examine the generalizability of the hypothesized SEM to multiple socio-economic factors, we conducted multi-group comparisons of SEMs for active recreation sport participation. We divided the sample to two groups: female respondents (n = 1023) and male respondents (n = 1878), and tested the SEMs between the two groups. We tested the SEMs using six types of models including unconstrained, measurement weights, structural weights, structural covariances, structural residuals, and measurement residuals, and selected the model with the highest levels of goodness-of-fit. Among the six models, the structural residual model was selected as the final model since it had the lowest AIC and ECVI. In the final SEM model, all goodness-of-fit indices met the standards of the SEM (Table 7).

The standardized coefficients of SEM for males and females are shown in Figures 3 and 4. In general, the results indicate that the SEM model can be accepted by both female and male groups, and no significant differences were detected for the standardized coefficient between two groups. The leisure opportunity constraints, intrapersonal constraints, facility-service management constraints, and interpersonal constraints were also the four most important perceived constraints for the male and female residents.

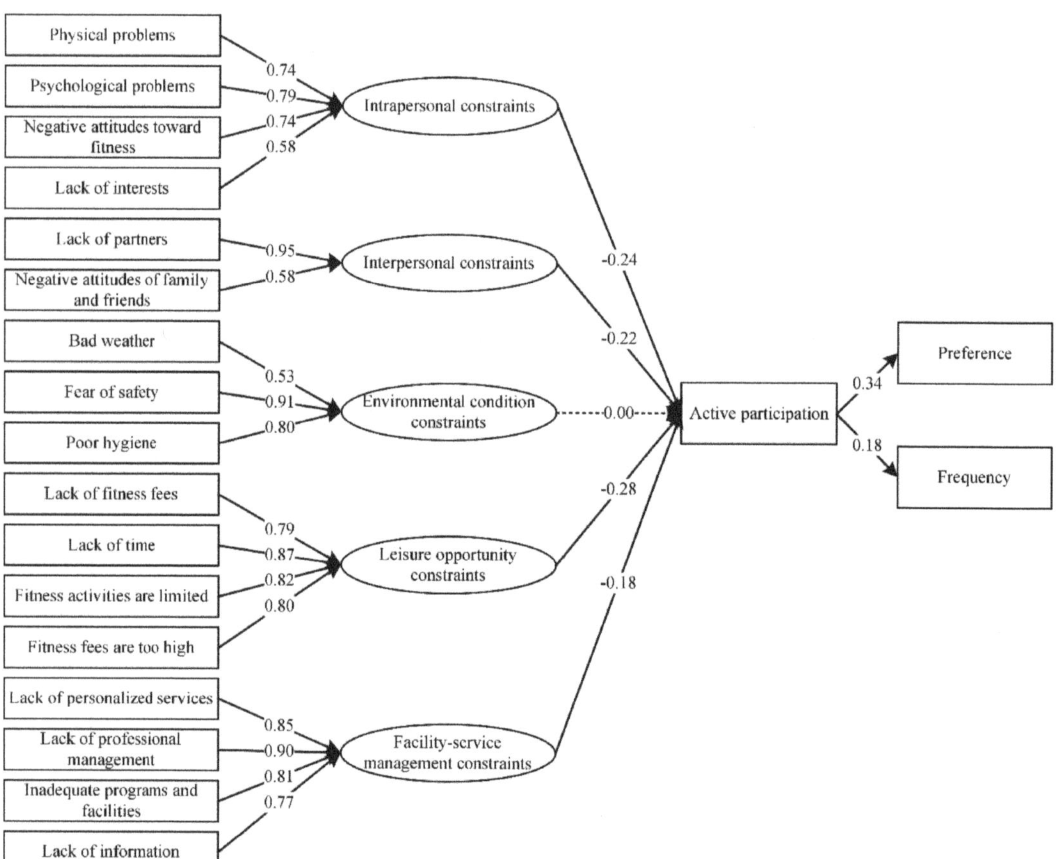

Figure 3. The path of standardized estimates for male groups in the structural residuals model.

Table 7. Summary of the goodness-of-fit indices for the structural residuals model in multi-group comparisons of SEMs.

Overall Fit Indices	Ideal Indices	Inspection Results	Test Results
Absolute fit indices			
χ^2	$p < 0.05$	5935.89 ($p = 0.000 < 0.05$)	Acceptable
RMSEA	<0.08	0.05	Acceptable
GFI	>0.90	0.90	Acceptable
AGFI	>0.90	0.90	Acceptable
Incremental fit indices			
NFI	>0.90	0.90	Acceptable
RFI	>0.90	0.90	Acceptable
IFI	>0.90	0.91	Acceptable
TLI(NNF1)	>0.90	0.90	Acceptable
CFI	>0.90	0.91	Acceptable
Parsimonious fit indices			
PGFI	>0.50	0.56	Acceptable
PNFI	>0.50	0.61	Acceptable
PCFI	>0.50	0.62	Acceptable
CN	>200	386	Acceptable
CMIN/DF	<2.00	17.06	Not accepted
AIC	The smaller the better	6379.89	Acceptable
ECVI	The smaller the better	1.10	Acceptable

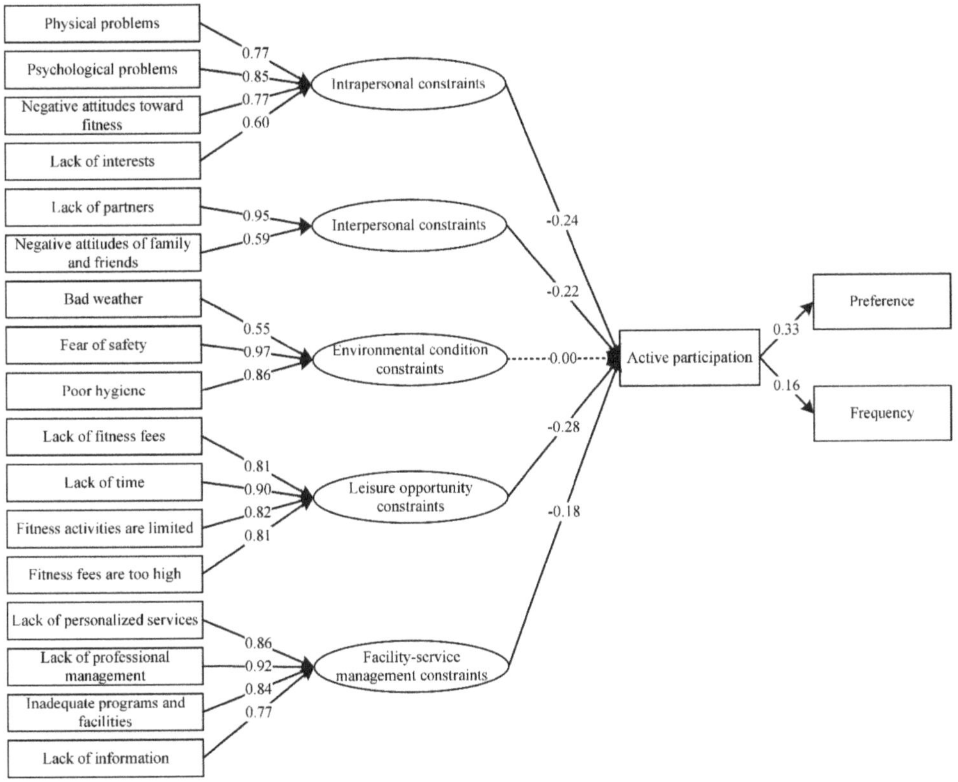

Figure 4. The path of the standardized estimates for female groups in structural residuals model.

5. Discussion and Conclusions

This study analyzed the perceived constraints of active recreational sport participation and tested the relationships between the perceived constraints and active recreational sport participation by urban residents in China. The findings provide support and expansive clarification of a conceptual model of leisure constraints [43], and also provide theoretical and practical implications to encourage recreational sport participation by urban residents in China. Theoretically, our study findings support the model of leisure constraints, and extend the Crawford's leisure constraint model (1991) to broader dimensions by highlighting the importance of leisure opportunities constraints, intrapersonal constraints, facility-service management constraints, and interpersonal constraints in the urban residents' active recreational sport participation. Aligned with Crawford's leisure constraint model [43], the structural constraints play an important role on limiting recreational sport participation, however, the effects of structural constraints on active recreational sport participation were primarily manifested in two sub-order dimensions in our study: leisure opportunity constraints and facility-service management constraints. The SEM model indicates that leisure opportunity constraints such as lack of time, fitness activities, or expensive fitness fees, could be the most significant factors that prohibit the active participation of urban residents in recreational sport activities. This result is aligned with findings in earlier studies that leisure opportunities and initiatives can mitigate the constraints for leisure activities, particularly for traditionally marginalized groups [63,64]. Urban areas, particularly urban areas in China, often have a high density of population and condense residential and industrial construction, making the leisure opportunities essential for urban residents to be able to or willing to actively participate in diverse recreational sport activities. Notably, this result highlights the necessity of leisure opportunities (e.g., perceived freedom, not busy, have free time, and multiple choice of fitness consumption) for active recreational sport participation by broader urban residents. As noted in earlier studies, developing second-order factors with the traditional three-dimensional (intrapersonal, interpersonal, and structural constraints) framework can be helpful in expanding the theory of leisure constraints [48]. Our study extended the generalizability of leisure constraint theory by developing five-dimensions perceived constraints and particularly tested the validity of the sub-dimensions by active recreational sport participation. The multi-group comparisons of SEMs indicate that the five-dimensional perceived constraints also exist in both female and male groups, and the same four constraints impacting active recreational sport participation can be generalized for female and male residents in urban China.

Aligned with Crawford's leisure constraint model [43], the SEM model suggested that intrapersonal and interpersonal constraints would limit the urban residents' active participation in recreational sport activities. For intrapersonal constraints, psychological problems and negative attitudes toward fitness were the most important perceived factors limiting active recreation sport participation, indicating that the psychological or cognitive issues, rather than the physical problems, prohibit the urban residents' active recreation sport participation to a large extent. For interpersonal constraints, the SEM model indicates that the lack of family support or partners can affect the active participation of urban resident' in recreational sports, however, the effect was minimal compared to the intrapersonal constraints. This finding is aligned with the findings in Godbey et al. [56], where the impacts of the interpersonal and intrapersonal constraints on leisure participation were mixed among different recreational settings. Social constructivism holds the view that the self is a relationship that is associated with a certain history and culture. Under the long-term influence of traditional Chinese culture characterized by Taoism and Confucianism, Chinese people have a sense of collective and relationship-oriented self. They are mostly influenced by others such as family and friends (i.e., Markus and Kitayama's (1991) [68] self-construal findings also stated that while Westerners were more likely to endorse an independent self (e.g., to value being unique), East Asians were more likely to endorse an interdependent self (e.g., to value fitting in). Our findings echo some researchers' findings (e.g., Chick et al. [50–52]; Liu and Walker [52]; Liang and Walker [69]) that cultural consonance can be a moderator between leisure constraints and leisure participation. For urban residents in China, interpersonal constraints may play important factors in indigenous Chinese concepts (e.g., collectivism; the effect of family and friends; social status and prestige).

Our study findings also suggest that facility-service management constraints can significantly limit the active participation of urban residents in recreational sport activities. Rather than the traditional leisure activities that rely on natural resources (hiking, mountain biking, fishing), recreational sport activities are highly dependent on the facilities and services, particularly indoor sporting activities. Inadequate and unprofessional management of the facilities, services, and information can be essential perceived barriers for the active participation of urban residents in recreational sport activities. The facility-driven nature of recreational sport activities highlights the need to add the specific dimension of facility-service management to overcome the urban residents' perceived constraints for active sport participation.

6. Management Implications

Our study findings also provide insightful guidance and management strategies for recreational sports managers and stakeholders. First, to address the leisure opportunity constraints, government agencies, and/or sport organizations could implement practical strategies such as providing more flexible operational schedules for sport activities, increasing a variety of personalized, engaging, and affordable sports leisure activities as well as promoting the strategic establishment or expansion of leisure activities and venues to encourage Chinese urban residents to actively participate in sport activities more frequently. From the perspective of intrapersonal constraints, inspiring the urban residents' enthusiasm for positive participation, enhancing the awareness about healthy lifestyles, and encouraging long-term commitment for physical exercise can be possible ways to increase active recreational sport participation.

Our results also indicate the importance of facility-service management in active recreational sport participation for Chinese urban residents. The inadequate management for recreational sport facilities and services may be related to the current priorities on material leisure space construction rather than service management quality in the past ten years. Based on our study findings, improving the environmental management levels, service quality, and attractive fitness programs and the convenience of fitness information would help attract more residents to active engage in recreational sport participation in China. This included specific elements such as

- Increasing the professional service capabilities of employees;
- Increasing the professional quality of coaches and their interpersonal communication skills;
- Promoting a personalized, diversified, and convenient service experience;
- Improving a harmony and user-friendly atmosphere that is full of mutual assistance and comfort;
- Building a leisure service information network for venue booking, fitness guidance, physical exercise analysis, physical fitness monitoring, and communication of recreational sport participation.

Moreover, "having a companion who exercises together", followed by "proactive support attitude of family (friends) to participation" are tackling strategies to overcome perceived constraints for active sport participation.

7. Limitations and Future Research

The study assessed the perceived constraints of active recreational sport participation in a statewide random sample of Chinese urban residents and also provided support for the four hypothesized relationships between the perceived constraints and active recreational sport participation. There were several study limitations. Future research with populations and activities in different cities would be needed to determine the universality of the findings identified. Furthermore, future studies might address the impacts of the COVID-19 pandemic on the constraints of recreational sport participation if the newest dataset is available.

Second, the construct structure is often believed to be ambiguous due to the intertwining relationships among leisure constraints [57]. Although this structural model is useful for analyzing the mutual and multiple relationships between the perceived constraint variables and active leisure participation, sample statistics could be produced that were poor estimates of the true population parameters. Our sample size (2901) to estimated parameters (36) ratio was 80.6 to 1, which was well above the minimum power needed for model estimation cited by structural equation modeling experts. We need to consider the sample size for the validation in future research.

Author Contributions: Conceptualization, L.L. and Q.L. (Qun Liu); Formal analysis, L.L. and Q.L. (Qin Luo); Methodology, L.L., X.X. and Q.L. (Qin Luo); Writing—original draft, L.L., Q.L. (Qun Liu), X.X., and Q.L. (Qin Luo); Writing—review & editing, L.L., Q.L. (Qun Liu), and X.X. All authors have read and agreed to the published version of the manuscript.

Funding: This research was funded by the National Natural Science Foundation of China (Grant ID: 41871146).

Institutional Review Board Statement: Not applicable.

Informed Consent Statement: Written informed consent was obtained from the respondents to publish this paper.

Data Availability Statement: The data presented in this study are available on request from the corresponding author.

Acknowledgments: We are very appreciative of the anonymous reviewers and the editors' constructive suggestions, and sincerely thank for Linda L. Caldwell from Department of Recreation, Park and Tourism Management, Pennsylvania State University, who had given us more suggestions in our studies. Also, we thank the sports institutions as well as the residents who participated in this study.

Conflicts of Interest: The authors declare no conflict of interest.

References

1. Pedersen, P.M.; Thibault, L. *Contemporary Sport Management*; Human Kinetics: Champaign, IL, USA, 2018.
2. Ding, G.; Zeng, S. Healthy cities' construction in the past 30 years in China:reviews on practice and research. *Mod. Urban Res.* **2020**, *4*, 2–8. (In Chinese)
3. Xu, A.; Liu, Z.; Lou, J. Study on the quality of the leisure cities in China. *World Reg. Stud.* **2020**, *29*, 856–866.
4. Yang, J.; Siri, J.G.; Remais, J.V.; Cheng, Q.; Zhang, H.; Chan, K.K.Y.; Sun, Z.; Zhao, Y.; Cong, N.; Li, X.; et al. The Tsinghua-Lancet Commission on Healthy Cities in China: Unlocking the power of cities for a healthy China. *Lancet* **2018**, *391*, 2140–2184. [CrossRef]
5. Chalip, L.; Schwab, K.; Dustin, D.S. Bridging the Sport and Recreation Divide. *Schole* **2010**, *25*, 1–10. [CrossRef]
6. Dixon, M.A. Contemporary sport management (3rd edition). *J. Sport Manag.* **2008**, *22*, 110–113. [CrossRef]
7. Mobily, K.E. Meanings of recreation and leisure among adolescents. *Leis. Stud.* **1989**, *8*, 11–23. [CrossRef]
8. Brechot, M.; Nueesch, S.; Franck, E. Does sports activity improve health? Representative evidence using local density of sports facilities as an instrument. *Appl. Econ.* **2017**, *49*, 4871–4884. [CrossRef]
9. Faria, F.; Howe, C.; Faria, R.; Andaki, A.; Marins, J.C.; Amorim, P.R. Impact of Recreational Sports Activities on Metabolic Syndrome Components in Adolescents. *Int. J. Environ. Res. Public Health* **2020**, *17*, 143. [CrossRef]
10. Mielke, G.I.; Bailey, T.G.; Burton, N.W.; Brown, W.J. Participation in sports/recreational activities and incidence of hypertension, diabetes, and obesity in adults. *Scand. J. Med. Sci. Sports* **2020**, *30*, 2390–2398. [CrossRef]
11. Su, C.L.; Lee, C.J.; Shinger, H.S. Effects of Involvement in Recreational Sports on Physical and Mental Health, Quality of Life of the Elderly. *Anthropologist* **2014**, *17*, 45–52. [CrossRef]
12. Tokarski, W.; Zarotis, G.F. The effect of recreational sports on human health. *IOSR J. Sports Phys. Educ.* **2020**, *7*, 25–33.
13. Chen, C.; Tsai, L.-T.; Lin, C.-F.; Huang, C.-C.; Chang, Y.-T.; Chen, R.-Y.; Lyu, S.-Y. Factors influencing interest in recreational sports participation and its rural-urban disparity. *PLoS ONE* **2017**, *12*, e0178052. [CrossRef] [PubMed]
14. Alexandris, K.; Stodolska, M. The Influence of Perceived Constraints on the Attitudes Toward Recreational Sport Participation. *Loisir Soc.* **2004**, *27*, 197–217. [CrossRef]
15. Dong, E.; Chick, G. Leisure Constraints in Six Chinese Cities. *Leis. Sci.* **2012**, *34*, 417–435. [CrossRef]
16. Crawford, D.W.; Godbey, G. Reconceptualizing barriers to family leisure. *Leis. Sci.* **1987**, *9*, 119–127. [CrossRef]
17. Manning, R.E. *Studies in Outdoor Recreation*; Oregon State University Press: Corvallis, OR, USA, 2011.

18. Xie, J.; Weybright, E.; Caldwell, L.; Wegner, L.; Smith, E. Parenting Practice, Leisure Experience, and Substance Use Among South African Adolescents. *J. Leis. Res.* **2020**, *51*, 36–55. [CrossRef]
19. Kerstetter; Deborah, L.; Zinn; Harry, C.; Graefe; Alan, R.; Chen, P.J. Perceived Constraints to State Park Visitation: A Comparison of Former-Users and Non-Users. *J. Park Recreat. Adm.* **2002**, *20*, 23–36.
20. Xiao, X.; Lee, K.J.; Larson, L. Who Visits U.S. National Parks (and Who Doesn't)? A National Study of Perceived Constraints and Vacation Preferences across Diverse Populations. *J. Leis. Res.* **2021**, *53*, 404–425. [CrossRef]
21. Borena, Y.G.; Shidaram, H.S.; Abdulkadir, Y.I. Association of sport and recreational facilities with adult residents' participation in leisure time physical activities in Addis Ababa, Ethiopia. *Sport Soc.* **2020**, *23*, 1163–1185. [CrossRef]
22. Fitzgerald, N.; Spaccarotella, K. Barriers to a Healthy Lifestyle: From Individuals to Public Policy—An Ecological Perspective. *J. Ext.* **2009**, *47*, 1FEA3.
23. Prins, R.G.; Oenema, A.; van der Horst, K.; Brug, J. Objective and perceived availability of physical activity opportunities: Differences in associations with physical activity behavior among urban adolescents. *Int. J. Behav. Nutr. Phys. Act.* **2009**, *6*, 70. [CrossRef] [PubMed]
24. Witten, K.; Hiscock, R.; Pearce, J.; Blakely, T. Neighbourhood access to open spaces and the physical activity of residents: A national study. *Prev. Med.* **2008**, *47*, 299–303. [CrossRef] [PubMed]
25. Anaza, E.; McDowell, J. An Investigation of Constraints Restricting Urban Nigerian Women from Participating in Recreational Sport Activities. *J. Leis. Res.* **2013**, *45*, 324–344. [CrossRef]
26. Wicker, P.; Hallmann, K.; Breuer, C. Micro and macro level determinants of sport participation. *Sport Bus. Manag. Int. J.* **2012**, *2*, 51–68. [CrossRef]
27. Hubbard, J.; Mannell, R.C. Testing competing models of the leisure constraint negotiation process in a corporate employee recreation setting. *Leis. Sci.* **2001**, *23*, 145–163. [CrossRef]
28. White, D.D. A Structural Model of Leisure Constraints Negotiation in Outdoor Recreation. *Leis. Sci.* **2008**, *30*, 342–359. [CrossRef]
29. Sivan, A.; Stebbins, R.A. Leisure education: Definition, aims, advocacy, and practices—Are we talking about the same thing(s)? *World Leis. J.* **2011**, *53*, 27–41. [CrossRef]
30. Wen, C.P.; Wai, J.P.M.; Tsai, M.K.; Yang, Y.C.; Cheng, T.Y.D.; Lee, M.-C.; Chan, H.T.; Tsao, C.K.; Tsai, S.P.; Wu, X. Minimum amount of physical activity for reduced mortality and extended life expectancy: A prospective cohort study. *Lancet* **2011**, *378*, 1244–1253. [CrossRef]
31. Ma, S.-M.; Ma, S.-C. Testing a Structural Model of Psychological Well-Being and Constraints Negotiation in Recreational Sports Participation in Individuals with Type 2 Diabetes. *Leis. Sci.* **2014**, *36*, 268–292. [CrossRef]
32. Russell, R.V. *Pastimes: The Context of Contemporary Leisure*, 7th ed.; Sagamore Venture Publishing: Urbana, IL, USA, 2020.
33. Spivey, L.M.; Hritz, N.M. A Longitudinal Study of Recreational Sport Participation and Constraints. *Recreat. Sport J.* **2013**, *37*, 14–28. [CrossRef]
34. Mueller, T.S. The recreational sport participation scale: Development, testing and practical application. *Int. J. Sport Manag. Mark.* **2012**, *12*, 144–158. [CrossRef]
35. Tsai, L.T.; Lo, F.E.; Yang, C.C.; Keller, J.J.; Lyu, S.Y. Gender differences in recreational sports participation among Taiwanese adults. *Int. J. Environ. Res. Public Health* **2015**, *12*, 829–840. [CrossRef] [PubMed]
36. Stodolska, M.; Shinew, K.; Floyd, M. *Race, Ethnicity, and Leisure*; Human Kinetics: Champaign, IL, USA, 2013.
37. Alexandris, K.; Tsorbatzoudis, C.; Grouios, G. Perceived constraints on recreational sport participation. *J. Leis. Res.* **2002**, *34*, 233–252. [CrossRef]
38. Kellstedt, D.K.; Schenkelberg, M.A.; Essay, A.M.; Von Seggern, M.J.; Rosenkranz, R.R.; Welk, G.J.; High, R.; Dzewaltowski, D.A. Youth sport participation and physical activity in rural communities. *Arch. Public Health* **2021**, *79*, 46. [CrossRef] [PubMed]
39. Chick, G.; Hsu, Y.C.; Yeh, C.K.; Hsieh, C.M.; Ramer, S.; Bae, S.Y.; Xue, L.; Dong, E. Cultural Consonance Mediates the Effects of Leisure Constraints on Leisure Satisfaction: A Reconceptualization and Replication. *Leis. Sci.* **2018**, *44*, 201–220. [CrossRef]
40. Chen, Q.; Liu, T. The effectiveness of community sports provision on social inclusion and public health in rural China. *Int. J. Environ. Res. Public Health* **2020**, *17*, 597. [CrossRef]
41. Wu, X.; Qin, X.; Zhou, H. Use of community spaces for sports and fitness—A case study of urban inhabitants in Shenzhen City, China. *Int. Rev. Sp. Plan. Sustain. Dev.* **2018**, *6*, 49–62. [CrossRef]
42. Jackson, E.L. In the eye of the beholder: A comment on Samdahl & Jekubovich (1997), "A critique of leisure constraints: Comparative analyses and understandings". *J. Leis. Res.* **1997**, *29*, 458–468.
43. Crawford, D.W.; Jackson, E.L.; Godbey, G. A Hierarchical Model of Leisure Constraints. *Leis. Sci.* **1991**, *13*, 309–320. [CrossRef]
44. Scott, D.; Munson, W. Perceived constraints to park usage among individuals with low incomes. *J. Park Recreat. Adm.* **1994**, *12*, 79–96.
45. Shores, K.A.; Scott, D.; Floyd, M.F. Constraints to outdoor recreation: A multiple hierarchy stratification perspective. *Leis. Sci.* **2007**, *29*, 227–246. [CrossRef]
46. Samdahl, D.M.; Jekubovich, N.J. A Critique of Leisure Constraints: Comparative Analyses and Understandings. *J. Leis. Res.* **1997**, *29*, 430–452. [CrossRef]
47. Jackson, E.L. Recognizing Patterns of Leisure Constraints—Results from Alternative Analyses. *J. Leis. Res.* **1993**, *25*, 129–149. [CrossRef]

48. Nyaupane, G.P.; Andereck, K.L. Understanding Travel Constraints: Application and Extension of a Leisure Constraints Model. *J. Travel Res.* **2007**, *46*, 433–439. [CrossRef]
49. Alexandris, K.; Tsormpatzoudis, C.; Bliatsou, P.; Grouios, G. Relationship between perceived constraints and commitment to recreational sport participation of university students in Greece. *Int. J. Sport Manag.* **2001**, *2*, 282–297.
50. Chick, G.; Hsu, Y.-C.; Yeh, C.-K.; Hsieh, C.-M. Leisure Constraints, Leisure Satisfaction, Life Satisfaction, and Self-Rated Health in Six Cities in Taiwan. *Leis. Sci.* **2015**, *37*, 232–251. [CrossRef]
51. Chick, G.; Dong, E.; Iarmolenko, S. Cultural consonance in leisure activities and self-rated health in six cities in China. *World Leis. J.* **2014**, *56*, 110–119. [CrossRef]
52. Liu, H.; Walker, G.J. The Effects of Urbanization, Motivation, and Constraint on Chinese People's Leisure-Time Physical Activity. *Leis. Sci.* **2015**, *37*, 458–478. [CrossRef]
53. Chen, Q. Comparison of the influencing factors of leisure sports activities of urban residents. *J. Jilin Inst. Phys. Educ.* **2012**, *28*, 44–46. (In Chinese)
54. Lin, M.; Bao, J.; Dong, E. Dancing in public spaces: An exploratory study on China's Grooving Grannies. *Leis. Stud.* **2020**, *39*, 545–557. [CrossRef]
55. Auster, C.J. Transcending potential antecedent leisure constraints: The case of women motorcycle operators. *J. Leis. Res.* **2001**, *33*, 272–298. [CrossRef]
56. Godbey, G.; Crawford, D.W.; Shen, X.S. Assessing hierarchical leisure constraints theory after two decades. *J. Leis. Res.* **2010**, *42*, 111–134. [CrossRef]
57. Scott, D. The problematic nature of participation in contract bridge—A qualitative study of group-related constraints. *Leis. Sci.* **1991**, *13*, 321–336. [CrossRef]
58. Shaw, S.M. Gender, leisure, and constraint—Towards a framework for the analysis of women's leisure. *J. Leis. Res.* **1994**, *26*, 8–22. [CrossRef]
59. Zhu, Z.; Lin, L.; Shi, L.; Wan, P. The influence of physical fitness leisure constraints and leisure participation of urban residents: An Empirical Analysis of Fuzhou. *Tour. Trib.* **2017**, *32*, 12. (In Chinese)
60. Wood, L.; Danylchuk, K. Constraints and Negotiation Processes in a Women's Recreational Sport Group. *J. Leis. Res.* **2012**, *44*, 463–485. [CrossRef]
61. Xiao, X.; Aultman-Hall, L.; Manning, R.; Voigt, B. The impact of spatial accessibility and perceived barriers on visitation to the US national park system. *J. Transp. Geogr.* **2018**, *68*, 205–214. [CrossRef]
62. Xiao, X.; Manning, R.; Perry, E.; Valliere, W. Public Awareness of and Visitation to National Parks by Racial/Ethnic Minorities. *Soc. Nat. Resour.* **2018**, *31*, 908–924. [CrossRef]
63. Xiao, X.; Perry, E.; Manning, R.; Krymkowski, D.; Valliere, W.; Reigner, N. Effects of Transportation on Racial/Ethnic Diversity of National Park Visitors. *Leis. Sci.* **2017**, *39*, 126–143. [CrossRef]
64. Perry, E.E.; Xiao, X.; Manning, R.E. Barrier or bridge? The role of transportation in national park visitation by racial and ethnic groups. *World Leis. J.* **2015**, *57*, 173–184. [CrossRef]
65. Guo, T.; Schneider, I. Measurement Properties and Cross-Cultural Equivalence of Negotiation with Outdoor Recreation Constraints. *J. Leis. Res.* **2015**, *47*, 125–153. [CrossRef]
66. Ito, E.; Walker, G.J.; Liang, H. A Systematic Review of Non-Western and Cross-Cultural/National Leisure Research. *J. Leis. Res.* **2014**, *46*, 226–239. [CrossRef]
67. Schneider, I.E. Leisure constraints and negotiation: Highlights from the journey past, present, and future. In *Leisure Matters: The State and Future of Leisure Studies*; Walker, G.J., Scott, D., Stodolska, M., Eds.; Venture: State College, PA, USA, 2016; pp. 151–161.
68. Markus, H.R.; Kitayama, S. Culture and the self: Implications for cognition, emotion, and motivation. *Psychol. Rev.* **1991**, *98*, 224–253. [CrossRef]
69. Liang, H.; Walker, G.J. Does "face" constrain Mainland Chinese people from starting new leisure activities? *Leis. Loisir* **2011**, *35*, 211–225. [CrossRef]

International Journal of
Environmental Research and Public Health

MDPI

Article

How Can Physical Inactivity in Girls Be Explained? A Socioecological Study in Public, Subsidized, and Private Schools

Rodrigo Soto-Lagos [1,*], Carolina Cortes-Varas [1], Solange Freire-Arancibia [1], María-Alejandra Energici [2] and Brent McDonald [3]

1 Faculty of Education and Social Sciences, Andres Bello University, Viña del Mar 2520000, Chile; a.cortesvaras@gmail.com (C.C.-V.); solangefreirearancibia@gmail.com (S.F.-A.)
2 Faculty of Psychology, Alberto Hurtado University, Santiago 9160000, Chile; menergic@uahurtado.cl
3 Institute for Health and Sport, Victoria University, Melbourne, VIC 3011, Australia; brent.mcdonald@vu.edu.au
* Correspondence: rodrigo.soto@unab.cl

Abstract: In the last few years, the World Health Organization has highlighted that physical inactivity is a global issue affecting women to a greater extent than men. Faced with this, different nation states have developed public policies to reduce physical inactivity at school; however, the biomedical and individualistic models used have generated widespread criticism, as figures remain the same. In the context of failed interventions on increasing levels of physical activity, this study utilizes a socioecological model to analyze and understand how physical inactivity is reproduced in girls in the Chilean education system. A qualitative study was implemented, as it allows a focus on the entailed meanings, context, and processes. Active semi-structured interviews were conducted with 40 groups comprising headmasters, teachers, non-teachers, students, and families. The results show that physical inactivity is linked to factors that go beyond the individualistic model; that is, consideration must include intrapersonal, interpersonal, organizational, community, and public policy dimensions. Furthermore, gender stereotypes gain relevance in physical education classes, in addition to friendships and family, teaching, and administrative work, access to safe play areas, use of spaces, and widespread cultural factors associated with men and women. This study concludes that the assessed gender differences should be approached from a pedagogical perspective beyond common sense, further reporting that the individualized explanation for physical inactivity is irrelevant to answer why women are more inactive than men.

Keywords: physical inactivity; gender; physical education; socioecological model; physical activities; girls; public policies

1. Introduction

Physical inactivity has been cited as the 4th leading cause of death worldwide [1], and in recent years, the World Health Organization (WHO) reported that this global issue is more frequent and severe in girls and women [2–5]. The WHO further stated that schools should promote physical practices, such as exercise and sports, to ensure that recommendations for daily physical activity are adopted and achieved in student populations [6].

Chile is no exception in relation to the population achieving the required levels of physical activity encouraged by public health guidelines. The 2017 National Health Survey [7] reported that 86.7% of people do not exercise at least 3 times per week and noted the worrying trend that 9 out of 10 women, and people from lower socioeconomic backgrounds, were deemed sedentary. Further, 96% of children with less than 8 years of schooling were also considered inactive.

The Ministry of Education generates actions to decrease physical inactivity at school. The National School and Scholarship Assistance Council (JUNAEB, for its Spanish acronym) presented the nutritional map of the country's educational institutions, indicating that 50% of students attending pre-kindergarten to 9th grade were overweight or obese, as a result of physical inactivity, among other causes [8]. To overcome this situation, JUNAEB promotes the programs "Escuelas Saludables para el Aprendizaje" (Healthy Schools for Learning) and "Contrapeso" (Counterweight), which are aimed at reducing physical inactivity and obesity. Meanwhile, the Ministry itself published the Guidelines and Considerations for School Physical Activity during the pandemic [9]. In December 2021, the Ministry of Sports declared that 78.5% of children aged 11–17 were physically inactive and highlighted that girls are the most affected group (84.9%) compared with boys (71.8%) [10].

In line with this problem, from 2014 onwards, all Chilean schools began to be evaluated through the education quality measurement system (SIMCE, Spanish abbreviation) regarding the promotion of healthy lifestyle habits in the school community [11]. Moreover, in 2015, the Ministry of Sports created the "Escuelas Deportivas Integrales" program (Comprehensive Sports Schools), which offered an increase in physical activity in public schools alongside professional mentoring by psychologists and nutritionists. Under Sebastián Piñera's government (2018–2022), this program changed its name to "Crecer En Movimiento" (Growing on the Move), maintaining the same intervention strategy.

Today, different schools across the country implement and/or create interventions aimed at reducing the population's physical inactivity. Therefore, educational institutions have become privileged spaces to affect behavioral changes in the physical activity of students [2,6]. In this context, a bill requiring Chilean schools to undertake 15 min of daily physical activity was passed (see: Boletín 11518-11), an initiative that has led to tension in the school communities, as not all of them have the resources to adopt this bill.

As for the public and private initiatives that have attempted to reduce physical inactivity, several studies [11–15] have shown that interventions focused on prompting individual behavioral changes concerning diet and amount of physical activity do not lead to significant changes.

Some explanations have noted that the discourse inspiring the development of healthcare policies is based on medicine and biomedicine [16], and that the actions suggested by them have focused on individuals [17]. This has been consistent with linear logic with respect to problems and solutions, as the idea that people should be responsible and make the correct choices to reduce physical inactivity in their lives has been established, which several authors [18,19] have called the moralization of everyday life, which ignores the various social determinants of health [1,12].

In agreement with the above, different studies have aimed to contribute to the project for the reduction of physical inactivity across the world. In this sense, Mielke et al. [20] highlight the fact that, except for only 8 of the 142 countries studied, women were more inactive than men, a situation that aligns with the Chilean figures.

As for the approach adopted to reduce physical inactivity, Westerbeek and Eime [21] suggest that a transition has been observed in the last few years regarding public policy models—from a sports-competition to a sports-recreation model that is fully integrated into individual's daily lives. The sports-recreation model is known as a comprehensive sports ecosystem because, and similar to Muzenda et al.'s [22] proposition, it considers trans-sectoral cooperation, and the incorporation of contributions from other sectors such as health, education, transportation, and urban planning to be essential.

Recent studies show that including children's preferences is crucial for them to acquire the habit of exercising. In other words, to achieve positive changes in public policies, children should be included in this process by listening to their opinions, and regarding them as active subjects capable of engaging in reality [23].

Considering the pandemic, several studies [24,25] mention that physical inactivity and sedentary behavior in children and youth increase as a result of COVID-19. This last study highlights that the gap between men and women remained stable during this period and that keeping schools open facilitates physical activity, which decreased when schools were closed. This suggests the relevance of school establishments regarding the promotion of physical activity in children and youth.

1.1. Physical Inactivity in Girls

Isorna et al. [26] indicated that the physical (in)activity of women is influenced by gender stereotypes that condition the pedagogical processes and students' aptitude. These processes affect personal interests and motivations, thus influencing their level of involvement in some physical activities.

Castejón and Gimenez [27] revealed that in physical education (PE) class, boys preferred sports, while girls opted for expressive activities, such as dancing. According to Alsarve [28], this could be associated with the masculinized approach used in these classes, as it highlights that the beliefs and views of masculinity and femininity are stereotyped. Based on this work, masculinity was linked to traits such as physical strength, roughness, and agility; conversely, however, feminine roles were related to household chores, fragility, rhythm, subordination, and weakness.

According to Alvariñas and Pazos [29], Curieses [30], and Mujica [31], these stereotypes threaten women's involvement in traditionally male-dominated disciplines and are justified by the idea of sports as an impractical and dangerous activity for women. Similarly, imagery has been constructed of women who engage in sports (either recreationally or competitively) as transgressing gender norms.

As for the role played by PE, several authors [29,30] express that this discipline is permeated by male and female stereotypes that are present at school, validating the differences between genders and thus affecting school culture. In this sense, Cameron and Humbert [32] indicated that this situation is closely related to the roles played by men and women in society, concretely representing this through the existing differentiation between sports designated as "male" or "female." In this way, gendered differences in PE and incidental physical activity (play) at school become naturalized to educators [33].

The above, according to Parri and Ceciliani [34], would translate into differential behaviors by teachers, conveyed in subtle and explicit manners through various learning expectations. The authors further indicate that the differential expectations also affect girls in key aspects related to their identity and self-esteem, negatively conditioning their engagement with physical activity, and pushing them into smaller spaces, instilling submission, and a lower acceptance of physical contact. In contrast, Fissette [35] explained that female students consider differential treatment and gender and sports-associated stereotypes to be unfair, contributing to the 'why' they drop out of sport and physical activity.

In line with this issue, Mayorga et al. [36] suggested that unequal treatment is one of the barriers perceived by teenagers when doing physical activity, subsequently influencing their habits as adults. Moreover, Sánchez et al. [37] stated that the role played by teachers and their behavior concerning gender is conditioned by the influence of other factors, such as socioeconomic, environmental, family, or cultural variables. For this reason, teachers face the challenge of integrating these variables into their work and promoting innovations in each class for students to feel involved in the educational process, rather than feeling excluded owing to their gender, abilities, or physical qualities.

In the same vein, a recent study conducted by Energici et al. [38] reported that the abovementioned situation may be explained by the reproduction of gender stereotypes created in and through the practice of physical activities. This study may be considered a radical criticism of the individualistic model for addressing physical inactivity, as it suggests that the factors affecting this problem go beyond individuals.

The concern with children's and adolescents' experiences of physical activity is the relationship between these experiences and lifelong engagement with physical activity [39]. The school and PE are likely to be important locations for these experiences. If PE is gendered to create negative experiences for girls, then the likelihood of physical activity in adulthood for women may be reduced [40].

1.2. The Socioecological Model

Criticism of the individualistic perspective that seeks to reduce physical inactivity at school has been identified in recent years. One critique suggests that this perspective has not considered that each educational reality has its own school culture, and that the provision of a standard measure may overshadow both the local problems and the strengths of a community to solve them [6]. Similarly, studies report that including health in PE has led to activities that children are reluctant to do [41], as well as triggered emotions that may result in a preventive pathologization of their everyday life [42], causing fear [43,44] and annoyance [45]—emotions that fail to bring about the change that public policies seek [46].

These studies considered the socioecological model developed by Bronfenbrenner [47], who aimed to make the various dimensions interacting in the continuance and promotion of several social problems visible, specifying the existence of a dependency between systems and agents, which, in turn, exert a great influence on individuals' behaviors and practices.

Specifically, research on physical inactivity from this approach includes studies conducted by other scholars [48–50]. McLeroy et al. [48] suggested an ecological model featuring five degrees of influence (at the intrapersonal, interpersonal, institutional, community, and public policy levels), which should be considered in any intervention promoting a reduction in physical inactivity, as proposed by the WHO. Sallis et al. [51] highlighted the environmental and political influences in four fields of active life (recreation, transportation, occupation, and home) and called for collaboration with policy researchers to improve the probability of translating research results into changes in the environments, professional practices, and public policies. Bauman et al. [52], for their part, focus on the areas of life wherein exercise is done (home, work, transportation, and leisure time) and mention that these are different according to the country, age, gender, ethnic origin, and socioeconomic status of each context.

In the last few years, different authors [53–57] have adopted this approach to assess physical inactivity. In a cross-sectional way, they indicate that at the intrapersonal level, gender, age, ethnic group, and self-concept are relevant aspects, while at the interpersonal level, the family environment and meeting with friends are key points to explain engagement in physical activities. As for organizations and schools, the role of teachers and principals should be emphasized, whereas at the community level, socioeconomic aspects, educational level, and screen time are factors affecting physical inactivity. From the public policy dimension, access to facilities and safe neighborhoods are crucial factors for individuals to undertake physical activity.

Taking into account the criticisms of the individualistic and biomedical approach to achieving any meaningful change in the physical activity levels of populations, especially in relation to gendered differences, our study seeks to assess the effects of the public policy agenda to increase physical activity in Chilean schools. We utilize a socioecological framework to engage with a variety of actors in schools to understand the complexities of implementing such agendas, especially in relation to the reproduction of physical inactivity in girls in educational settings.

2. Materials and Methods

2.1. Methodology

This study is based on Sparkes and Smith's [58] postulates regarding qualitative research. The authors claim that this type of study must focus on the meanings, context, and processes that condition the issue that is the object of research. In this case, knowledge is built based on the opinions and experiences of the individuals affected by the public policies that seek to reduce physical inactivity in Chilean schools.

2.2. Participants

A theoretical sampling of schools was carried out with the understanding that all public, subsidized, and private establishments have been invited to carry out actions to reduce physical inactivity. In this context, based on the institutional relationship of the university sponsoring this research, three schools were invited for each type of administration that exists in Chile. The invitation was made directly to the email of each director, who invited the rest of the educational community.

The sample comprised eight schools: three public (all of primary level), two subsidized (both with primary and secondary level), and three private (one primary level and two primary and secondary levels). Five roles were identified in each one, which led to the development of a sample including principals (N = 31), teachers (N = 54), non-teachers (N = 37), students (N = 59), and families (N = 43). The participants came from the same organizations that agreed to participate. Access to the participants was through the management teams, who invited them, and they freely agreed to participate in the interviews. Likewise, the directors were asked to ensure parity between men and women in the calls.

It should be noted that the three types of schools have a director, but they are managed by a management team made by the director, vice director, curricular manager, and behavior manager. In the call for participants, the teams were invited all together because the decisions of the Chilean schools were taken in groups. The teachers were from PE and from other subsectors, as the practices to reduce physical inactivity affect the community, and all teachers can have an opinion about it. The non-teaching staff were administrative staff, support professionals (psychologists, social workers, speech therapists), and auxiliary and cleaning staff; they were included in the interviews in the understanding that practices to reduce physical inactivity affect the community and because their experience could add more layers and nuance on the topic. The students who participated, at the time of the interviews, were between seventh grade of elementary school (11–12 years old) and 4th grade of secondary school (17 years old). In families, not only fathers and mothers were invited, but also caregivers, who in some interviews were grandparents and uncles. Students and families were not always related.

In total, 40 group interviews were conducted, totaling 224 individuals participating in the study. All participants were invited by the manager team of each school, and their participation in the research was voluntary. Public establishments were located in the Metropolitan and Valparaíso region, whereas subsidized schools were situated in the region of Valparaíso and O'Higgins, and private institutes were in the Valparaíso and Magallanes areas.

To contribute to the understanding of the Chilean context in economic terms, public schools depend exclusively on the state for funding. The subsidized schools receive a monthly amount of public money for each student, and they have the option of receiving money from the families; that is, they receive public and private resources. Private schools are only maintained with the contribution of families. As for the curriculum, all schools must meet the minimum content proposed by the Ministry of Education. However, if some want to teach more content, they can do so (for example, languages, science, or other sports). Private schools are most likely to teach more content.

2.3. Data Production

Data were obtained from semi-structured active–reflective group interviews [59,60]. Considering group diversity, the research team asked each administrative team to manage the participants, who, in turn, voluntarily and freely consented to take part in this study.

The interviews were divided into three sections. The first delved into the work of each position within the school community. For example, tell us about your work and include all the information you consider relevant to understand what you do in this school. The second section asked about their experience with public policies aimed at reducing physical inactivity. For example, what actions do you carry out as an establishment to reduce physical inactivity? Do you have any link with a public service to reduce physical inactivity in your school? Finally, the third section sought information on the complexities observed by each role when trying to reduce physical inactivity at school, for example: How do you deal with physical inactivity in your establishment? What are the complexities experienced in increasing PA in your school? Do gender, socioeconomic level, cultural background, and educational level play any role? It is worth noting that, in view of the COVID-19 pandemic, most interviews were conducted via Zoom. Each interview lasted for around 45–60 min.

2.4. Analysis

To perform the analysis, the dimensions of the abovementioned socioecological model were used [61]. This proposal was divided into five aspects: the intrapersonal, interpersonal, organizational, community, and public policy levels. It is worth highlighting that considerable attention has been given to gender dimensions, as, according to what has been stated earlier, girls and women embody the most worrisome figures concerning physical inactivity.

The premises of the discourse analysis were followed to perform the analysis itself [62–65]. In line with these ideas and the socioecological model, inductive logic was adopted [66–68], in addition to deductive logic, from the categories provided by the model. To conduct the interpretative task, Moreno, Rivera, and Trigueros' study was considered [69].

For the validation of the research results, transferability [70] and representativeness [71] criteria were used. Similarly, all bioethical guidelines proposed by the Bioethics Committee of the Andrés Bello University were followed.

3. Results

The results of this study are presented after performing the analyses, following the intrapersonal, interpersonal, organizational, community, and public policies referred to in the socioecological model.

This study allowed for the gender-based assessment of physical activities that different educational actors (principals, teachers, non-teachers, students, and family) promote to reduce physical inactivity at school.

3.1. Intrapersonal Level

The intrapersonal level considers the biological and psychological factors that influence an individual's behavior. Based on the data obtained, the educational establishments under study show that physical inactivity in children is conditioned by physical and emotional changes that can be explained by their life cycles. In a cross-sectional way, all educational actors indicate that no play differences are observed in children aged 5–11 years (1st–6th grade), but boys and girls aged 11 and 12 go through a transition point regarding their engagement in this practice, which was attributed to the onset of puberty and subsequent breast development and menstruation in girls. Changes due to puberty were seen as a reason why girls disengaged with PE classes, sports, and physical activities at school owing to the emotional changes generated by these physical and social changes.

Teachers and principals attribute girls' lack of motivation to the effects of adolescence and puberty. Although this is a common situation for most students, "not all of them" experience decreased motivation in class.

> *In sixth, seventh, eighth grades (. . .) we usually see unmotivated girls in class, and boys always seem to be more involved, so something goes on during said maturity, adolescence, and puberty cycle, when girls lose motivation in their physical education classes. This is not the case for all of them, but in general. I have experience teaching at all levels, and we always see a decrease in the girls' engagement in [high school].*
>
> *(Subsidized School No. 2, Teacher)*

In the excerpt above, girls' decreased involvement is the result of their life cycle, a situation "they undergo during their maturity process"; furthermore, the teacher expresses that no differences in the involvement between girls and boys can be observed in the first school cycle (1st–5th grade), as is the case when they reach sixth grade, and onward. The teacher indicates that "their involvement always decreases slightly in [high school]," an expression that normalizes the students' attitudes, behaviors, and emotions, without making the social dimension of the teaching-learning process visible.

In connection with the above, another aspect that turned out to be relevant in the intrapersonal dimension was the biological differences between men and women. According to the students themselves, before adolescence, no physical differences can be seen between them, but as they grow, the characteristics that make teachers draw a distinction between the difficulty/weight of exercises for men and women emerge, as can be noted in the following excerpt.

> *Student No. 2: Because of the biological differences between men and women.*
>
> *Interviewer: I see... and what are said differences like?*
>
> *Student No. 3: Different muscle mass; ours is lower than boys.*
>
> *Student No. 2: As already mentioned, it varied based on our age, as you could say that there are not so many differences in terms of school development when we are young. As we reach eighth year, boys and girls begin doing different exercises.*
>
> *Student No. 3: So, in basic education grades, boys and girls are asked to "do 10 crunches," but in middle school, girls are told to do 30 push-ups, for example, whereas boys are asked to do 40 of them, or something like that.*
>
> *(Private School No. 2, Students)*

In view of the differences between boys and girls, students highlight that "biological" distinctions can be identified in the PE class, associated with a "different muscle mass," making reference to the fact that women are not as strong as men. Based on this role, they agree that when younger children perform the same activities, but after eighth grade, contrasts become more noticeable, for example, regarding demands. The expression "in middle school, they are asked to . . . " reveals that the requests are different for boys and girls, as the latter, for instance, are requested to do 30 push-ups, whereas boys must do 40. While this situation can seem natural to them, it can be regarded as an externally imposed limitation, given that expectations in terms of demand come from teachers who "tell you" the amount of exercise to be done.

Another relevant aspect that may account for the low involvement of girls in PE or sports classes is menstruation and breast development.

> *Student No. 1: Besides, another thing that people do not talk about much . . . of course, women menstruate once a month so, in some classes, you cannot clearly ask a girl who is on her period to run 15 min. At least I consider it to be really uncomfortable, to run and feel you can stain your clothes. I am new; I entered the school in first grade, and I barely know my peers, so the first class together was really uncomfortable; I was on my period, and it was really difficult, not knowing my partners, and all that . . .*
>
> *(Private School No. 2, Students)*

In view of the girls' opinion, this seems to be taboo, as this is not something that people "talk about" in face-to-face classes. Being on their menstrual cycle causes discomfort in female students, affecting their participation in physical activities, as this is a subject rarely addressed. Girls are not sufficiently confident to talk about it with their peers or teachers.

As indicated in the excerpt, menstruation is an issue that generates concern in girls, which is enhanced when they are "new" students, as they are not close enough to their peers. This would lead to different emotions, and getting involved in class becomes a "difficult" and "uncomfortable" situation that requires building confidence to overcome it. This presents a situation that should be explored beyond the common sense of students and educational actors.

Based on their experience, teachers suggest that breast development is a situation associated with shame, an emotion that students experience when they feel that they are being observed or criticized during PE class:

> *Teacher No. 3: Maybe, as they are going through a growth stage, they feel more ashamed if they have bigger breasts, and aspects like that; they do not want to be exposed in front of others or criticized, I think.*
>
> *Teacher No. 1: They seem to be insecure about their physical aspect, you know? About their appearance . . . [they feel insecure]*
>
> *Teacher No. 2: [And frequently, in the second course] that is really common, girls are really insecure, and in all senses, when they have to take part in activities, if they have to sing or move, there is little involvement from them.*
>
> *(Public School No. 1, Teachers)*

Therefore, according to the data obtained, physical changes, such as breast development and menstruation, are associated with non-positive emotions in the PE class. This occurs in the three types of education administration (public, subsidized, and private), wherein emotions such as insecurity, shame, and lack of self-esteem and self-acceptance develop, evident from the concern about their body and, more specifically, about their peers' opinions of them.

> *Student: Yes, I remember that in other years, and even before COVID, girls in dressing rooms were more concerned about looking good rather than being worried about having shoes, for instance, or they did not want to exercise wearing these leggings as people would be looking at them, or . . . stuff like that. I believe that these effects girls' performance because I've never seen differences made by the establishment or teachers*
>
> *(Subsidized School No. 2, Student)*

The quote above shows that dynamics are developed in PE classes that, although they may concern biological aspects associated with development stages, agree with the relationships built between peers. For instance, in the statement wherein a student says that she does not want to exercise wearing leggings, as people would be looking at her, she gives a social justification that may explain the high rates of physical inactivity in women, which is related to the fear of exercising owing to the opinion that other individuals may have about their bodies.

The above statements made by teachers and principals can be explained as self-esteem problems, which may lead to insecurity. During the pandemic, self-esteem problems became evident as girls attended lessons, but their cameras were switched off.

> *As for girls' drop out, if I consider the stage, age of students, and girls who become judgmental, self-esteem is crucial to prevent this issue. Unfortunately, their self-esteem makes them insecure, and this lack of security is evident now in the light of the pandemic, when we insist on asking them to switch their cameras on, and they try to avoid showing themselves, because they fail to accept their bodies. So, this becomes a key issue when they stop doing physical activity, showing themselves, or taking care of themselves*
>
> *(Public School No. 1, Teacher)*

The excerpt above reports that the insecurities identified in students—illustrated with expressions such as "they avoid showing themselves," "they do not switch their cameras on," and "they do not accept their bodies"—may be the reasons why they stop doing physical activity, showing themselves, and, thus, stop "caring about themselves." This passage also provides a social and pedagogical explanation to address inactivity in women and in school in general.

3.2. Interpersonal Level

The next dimension developed within the socioecological model is interpersonal, associated with social networks (formal and informal) and social support systems, including family and friends.

From the data obtained, students make a difference between their involvement in face-to-face physical education classes and those delivered via digital platforms as a result of the COVID-19 pandemic. The first was associated with fun and positive emotions, whereas the online format was linked to being alone and a lack of interaction with peers—a non-positive perception.

Student No. 2: Yes, face-to-face classes were funnier because we were together . . . we always run at the beginning, while at the end we played games, so physical education classes were really fun under said modality.

Interviewer: And what are classes like now?

Student No. 2: Now . . . well, the virtual class is good too, but . . . not as fun as it was before because you are alone, and you don't speak to almost anybody, so . . . it's okay, but face-to-face classes are better.

(Private School No. 3, Students)

When pointing out that "we were together," the student highlights meeting with peers as the reason for "fun" in the PE class. Similarly, this positive emotion is linked to the games played at the end of the class, which are positively associated with face-to-face modality and gathering with friends. For their part, virtual lessons were related to being alone and unable to talk to anyone, aspects that would decrease the motivation that the group feels over individual and lonely practice.

In the same vein, a student from another type of establishment states that if he needs help during the virtual class, he never asks for it. However, in face-to-face lessons, "he turns to a friend for help."

Student No. 1: Another could be when we want to get help, but do not feel confident, so we just avoid doing it in online lessons (. . .) In face-to-face classes, if you do not feel sure about something, you can ask a friend for help, who acts as a companion.

(Subsidized School No. 2, Students)

This excerpt highlights that social support from friends in PE classes is relevant for students. A significant figure accompanying the student, such as a friend, can help students ask for help and perform activities that can be regarded as challenging.

With regard to family support, different experiences were observed in face-to-face and online lessons. Parents mentioned that virtual lessons led to less positive emotions regarding participation, and technology was identified as a challenge for families, as the link with digital devices increased with this modality. According to a guardian, sedentary behavior as a result of technology was greater in times of COVID but even higher in women than men.

Parent No. 1: My little son (. . .) for example, I have a treadmill, and he turns it on by himself, starts running, jumps on the trampoline . . . he is always looking for something to do, because he is not the kind of child that can be entertained with a cell phone or the TV. Thank God! he is not the kind of child who keeps quiet sitting, no . . . he is always in the backyard, playing with the dog; he is restless. This is not the case with girls, who play with their phones, use TikTok, etc. It's difficult for me to take my daughter away from the TV, cell phone . . . but yes, I can tell the difference between a girl and a boy, and it is worse when they are children of different ages.

(Public School No. 1, family member).

In the above statement, a scenario is built wherein the motivation for physical exercise varies between men and women, and this could be conditioned by the development stage, as already mentioned. At this point, a teacher suggests that families play a key role in promoting physical activities and sports in boys and girls.

I think this is a cultural matter, I don't know ... I still believe physical activity is not promoted by families in the same way for girls or boys . . . as with soccer, for instance, nowadays, girls are highly motivated to play soccer, but it is not natural for us to understand that a girl may like to do a sport, like girls who like doing sports or exercising are really peculiar. The case of men is more general . . . those who like doing physical activity. But I do believe that both genders have reduced their willingness to exercise, and I think this can be partially explained by their sedentary behavior.

(Public School No. 2, Teacher)

The expression "physical activity is not promoted by families in the same way for girls or boys" shows that men and women are encouraged to exercise in different ways. Although the number of girls doing sports is growing, the teacher highlights that "girls who like sports are peculiar," thus reinforcing the idea that they may be less motivated than their male peers. Nonetheless, according to the teacher, "both have decreased their willingness to do physical activity," which poses a challenge for schools and families as sedentary behaviors increase in the pandemic context.

3.3. Organizational Level

This dimension refers to the influence of the school, especially from teachers and principals. Based on the data assessed, the relationship with teachers is notably a positive factor in promoting physical activity. Similarly, the decisions made by the administrative team concerning the sports practiced in the school community are relevant, as are whether they make the decision to make a difference between girls and boys.

With regard to principals, the data assessed present this group as strategic for intervention purposes in terms of physical inactivity at school. This is because the measures adopted by this group will influence the experiences of many students, as well as the community as a whole. An example of the decisions made concerning the sports to be promoted in their schools is as follows:

> *The problem is that this was originally a men's school, so soccer at school has always been a male thing . . . for example, even during breaks . . . And this is the case of basketball too, but not of other (x) ... activities or sports that have been implemented later. In fact, girls began to play sports, and later the course included girls playing soccer. Track, for example, has always been considered to be more feminine, if I am not mistaken, right? And in fact, girls . . . always perform well, so to speak.*
>
> *(Private School No. 3, Principals)*

This quotation from the administrative team notes that the physical activities mostly promoted by educational establishments are sports, and these, in turn, have a historical and cultural burden that takes root in school communities. In this case, the burden is associated with gender, as soccer and basketball are related to men, whereas track is more linked to women. This would affect the school community in general by offering differential possibilities to students. However, some girls began to play soccer, indicating that gender-based sports are not sensible to students.

Although several educational establishments have been making progress in the integration of women into sports, an aftertaste is still perceived regarding the male-oriented perspective, as shown in the following paragraph:

> *Student No. 1: When I played basketball, when lessons were face-to-face, I remember that there were not so many balls for girls, as we use different balls. Boys for instance, use No. 7 and girls No. 6 balls, and sometimes there were no No. 6 balls for all of them, and good ones, because some were made of a material that not everyone likes. So we had to use a smaller ball, a No. 5, or use balls for boys (No. 7). That was the negative thing that often happened.*
>
> *(Private School No. 2, Students)*

The above excerpt highlights that access to sports material provided by the educational establishment is an issue that can further affect students' motivation to play sports and, therefore, the establishment's physical inactivity figures.

As for the relationship with teachers, it was reported that once students, especially girls, reach sixth grade, they tend to be less involved in the physical education class, as they feel their bodies are more exposed and the menstrual cycle is crucial in that connection. At this point, it was noted that this moment of the menstrual period could be addressed with a supportive bond between the teacher and the students, as indicated in the following excerpt.

Student No. 2: But teachers are flexible, I mean, the good thing is that our teacher is a woman, so if we tell her that we are on our period, and ask if we can sit down, she agrees, so she is more flexible with that, of course.

(Private School No. 2, Students)

This flexibility from the PE teacher can be perceived as empathy toward students, as "a female teacher" can understand what students go through during their menstrual cycle. When a teacher's gender is emphasized, students highlight that male teachers have fewer possibilities of empathizing with them, a situation that opens up the possibility for male teachers to develop pedagogical tools to understand and empathize with this situation.

Another factor to consider is the teacher's practice, which may be mediated by their expectations with regard to what men and women can do in terms of physical demands. The data assessed accounted for the differentiation and categorization of physical exercises by gender, a practice that is not enjoyed by students, as can be seen in the following excerpt.

Student No. 1: And physical education classes are mixed-sex. What happened to me in the other school is that we were divided into male and female groups, rather than into courses. We were separated and, if the class was small, they blended seventh and eighth grades together, for instance. Or in case of larger classes, eighth grade A and B were grouped together, but boys and girls did not exercise together. And here the case was totally the opposite, being all together. There was no differentiation between strength exercises (for boys), track (for girls) as they did in my former school.

Student No. 2: The difficulty of the exercise only depends on the ability of each individual, regardless the gender.

(Private School No. 1, Students)

The quote shows a comparison between two types of PE classes: one that makes a distinction between boys and girls, and another that does not do so. Student No. 1 highlights that mixed-sex classes are "a totally different thing," which is in contrast with the gender separation that she experienced in the other school. This comparison shows that both methods coexist in our time, leading to various effects on individuals. In view of this, the expression "the difficulty of the exercise only depends on the ability of each individual, regardless of gender" explicitly indicates that the differentiation in PE class should be based on the difficulty of an exercise for each individual, rather than the assumption that boys will do "strength exercises" while girls would be engaged in "gymnastics."

The data obtained showed different aspects of facilities. In this sense, the use of educational establishment areas was significant.

Teacher No. 1: One remark about that: I agree with Rosita, who speaks about the interest of girls at that age, but if we take into account the physical distribution of every educational establishment, and we take a look at fields, which are great areas … (Who uses the field?) Which is the group that makes use of the field?

Several teachers: [Boys]

Teacher No. 1: [boys], who play soccer, exactly, so girls stand at the sides. Have you noticed that? Girls are always at the side of the fields, so stereotypes also begin there. We are always fostering our reduction as women in sports, even in the distribution of the physical area available.

(Public School No. 1, Teachers)

In this sense, a very important situation that is not so widely acknowledged is the use of facilities. Although students' access to facilities is relevant, their use is equally significant. Data reveal that these areas are mostly used by boys who play soccer to the detriment of other potential activities and games. This situation occurs in both public and private spaces, thus suggesting that the spaces available to play, such as the backyard and break areas, are not democratically distributed between boys and girls and those who do not wish to play soccer.

3.4. Community Level

The community dimension refers to the services and relationships between organizations, including the safety of the neighborhood and the accessibility of facilities crucial in reducing physical inactivity.

With regard to safety, the risk level identified in a neighborhood is considered relevant when deciding to exercise in a square.

> *Well, I don't know, the people who cannot afford a ... well, one says "you could go exercise in the square's sports area," but it depends on the area where you live, because if the square of your neighborhood is very insecure, you will not go there to play sports in the morning. I mean, there are lots of factors that fall outside the policies that this or previous administrations have been able to execute.*
>
> *(Private School No. 3, Teachers)*

Based on the above, a teacher highlights the "economic access" of individuals, as this determines whether an individual is "playing sports in the square." This conditioning factor is linked to the sense of security in public areas, which suggests that physical inactivity may be associated with factors that go beyond the individual dimension, something that would "fall outside the policies," regardless of the government in power.

As for access to facilities, the possibility of playing sports or different physical activities in squares is also regarded as a relevant aspect.

> *Interviewee No. 5: There should be more just open grounds, or maybe a larger amount of fitness equipment in squares, I don't know. In most squares, there is fitness equipment or areas to play sports. Yes, maybe if we had more open grounds or stuff like that to play more sports, or maybe more clubs to be enrolled in within the municipality, in different sports, not just soccer teams.*
>
> *(Public School No. 1, Students)*

With regard to what has been stated above, students mention their need to have more squares available, and the expression "not just soccer" highlights that they want areas that allow them to play "different sports." This situation is relevant, especially in the public system, as access to sports and physical activities outside school is conditioned, as indicated below, by each family's economic access. In this sense, from a social justice perspective, the public area should be one to challenge inequalities in access to physical activities, something that cannot be achieved.

3.5. Public Policy Level

The public policy level considers national and local initiatives in addition to laws that may have an impact on individuals' physical inactivity. The data assessed show that standardized testing, PE curriculum, and education in general, and several cultural aspects that public policies do not critically analyze, have a role at school, influencing physical inactivity. The following excerpt delves into this:

> *How ashamed girls were and, based on objective data, the other SIMCE indicators, which also measure academic self-esteem, we found that their self-esteem was really low, especially in the second cycle, so these self-esteem workshops were created (...) Self-esteem is closely related to physical activity so, as we said earlier, if girls ... there are high rates of obesity at school, and they feel fat and try to hide their bodies. This is why they do not want to do physical activity, so that would be a subject to research too.*
>
> *(Public School No. 1, Teachers)*

Another relevant aspect that the above quote makes reference to deals with the standardized SIMCE test, which reveals that self-esteem is related to doing physical activity. In specific terms, teachers build a local correlation of the results of this test, mentioning that the "self-esteem" indicator is objectively low, which would guide the decisions made by the school. They particularly associate self-esteem with obesity, indicating that because there is low self-esteem and high obesity rates, involvement in PE classes will decrease.

In relation to the above, public education establishments are those that notoriously adopt more state plans and programs, turning them into the main recipients of public policies. In this context, the fact that a centralized and standardized program developed by the Ministry of Health was adopted by an educational establishment has been raised as a problem by an administrative team, as this would lead to difficulties in the school community.

> *Interviewee No. 1: Sure, this was developed by the MINSAL (Ministry of Health), and there were children who have been examined at the doctor's office, diagnosed with this ... with obesity, for instance, so it was mandatory for them to be in the program. And they felt like "I am in the program because I am fat." So we wanted to change that view and extend our invitation for every big boy and girl who wanted to be part of the program, so that every interested person could be part of it.*
>
> *(Public School No. 1, Principals)*

The above paragraph shows that administrative teams regulate public policies that seek to help their overweight students by implementing local criteria that aim not to differentiate the recipients chosen by the health service, as prioritized children said, "I am in this program because I am fat," which would lead to school dynamics that may be perceived as negative to them. For this reason, they made the decision to "change that view, and extend the invitation to everyone" in order to involve the educational community and avoid promoting an individualization of neither the problem nor the solution.

Although public policies condition the actions that may be implemented by schools and individuals, the data also showed that there are given roles in society that are both targeted at men and women, and their promotion through the communication media affects physical activity rates.

> *Interviewee No. 1: I also believe there is a decrease that goes beyond the school in particular, but is more related to society in general, where the role that women can play is circumscribed, delimited, previously demarcated and, therefore, they never break ground, no ... unlike boys, who are more encouraged to play sports. Outstanding sportsmen portrayed by the media are generally men; women who stand out in sports or (x) highlighted by the press are always a few.*
>
> *(Private School No. 1, Principals)*

This quote indicates that the sociocultural dimension can also play a part in physical inactivity at school, as there are roles for women that "are circumscribed, delimited, previously demarcated," and these guidelines are linked to aspects that are not related to sports and physical activities. Therefore, if a girl wants to engage in physical activity, she will be breaking social grounds that are difficult to change. Furthermore, the fact that the media highlights sports figures who "are generally men" accounts for the lack of female role models for girls to identify with.

4. Discussion

The results of this analysis are in line with the WHO diagnosis regarding physical inactivity in girls and women [2–5]. In a cross-sectional manner, all educational actors and types of schools agree that girls are more inactive than boys. This situation is also consistent with the information obtained in Chile by the Ministries of Health and Sports, which suggests that girls are more inactive than boys [7,10].

Concerning the educational actors' assessment method for physical inactivity, they also agree that it is a problem with more dimensions than just individual agency, which is in line with the criticism of the biomedical model adopted by public policies [6,16,17].

These criticisms are grounded in the evaluation of physical inactivity using the socioecological model, as there is consensus that this is a complex issue, and attempting to solve it based on individual behavioral change will not succeed [18,19]. In this sense, our results state that, at the intrapersonal level, the dimensions explicitly affecting physical inactivity are gender, self-esteem, and age. Ethnic origin was not a problem mentioned in the interviews conducted, which suggests a discrepancy with several studies [56].

As for the interpersonal level, the results are consistent with those of Hu et al.'s [56] study because friends and family are relevant factors when doing physical activity. In this regard, students make a difference between their involvement in face-to-face PE classes and those delivered via digital platforms as a result of the COVID-19 pandemic. The first modality was associated with fun and positive emotions, whereas online classes were linked to less positive feelings. Another significant aspect is the fact that, owing to the pandemic, virtual classes increased the use of electronic devices at home, which was considered a problem by families.

At the organizational level, teachers' support has been shown to promote motivation in boys and girls in PE classes, which aligns with the study carried out by Hu et al. [51]. In this sense, it is worth mentioning that PE classes are stereotyped [26,28]. Similarly, this study's findings are consistent with those of Castejón and Gimenez's study, which indicated that girls prefer dancing-related activities, whereas boys choose sports [27]. Nonetheless, these decisions are conditioned by the choices made by adults (principals and teachers) without asking the students about their preferences first [23]. When students give their opinions, they state that they prefer a mixed-sex class, with no gender differences [32,34].

At this point, data encourage us to develop pedagogical tools to address the menstrual cycle in PE classes because, so far, common sense has prevailed both from the students and the professionals working at schools. This aspect would require deeper scientific research.

At the community level, it can be seen that the access to and use of the establishments' shared areas are relevant for engaging in physical activity. For access, it is indicated that safety and the type of fitness equipment available in public squares are important for individuals. Concerning the use of space, the data show that areas are mostly used by boys in their soccer practice over girls or other activities. This can be linked to the study conducted by Hidalgo and Almonacid [71], which indicates that the main difference between boys and girls is the use of physical space for playing purposes. They also state that girls show self-marginalization attitudes, giving more prominence to boys, who tend to play soccer in common areas.

As for the last level, the results show that public policy focuses on the individual, which aligns with the criticisms made earlier [17–19]. In this vein, schools tend to regulate public policies for them to be consistent with their institutional identity, which is often more collective than individual.

5. Conclusions

In relation to the aim of this study, the socioecological model provides an alternative explanation and insight into how physical inactivity is reproduced in girls from the experiences of public, subsidized, and private schools in Chile. In this sense, it is possible to conclude that physical inactivity is conditioned by factors consistent with the socioecological model. It can be stated that women are more physically inactive than men as an effect of sociocultural factors, and that these gendered relationships with physical activity are developed in the education system. These factors are not natural and can be transformed in schools as well as from public policies. Aspects such as social construction of growth stages, gender stereotypes in PE and sports classes, access to safe squares, emotions, and public policies are aspects that can be transformed. It should be clarified that the results of this study represent public, subsidized, and private schools since the factors indicated are experienced by all the people who live in the country.

Although this research only sought to analyze how physical inactivity in girls is reproduced from school institutions, some practical implications that can collaborate in the solution of physical inactivity in girls can be identified. The first is linked to schools, understanding that management teams, teachers, and families can coordinate so that physical activity can become part of everyday life for both boys and girls. For example, workshops could be held that include children and families, or establishments could be opened after PE classes, such as on weekends. The second action is linked to policy makers. They could also adopt socioecological models to shape their work and generate actions to listen to the students and promote debate around the differences in gender that are promoted in Chilean society. Likewise, they could include in their analyses the local and territorial school cultures so that the activities are relevant in territorial terms.

To conclude, this study necessitates the continuation of scientific exploration of three areas. First, the menstrual cycle and its relationship to PE class, considering how girls indicated that they need greater confidence and openness to talk about these topics and that they feel their female teachers are more open to dialogue than male coaches. The second topic is gender separation in PE classes, as several establishments still preserve the idea that several sports are for men and others are for women. Furthermore, most students stated that they prefer mixed-sex PE classes. Finally, another issue that would be interesting to address is the effect of technology on family dynamics, as parents mentioned that due to the COVID-19 pandemic, their children were more connected to technology, thus increasing family conflicts. Policy interventions in educational settings to increase physical activity and improve public health based on an individualistic biomedical approach have failed to achieve their aims in the Chilean context; indeed, they may have contributed to even greater inequalities in physical activity based on gender. This research indicates a need to move to a socioecological model to adequately address the continuing inequality in physical activity for girls and women.

Author Contributions: Conceptualization, R.S.-L., C.C.-V., S.F.-A., M.-A.E. and B.M.; Data curation, R.S.-L.; Formal analysis, R.S.-L., C.C.-V., S.F.-A. and M.-A.E.; Funding acquisition, R.S.-L.; Investigation, R.S.-L., C.C.-V. and S.F.-A.; Methodology, R.S.-L., C.C.-V. and S.F.-A.; Writing—original draft, R.S.-L., C.C.-V. and S.F.-A.; Writing—review & editing, R.S.-L., C.C.-V., S.F.-A., M.-A.E. and B.M. All authors have read and agreed to the published version of the manuscript.

Funding: This research was funded by the National Agency of Research and Development (ANID), Fondecyt 11191188.

Institutional Review Board Statement: The study was conducted in accordance with the Declaration of Helsinki and approved by the BioEthics Committee of Andres Bello University (027/2019 and date of approval: 26 November 2019) for studies involving humans.

Informed Consent Statement: Informed consent was obtained from all subjects involved in the study.

Data Availability Statement: Not applicable.

Acknowledgments: The authors acknowledge the Vice Rectory of Research and Doctorate from Andres Bello University for support in the translation process of this paper.

Conflicts of Interest: The authors declare no conflict of interest.

References

1. Kohl, H.W.; Craig, C.L.; Lambert, E.V.; Inoue, S.; Alkandari, J.R.; Leetongin, G.; Kahlmeier, S. The pandemic of physical inactivity: Global action for public health. *Lancet* **2012**, *380*, 294–305. [CrossRef]
2. World Health Organization. *World Health Organization Global Strategy on Diet. Physical Activity and Health*; World Health Organization: Geneva, Switzerland, 2004.
3. World Health Organization. *World Health Organization Global Status Report on Non-Communicable Diseases*; World Health Organization: Geneva, Switzerland, 2010.
4. World Health Organization. *World Health Organization Global Recommendations on Physical Activity for Health*; World Health Organization: Geneva, Switzerland, 2010.
5. World Health Organization. *World Health Organization Global Action Plan on Physical Activity 2018–2030: More Active People for a Healthier World*; World Health Organization: Geneva, Switzerland, 2018.
6. Soto-Lagos, R. Deporte y Actividad Física Como Herramientas para la Estandarización de la Salud Global: La Dietética de la Organización Mundial de la Salud [Sports and Physical Activity as Tools for Standardizing Global Health: The World Health Organization's Diet]. In *Encontrando el Futuro de los Estudios Sociales y Culturales sobre Deporte [Looking for the Future of Social and Cultural Studies on Sports]*; Mora, B., Ed.; University of the Republic: Montevideo, Uruguay, 2018.
7. Ministry of Health Chile. *National Health Survey*; Ministry of Health Chile: Santiago, Chile, 2017.
8. Ministry of Education. National School and Scholarship Assistance Council Chile. Healthy Schools for Learning. 2018. Available online: https://www.junaeb.cl/escuelas-saludables-para-el-aprendizaje-2 (accessed on 1 March 2019).

9. Ministry of Education Chile. Guidelines and Considerations for School Physical Activity during a Pandemic. 2021. Available online: https://formacionintegral.mineduc.cl/wp-content/uploads/2021/11/orientaciones-para-actividad-fisica-en-pandemia.pdf (accessed on 1 March 2022).
10. Ministry of Sports Chile. National Physical Activity and Sports Survey with Children Aged 5–17. 2021. Available online: https://cdn.digital.gob.cl/public_files/Campa%C3%B1as/Cuenta-P%C3%BAblica-2020/CP-sectoriales/23-2020-SECTORIAL-MINISTERIO-DEL-DEPORTE.pdf (accessed on 15 January 2022).
11. Ministry of Education. Chile. SIMCE Technical Report. 2014. Available online: http://archivos.agenciaeducacion.cl/InformeTecnicoSimce_2014.pdf (accessed on 1 March 2019).
12. Kay, T. Bodies of knowledge: Connecting the evidence bases on physical activity and health inequalities. *Int. J. Sport Policy Politics* **2016**, *8*, 539–557. [CrossRef]
13. Ferrer, M. Reflexiones sobre la Concepción De Salud Como responsabilidad individual. Construyendo bioética en salud pública [Insights on the Idea of Health as Individual Responsibility. Building Bioethics in Public Health]. In *Bioética y Sociedad en Latinoamérica [Bioethics and Society in Latin America]*; León, F.J., Ed.; Fundación Interamericana Ciencia y Vida: Santiago, Chile, 2011; pp. 115–122.
14. Edmundo Granda Ugalde. La Salud y la Vida. [Health and Life]; Quito, Ecuador. 2011. Available online: https://pesquisa.bvsalud.org/ripsa/resource/pt/biblio-911885 (accessed on 19 May 2022).
15. Pedraza, Z. Movimiento y estética para estilos de vida saludable [Movement and Esthetics for Healthy Lifestyles]. *Rev. Méd. Risaralda* **2012**, *12*, 50–55. [CrossRef]
16. Pedraza, Z. La estrategia higiénica: Movimiento y regeneración [The Hygienic Strategy: Movement and Regeneration]. *Educ. Fís. Deporte* **2011**, *30*, 445–456.
17. Tirado, F.; Gálvez, A.; Castillo, J. Movimiento y regímenes de vitalidad. La Nueva organización de la vida en la biomedicina [Movement and Regimes of Vitality. The New Organization of Life in Biomedicine]. *Política Soc.* **2012**, *49*, 571–590. [CrossRef]
18. Lamelas, V.S. La persona y el Estado como agentes de responsabilidad para la producción de sociedades saludables: Análisis temático desde la perspectiva de profesionales de la salud en Cataluña (España) [The Individual and the State as Agents Responsible for the Production of Healthy Societies: A Thematic Analysis from the Perspective of Healthcare Professionals in Catalunya (Spain)]. *Salud Colect.* **2017**, *13*, 45–61. [CrossRef]
19. Bagrichevsky, M.; Castiel, L.D.; Vasconcellos-Silva, P.R.; Estevão, A. Discursos sobre comportamento de risco à saúde e a moralização da vida cotidiana [Discourses about Health Risk Behaviour and the Moralization of the Everyday Life]. *Ciênc. Saúde Coletiva* **2010**, *15* (Suppl. 1), 1699–1708. [CrossRef]
20. Castiel, L.D.; Santos, M.; Ribeiro De Moraes, D. Os riscos e a promoção do autocontrole na saúde alimentar: Moralismo, biopolítica e crítica parresiasta. *Ciênc. Saúde Coletiva* **2014**, *19*, 523–532. [CrossRef]
21. Mielke, G.I.; Crochemore, M.; da Silva, I.; Kolbe-Alexander, T.L.; Brown, W.J. Shifting the Physical Inactivity Curve Worldwide by Closing the Gender Gap. *Sports Med.* **2018**, *48*, 481–489. [CrossRef]
22. Westerbeek, H.; Eime, R. The Physical Activity and Sport Participation Framework—A Policy Model Toward Being Physically Active Across the Lifespan. *Front. Sports Act. Living* **2021**, *3*, 1–11. [CrossRef]
23. Muzenda, T.; Shung-King, M.; Lambert, E.V.; Brugulat Panés, A.; Weimann, A.; McCreedy, N.; Tatah, L.; Mapa-Tassou, C.; Govia, I.; Were, V.; et al. Three Growth Spurts in Global Physical Activity Policies Between 2000 and 2019: A Policy Document Analysis. *Int. J. Environ. Res. Public Health* **2022**, *19*, 3819. [CrossRef]
24. Frömel, K.; Groffik, D.; Kudláček, M.; Šafář, M.; Zwierzchowska, A.; Mitáš, J. The Differences in Physical Activity Preferences and Practices Among High Versus Low Active Adolescents in Secondary Schools. *Sustainability* **2022**, *14*, 891. [CrossRef]
25. Dallolio, L.; Marini, S.; Masini, A.; Toselli, S.; Stagni, R.; Bisi, M.C.; Gori, D.; Tessari, A.; Sansavini, A.; Lanari, M.; et al. The Impact of COVID-19 on Physical Activity Behaviour in Italian Primary School Children: A Comparison Before and During Pandemic Considering Gender Differences. *BMC Public Health* **2022**, *22*, 52. [CrossRef]
26. Chen, S.; Wang, B.; Imagbe, S.; Gu, X.; Androzzi, J.; Liu, Y.; Yli-Piipari, S.R.; Hu, G.; Staiano, A.E. Adolescents' Behaviors, Fitness, and Knowledge Related to Active Living Before and During the COVID-19 Pandemic: A Repeated Cross-Sectional Analysis. *Int. J. Environ. Res. Public Health* **2022**, *19*, 2560. [CrossRef]
27. Isorna, F.; Ruiz, F.; Rial, A. Variables predictoras del abandono de la práctica físico-deportiva en adolescentes. [Predictor Variables for Dropping out of Physical Sports Activity by Teenagers]. *Cult. Cienc. Deporte* **2013**, *8*, 93–102. [CrossRef]
28. Castejón, F.J.; Giménez, F.J. Teachers' Perceptions of Physical Education Content and Influences on Gender Differences. *Mot. Rev. Educ. Física* **2015**, *21*, 375–385. [CrossRef]
29. Alsarve, D. Addressing Gender Equality: Enactments of Gender and Hegemony in the Educational Textbooks Used in Swedish Sports Coaching and Educational Programmes. *Sport Educ. Soc.* **2018**, *23*, 840–852. [CrossRef]
30. Alvariñas-Villaverde, M.; Pazos-González, M. Estereotipos de género en Educación Física, una revisión centrada en el alumnado [Gender Stereotypes in Physical Education: A Student-Centered Review]. *Rev. Electrón. Investig. Educ.* **2017**, *20*, 154–163. [CrossRef]
31. Curieses, P. Por una escuela inclusiva. Las fronteras del género [Towards Inclusion in Education. Gendered Borders]. *Rev. Int. Educ. Para Justicia Soc.* **2017**, *6*, 63–79. [CrossRef]

32. Mujica Johnson, F.N. Educación Física crítica: Un enfoque fundamental para la igualdad de género y la inclusión educativa en Chile [Critical Physical Education: A Fundamental Approach to Gender Equality and Educational Inclusion in Chile]. *Rev. Infanc. Educ. Aprendiz.* **2019**, *6*, 1–17. [CrossRef]
33. Van der Smee, C.; McDonald, B.; Spaaij, R. 'I play on a club team': Examining the development of the physically active habitus in early primary education. *Sport Educ. Soc.* **2022**, 1–15. [CrossRef]
34. Monforte, J.; Colomer, J. Como una chica: Un estudio provocativo sobre estereotipos de género en educación física [Like a Girl: A Provocative Study on Gender Stereotypes in Physical Education]. *Retos Nuevas Tend. Educ. Fís. Deporte Recreación* **2019**, *36*, 74–79. [CrossRef]
35. Cameron, N.; Humbert, L. 'Strong Girls' in Physical Education: Opportunities for Social Justice Education. *Sport Educ. Soc.* **2020**, *25*, 249–260. [CrossRef]
36. Parri, M.; Ceciliani, A. Best Practice in PE for Gender Equity—A Review. *J. Phys. Educ. Sport* **2019**, *19*, 1943–1952. [CrossRef]
37. Fisette, J.L. 'Are You Listening?': Adolescent Girls Voice How They Negotiate Self-Identified Barriers to Their Success and Survival in Physical Education. *Phys. Educ. Sport Pedagog.* **2013**, *18*, 184–203. [CrossRef]
38. Mayorga, D.; Parra, M.; Viciana, J. Condición física, actividad física, conducta sedentaria y predictores psicológicos en adolescentes chilenos: Diferencias por género. [Physical Fitness, Physical Activity, Sedentary Behavior and Psychological Predictors in Chilean Adolescents: Differences by Gender]. *Cult. Cienc. Deporte* **2019**, *14*, 233–241. [CrossRef]
39. Penney, D.; Jess, M. Physical education and physically active lives: A lifelong approach to curriculum development. *Sport Educ. Soc.* **2004**, *9*, 269–287. [CrossRef]
40. Sánchez, C.; Chiva, O.; Ruiz, J. Estereotipos de género y educación física en educación secundaria [Gender Stereotypes and Physical Education in Secondary School]. *Rev. Int. Cienc. Soc. Act. Fís. Juego Deporte.* 2016. Available online: http://hdl.handle.net/10234/167283 (accessed on 1 March 2019).
41. Metcalfe, S. Adolescent constructions of gendered identities: The role of sport and (physical) education. *Sport Educ. Soc.* **2018**, *23*, 681–693. [CrossRef]
42. Energici, M.; Schöngut-Grollmus, N.; Soto-Lagos, R. Aesthetic/Affective Norms of Femininity: An Obstacle to Women's Performance of Exercise. *Int. Rev. Sociol. Sport* **2021**, *56*, 1070–1086. [CrossRef]
43. Walters, S.R.; Payne, D.; Schluter, P.J.; Thomson, R.W. 'It Just Makes you Feel Invincible': A Foucauldian Analysis of Children's Experiences of Organized Team Sports. *Sport Educ. Soc.* **2015**, *20*, 241–257. [CrossRef]
44. De la Villa Moral, M. Crítica a la Visión Dominante de Salud-Enfermedad desde la Psicología Social de la Salud. Patologización Preventiva de la Vida Cotidiana [A Critique to the Dominant View of Health-Disease from the Social Psychology of Health. Preventive Pathologizing of Daily Life]. *Boletín Psicol.* **2008**, *94*, 85–104.
45. Gómez, R.A. La Salud, una metáfora biopolítica del temor a la muerte Lectura desde las epistemologías locales [Health, a Biopolitical Metaphor of Fear for Death. An Interpretation from Local Epistemologies]. *Cienc. Forenses Salud* **2015**, *9*, 129–148. [CrossRef]
46. Gagnon, M.; Jacob, J.D.; Holmes, D. Governing Through (In)Security: A Critical Analysis of a Fear-Based Public Health Campaign. *Crit. Public Health* **2010**, *20*, 245–256. [CrossRef]
47. Lupton, D. *Revolting Bodies: The Pedagogy of Disgust in Public Health Campaigns*; Sydney Health & Society Group Working Paper; Sydney Health & Society Group: Sydney, Australia, 2013; p. 3.
48. Soto-Lagos, R.; Deporte, P. Corporales, vida saludable y buen vivir: Un Análisis crítico para una nueva praxis [Sports, Physical Activities, Healthy Lifestyle and Good Living: A Critical Analysis for a New Practice]. *J. Lat. Am. Socio-Cult. Stud. Sport* **2018**, *9*, 29–44.
49. Bronfenbrenner, U. *La ecología del desarrollo humano. Experimentos en Entornos Naturales y Diseñados [The Ecology of Human Development. Experiments in Natural and Designed Environments] Cognición y Desarrollo Humano*; Paidós: Barcelona, Spain, 1987.
50. McLeroy, K.R.; Bibeau, D.; Steckler, A.; Glanz, K. An Ecological Perspective on Health Promotion Programs. *Health Educ. Q.* **1988**, *15*, 351–377. [CrossRef]
51. Sallis, J.F.; Cervero, R.B.; Ascher, W.; Henderson, K.A.; Kraft, M.K.; Kerr, J. An Ecological Approach to Creating Active Living Communities. *Annu. Rev. Public Health* **2006**, *27*, 297–322. [CrossRef]
52. Bauman, A.; Reis, R.; Sallis, J.; Wells, J.; Loos, R.; Brian, M. Correlates of Physical Activity: Why Are Some People Physically Active and Others Not? *Phys. Act.* **2012**, *2*, 258–271. [CrossRef]
53. Falco, C.; Samda, O.; Estevan, I.; Álvarez, O. Estructuración de la Estrategia para Organizar Actividades Físico-Deportivas y Recreativas [Structuring the Strategy for the Organization of Physical-Sports and Recreational Activities]. *Rev. Iberoam. Psicol. Ejerc. Deporte* **2013**, *8*, 373–391.
54. Vidal-Conti, J. Identificación de predictores de actividad física en escolares según el modelo socio-ecológico mediante un análisis multifactorial [Identifying Physical Activity Predictors in Schoolchildren Based on the Socioecological Model through a Multiple Factor Analysis]. *Cult. Cienc. Deporte* **2015**, *31*, 51–59.
55. El-Ammari, A.; El Kazdouh, H.; Bouftini, S.; El Fakir, S.; El Achhab, Y. Level and potential social-ecological factors associated with physical inactivity and sedentary behavior among Moroccan school-age adolescents: A cross-sectional study. *Environ. Health Prev. Med.* **2017**, *22*, 47. [CrossRef]

56. Hu, D.; Zhou, S.; Crowley-McHattan, Z.J.; Liu, Z. Factors That Influence Participation in Physical Activity in School-aged Children and Adolescents: A Systematic Review from the Social Ecological Model Perspective. *Int. J. Environ. Res. Public Health* **2021**, *18*, 3147. [CrossRef]
57. Knight, R.L.; McNarry, M.A.; Runacres, A.W.; Shelley, J.; Sheeran, L.; Mackintosh, K.A. Moving Forward: Understanding Correlates of Physical Activity and Sedentary Behaviour During COVID-19 in Children and Adolescents—An Integrative Review and Socioecological Approach. *Int. J. Environ. Res. Public Health* **2022**, *19*, 1044. [CrossRef]
58. Sparkes, A.; Smith, B. *Qualitative Research Methods in Sport, Exercise and Health. From Process to Product*; Routledge: London, UK; New York, NY, USA, 2014.
59. Holstein, J.; Gubrium, J. *The Active Interview*; SAGE: London, UK, 1995.
60. Denzin, N.K. The Reflexive Interview and a Performative Social Science. *Qual. Res.* **2001**, *1*, 23–46. [CrossRef]
61. Iñiguez, L.; Antaki, C. "El análisis del discurso en psicología Social" [Discourse Analysis in Social Psychology]. *Boletín De Psicol.* **1994**, *44*, 57–75.
62. Ibáñez, T.; Iñiguez, L. "Aspectos metodológicos de la Psicología Social aplicada" [Methodological Aspects of Applied Social Psychology]. In *Psicología Social Aplicada*; Alvaro, J.L., Torregrosa, J.R., Garrido, A., Eds.; McGraw-Hill: Madrid, Spain, 1996.
63. Potter, J.; Wetherell, M. Discourse and Social Psychology Quinlan, E. Conspicuous Invisibility. Shadowing as a Data Collection Strategy. *Qual. Inq.* **2008**, *14*, 1480–1499.
64. Wetherell, M.; Taylor, S.; Simeneon, Y. *Discourse as Data: A Guide for Analysis*; SAGE: London, UK, 2001.
65. Graham, G. *El Análisis de Datos Cualitativos en Investigación Cualitativa [The Analysis of Qualitative Data in Qualitative Research]*; Morata: Madrid, Spain, 2012.
66. Glaser, B.G.; Strauss, A.L.; Strutzel, E. The Discovery of Grounded Theory: Strategies for Qualitative Research. *Nurs. Res.* **1968**, *17*, 364. [CrossRef]
67. Strauss, A.; Corbin, J. *Basics of Qualitative Research: Techniques and Procedure*; University of Antioquia: Medellín, Colombia, 2002.
68. Moreno, A.; Rivera, E.; Trigueros, C. Sistema de medición de la calidad de la educación física chilena: Un análisis crítico [A Measuring System for the Quality of Chilean Physical Education]. *Movimento* **2014**, *20*, 145–167. [CrossRef]
69. Lincoln, Y.; Guba, E. *Paradigmatic Controversias, Contradiction and Emerging Confluences*; The Landscape of Qualitative Research. Theories and Issues; Denzin, N.K., Lincoln, Y.S., Eds.; SAGE: Thousand Oaks, CA, USA, 2003.
70. Sisto, V.; Fardella, C. Narrándose en la Flexibilidad. Un Análisis Narrativo Discursivo de la Identidad en Tiempos de Flexibilidad Laboral [A Narration in Flexibility. A Narrative Speech Identity Analysis in Times of Labor Flexibility]. *Rev. Psicol.* **2008**, *17*, 59–80.
71. Hidalgo, T.; Almonacid, A. Estereotipos de género en las clases de educación física [Gender Stereotypes in Physical Education Classes]. *Rev. Mot. Hum.* **2014**, *15*, 86–95.

International Journal of
Environmental Research and Public Health

MDPI

Article

Gender and Age Differences in Performance of Over 70,000 Chinese Finishers in the Half- and Full-Marathon Events

San-Jun Yang [1], Fan Yang [1,2,*], Yuan Gao [3], Yan-Feng Su [4], Wei Sun [4], Sheng-Wei Jia [2], Yu Wang [5,*] and Wing-Kai Lam [6,*]

1 Department of Physical Education and Research, China University of Mining and Technology—Beijing, Beijing 100083, China; 108947@cumtb.edu.cn
2 Li Ning Sports Science Research Center, Li Ning (China) Sports Goods Company Limited, Beijing 101111, China; jiashengwei@li-ning.com.cn
3 School of Physical Education, Yanshan University, Qinhuangdao 066004, China; gaoyuan1107@163.com
4 School of Physical Education and Coaching, Shanghai University of Sport, Shanghai 200438, China; suhui0909@163.com (Y.-F.S.); sunwei1@sus.edu.cn (W.S.)
5 School of Kinesiology and Health, Capital University of Physical Education and Sports, Beijing 100091, China
6 Sports Information and External Affairs Centre, Hong Kong Sports Institute, Sha Tin, Hong Kong
* Correspondence: yangfan6@li-ning.com.cn (F.Y.); wangyu@cupes.edu.cn (Y.W.); gilbert.lam@connect.polyu.hk (W.-K.L.); Tel.: +86-189-11326682 (F.Y.); +86-135-01126242 (Y.W.); +86-186-11783188 (W.-K.L.)

Abstract: (1) Background: The aim of the present study was to examine the characteristics of over 70,000 long-distance finishers over the last four years in Chinese half- and full-marathon events; (2) Methods: The available data of all finishers (n = 73,485; women, n = 17,134; men, n = 56,351) who performed half- and full-marathon events in Hangzhou from 2016 to 2019 were further analyzed for the characteristics of gender, age and average running speed; (3) Results: The total men-to-women ratio was the lowest in the half-marathon event (1.86) and the highest in the full-marathon event (17.42). Faster running performance in males than in females and faster average running speed in short-distance runners were shown. Gender and race distance were observed to have the most significant effects on average running speed ($p < 0.01$). For both male and female finishers, the slowest running speed was shown in older age groups ($p < 0.01$) during the full marathon. Our results indicated that the gender difference in performance was attenuated in the longer race distances and older age groups; (4) Conclusions: Understanding the participation and performances across different running distances would provide insights into physiological and biomechanical characteristics for training protocols and sports gear development in different groups.

Keywords: gender; men-to-women ratio; marathon; age; running speed

1. Introduction

The health benefits of endurance exercise might partially explain the increase in participation in marathon races during the last decades [1]. In recent years, marathon running has been considered a globally popular physical activity that can cater to the various healthy lifestyle needs of urban residents [2,3]. This running boom has gradually spread around the world. Well-known New York, London, Paris, and Berlin marathon events all had between 30,000 and 40,000 finishers [4]. While distance running used to be a male-dominated sport, today females account for 43% of marathon runners in the USA [5]. Marathon events have developed later in China than in Western countries. The number of marathon events held in China increased from 12 to 53 between 2010 and 2014 [6] to approximately 1100 in 2017 [7], which involved nearly 5 million participants and increased to over 2.2 million participants from 2016 to 2017 [7]. The number further increased to a total of 1900 events in 2019 [1]. The growing popularity of running has inspired a large amount of research on running biomechanics, performance and sport gears in the past decades [8]. Studies have found that proper pace can effectively reduce the risk of musculoskeletal injury [9], and different running strategies should be used in long-distance running according to gender, age and the event the runner is training for [10]. Moreover, differences in running biomechanics between Chinese men and women were observed, with female runners showing greater range of motion in the hip and knee joints, and a smaller shoe-to-ground angle during the heel touch-down phase. This is believed to be a form of self-regulation that women use to reduce the impact of landing, and men rely more on the performance of their shoes to achieve the purpose of buffering [11].

Following the increase in female participation in distance running [12], investigations into gender differences in running mechanics were intensified in the Western world [12–14]. The gender difference studies indicated clear differences in females' body fat and running speed [3], resulting in distinct movement characteristics and injury etiology. Nikolaidis et al. studied the performance and age composition of different genders during marathons, where they found that women achieved their best marathon race time ~5 years earlier in life compared to men. Women's participation increased disproportionately to men's participation, leading to an increase in the ratio of men to women [15]. In addition, more and more seniors are joining in marathon races [16]. The sex gap between elite female marathon racers and elite male runners may have reached its limit [17]. The age structure of most male marathon runners is larger and older than that of females (male: 40–44 years; female: 30–34 years) [18].

Although studies have been conducted on anthropometry, physiology and training characteristics have improved our understanding of the predictors of race time [19], as well as age- and gender-related differences in pacing during endurance running [20–23]. While Western counterparts have been extensively analyzed regarding their running characteristics, little attention has been paid to the Chinese population. Several articles have shown differences in running between Chinese and Western populations; one study found that, compared with Western women, Chinese women use the medial forefoot more during the push-off phase of running [24]. Western female runners have greater ankle valgus angles than males, while there is no significant difference between Chinese females and males [25]. Thus, research findings obtained from Western runners may not be directly applicable to the Chinese population because of racial differences. The present study examined trends of the men-to-women ratio, number of finishers and performances by gender and age groups across four years in half- and full-marathon events, respectively. It was expected that there would be a different men-to-women ratio and different performances across different running events. The comparison could help to better understand potential training requirements for both elite and recreational runners of different age groups, as well as to effectively estimate the demand of running shoes for different gender and age groups. To optimize female performance and health in sport, we need to include women in our analyses in order to better understand peculiarities that may exist in physiology. Therefore, we are happy to enrich the existing pool of knowledge with more data on female participation and performance in marathon racing. Understanding the participation and performance across different running distances (half- and full-marathon events) would provide insights into the physiological and biomechanical characteristics for training protocols for different gender and age groups.

2. Materials and Methods

2.1. Participants and Data Acquisition

The complete marathon event data for this study were officially obtained from Hangzhou Marathon Organizing Committee (https://www.hzim.org) [26]. The records were collected from all half marathons and full marathons between 2016 and 2019, and were officially certified by the World Athletics Organization. The Hangzhou marathon event included both full and half marathons and runs. Regretfully, the Hangzhou marathon event has been suspended due to the spread of COVID-19 in 2019. The study data included participants who completed the race in the appropriate amount of time. Age and gender information was provided for the period of 4 years. Ultimately, the study included a total of 73,485 participants (male, n = 56,351; female, n = 17,134).

2.2. Procedures

Age intervals of five years were selected to represent age groups among younger and older finishers in their categories. All runners over 71 years old were placed in one category, as there were only a few male runners in the oldest age group, while the oldest male runner was 74 years old. In total, the finishers were classified into 11 age groups; 21–25, 26–30, 31–35, 36–40, 41–45, 45–50, 51–55, 56–60, 61–65, 66–70 and 71+ years. Changes in gender participation are described by the men-to-women ratio (MWR, the quotient of males divided by female completers) [27].

2.3. Statistical Analysis

The official race time (i.e., accurate in seconds) was obtained for all finishers in both races. The average running speed in km/h was calculated using the final race time (h) divided by race distance (km) to allow comparison of performances between two long-distance races. All descriptive statistics were reported as mean and standard deviation. Prior to statistical analyses, data distribution normality was verified by visual inspection of histograms and QQ plots [18]. To assess age and gender distribution among finishers in the half- and full-marathon events, a chi-square test (χ^2) was performed. Statistical differences in marathon performance between 11 age groups and two events were observed. Meanwhile, their interactions were calculated using a two-way ANOVA, post hoc with Bonferroni-corrected tests, and the significance level was controlled at 0.05. All data were organized and summarized using Microsoft Office Excel 2019 (Microsoft Corporation, Redmond, WA, USA) and statistical testing was performed using SPSS 20.0 (IBM, Armonk, NY, USA).

3. Results

3.1. Participation by Gender, Race Distance, and Age Group

The MWR as well as the total number of male and female finishers in each age group and race distance are presented in Table 1.

Table 1. Distribution of male and female finishers in each age group and race distance.

	Half-Marathon				Full-Marathon			
Age Groups	**Males**	**Females**	**Total**	**MWR**	**Males**	**Females**	**Total**	**MWR**
21–25	940	505	1445	1.86	639	158	797	4.04
26–30	3667	2166	5833	1.69	3046	714	3760	4.27
31–35	4381	2063	6444	2.12	5110	1073	6183	4.76
36–40	4360	1712	6072	2.55	6274	1249	7523	5.02
41–45	3514	1538	5052	2.28	6733	1325	8058	5.08
46–50	2820	1404	4224	2.01	6573	1386	7959	4.74
51–55	1428	633	2061	2.26	3569	678	4247	5.26
56–60	618	179	797	3.45	1540	193	1733	7.98
61–65	208	47	255	4.43	502	64	566	7.84
66–70	111	20	131	5.55	209	12	221	17.42
71+	28	0	28	-	18	0	18	-
Total	22,075	10,267	32,342	2.15	34,213	6852	41,065	4.99

MWR = men-to-women ratio.

The total MWR was 2.15 and 4.99 in the half and full marathon, respectively. A gender × race distance association in participation was shown (χ^2 = 2294.505, p < 0.01, φ = 0.177). A gender × age group association in participation was observed in the half marathon (χ^2 = 89.091, p < 0.01, φ = 0.081) and in the full marathon (χ^2 = 53.431, p < 0.01, φ = 0.050). Furthermore, a race distance × age group association in participation was shown for male finishers (χ^2 = 1687.054, $p < 0.01$, φ = 0.187) and for female finishers (χ^2 = 600.388, $p < 0.01$, φ = 0.197) of different age groups. In the half marathon, the lowest MWR was observed in the age group of 26–30 years (1.69), whereas the highest MWR was observed in the age group of 36–40 years (6.12). In the full marathon, the lowest MWR was observed in the youngest age group (4.04), whereas the highest MWR was observed in the age group of 66–70 years (17.41).

3.2. Performance (Average Running Speed)

3.2.1. Overall Effects

The two-way ANOVA showed significant effects of gender [$F_{(1, 73,365)} = 612.757$, $p < 0.001$] and race distance [$F_{(1, 73,365)} = 7.914$, $p < 0.005$], as well as age group [$F_{(10, 73,365)} = 119.550$, $p < 0.001$]. Moreover, we found significant interactions for age group × race distance [$F_{(10, 73,365)} = 3.763$, $p < 0.001$], while no interaction was observed for gender × race distance [$F_{(1, 73,365)} = 3.270$, $p = 0.071$] and for gender × age group [$F_{(9, 73,365)} = 1.329$, $p = 0.216$].

3.2.2. Performance by Gender and Race Distance

A significant effect of gender on average running speed is shown ($p < 0.001$) in Figure 1, where male finishers (with the performance of 10.03 ± 1.67 km/h) were faster than female finishers (with the performance of 9.08 ± 1.27 km/h). In addition, a significant effect of race distance on average running speed was observed ($p < 0.001$). Figure 1 also shows that performance in the full-marathon event (9.95 ± 1.71 km/h) was faster than that in the half-marathon event (9.63 ± 1.53 km/h).

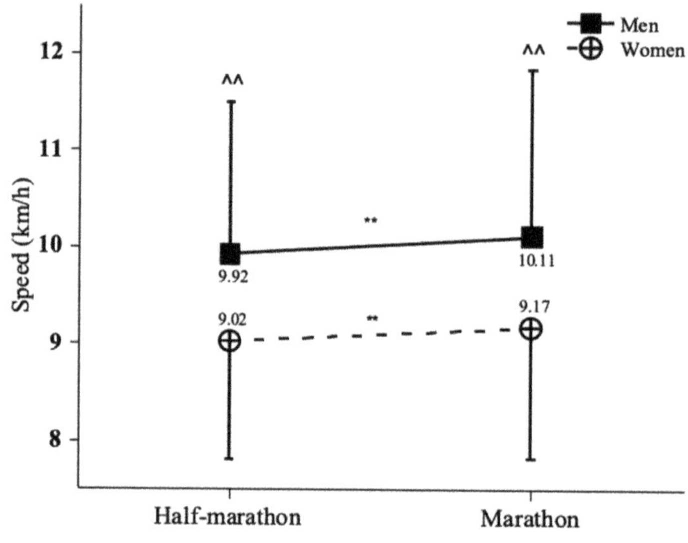

Figure 1. Race speed by race distance and gender. Error bars represent standard deviations. ^^ $p < 0.001$; ** $p < 0.001$.

No gender × race distance interaction on average running speed was found ($p > 0.05$), while the gender difference was lower in the half-marathon event (+9.98%) than in the full-marathon event (+10.25%). Half-marathon finishers were slower than full-marathon finishers among females (9.02 ± 1.22 versus 9.17 ± 1.35 km/h, respectively, $p < 0.001$), as well as among males (9.92 ± 1.57 versus 10.11 ± 1.73 km/h, respectively, $p < 0.001$).

3.2.3. Performance by Age Group and Race Distance

The age group × race distance interaction had a significant effect on average running speed ($p < 0.001$). Under closer examination of the performance, male finishers had the fastest average running speed of 10.33 ± 1.60 km/h, while female finishers had the slowest average running speed of 8.54 ± 1.03 km/h, regardless of the type of event.

In the half-marathon event, the fastest male age group was 61–65 years (average running speed of 10.32 ± 1.45 km/h), while the slowest male age group was 26–30 years (average running speed of 9.61 ± 1.57 km/h). In the full-marathon event, the male finishers had the fastest speed of 10.39 ± 1.62 km/h in the 46–50 age interval and the slowest speed of 9.16 ± 1.18 km/h in the 71+ age interval (Figure 2a).

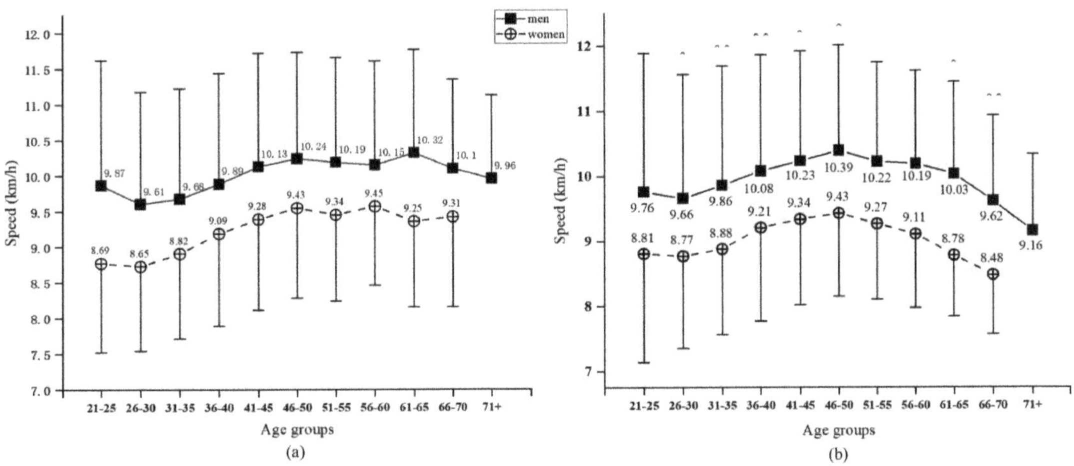

Figure 2. Race speed by age group and gender in the half-marathon event (**a**) and in the full-marathon event (**b**). Error bars represent standard deviations. ^^ $p < 0.01$; ^ $p < 0.05$.

In the half-marathon event, female finishers had the fastest average running speed of 9.61 ± 1.21 km/h in the 66–70 age interval, but the slowest average running speed of 8.65 ± 1.13 km/h in the 26–30 age group. In the full-marathon event, the fastest female finisher was observed in the 46–50 age group (9.43 ± 1.28 km/h), while the slowest female was in the 66–70 age group (8.48 ± 0.91 km/h) (Figure 2b).

3.2.4. Performance by Gender and Age Group

Although the main effect of gender × age group interaction on the average running speed ($p = 0.216$) was obtained, Bonferroni post hoc comparisons revealed a significant difference (Table 2).

In both male and female finishers, there was a significant difference between the age group of 21–25 years and the age group of 36–60 years ($p < 0.01$), as well as the age group of 61–55 years ($p < 0.05$). The same difference was found in the age groups of 26–30 years and 31–65 years ($p < 0.01$).

There was also a difference in the average running speed between age groups of 31–35 years, 36–60 years ($p < 0.01$) and 61–55 years ($p < 0.05$). Another significant difference was observed between the 36–40 age interval and the 41–55 age interval ($p < 0.01$). The performance of the 46–50 age interval showed a significant difference with the 41–45 age interval ($p < 0.01$) and the 51–55 age interval ($p < 0.01$).

Table 2. Bonferroni post hoc tests of age groups.

Age Groups	21–25	26–30	31–35	36–40	41–45	46–50	51–55	56–60	61–65	66–70	71+
21–25	-	-	-	**	**	**	**	**	*	-	-
26–30	-	-	**	**	**	**	**	**	**	-	-
31–35	-	##	-	**	**	**	**	**	*	-	-
36–40	##	##	##	-	**	**	**	-	-	-	-
41–45	##	##	##	##	-	**	-	-	-	-	-
46–50	##	##	##	##	##	-	**	-	-	-	-
51–55	##	##	##	##		##	-	-	-	-	-
56–60	##	##	##	-	-	-	-	-	-	-	-
61–65	#	##	#	-	-	-	-	-	-	-	-
66–70	-	-	-	-	-	-	-	-	-	-	-
71+	-	-	-	-	-	-	-	-	-	-	-

* represent male, # represent female, ** or ## $p < 0.01$; * or # $p < 0.05$.

4. Discussion

The aim of this study was to assess the age, gender and average speed characteristics of over 70,000 long-distance finishers over the last four years.

We found that the 31–35 and 36–40 age groups had the largest number of male finishers in the half-marathon event, while the 26–30 and 36–40 age groups had the largest number of female finishers. These findings are partly in agreement with previous studies, which reported that, regardless of gender, the largest number of finishers was found in the 24–34 age group [28]. In addition, a study conducted in Switzerland found that the two largest numbers of full-marathon finishers were in the age ranges 40–44 and 45–49 in men, but 35–39 and 40–44 in women; this study also reported that most half-marathon participants were 30–34 years old and 45–49 years old in men, but 25–29 years old and 30–34 years old in women [29]. Although there are differences among age groups in Asian and European populations, over 30 years of age appeared to be the dominant age in participants in long-distance running, which may be related to the relationship with physical needs, social influences and disposable time [30]. The study showed that the largest age group participating in full marathon events was usually older than the half-marathon runners. Such results may be due to older runners being more emotionally stable and responsible than younger people [31].

In terms of the number of finishers by race distance, there were ~1.3 times more marathon runners than half-marathon runners, which is not in agreement with the previous findings. The reason for this phenomenon may be that the marathon organizing committee limited the number of half-marathon runners during the registration period. In Switzerland, the total number of half-marathon runners was about 2.6 times higher than the marathon runners between 2000 and 2010 [32]. In Greece, the total number of half-marathon runners was about 3.5 times higher than that in the Oslo Marathon between 2008 and 2018 [28]. This could be explained by the fact that the registered number of half-marathon events is substantially lower than the full-marathon events held in China [33].

It is not difficult to understand the phenomenon that the number of people who finish the half marathon is higher than the number of people who finish the full marathon. The demand for physical fitness in the full marathon is undoubtedly higher. Running long distances can lead to dehydration, damage to muscle tissue and an increase in body temperature, which must be more difficult to overcome during a full marathon [34]. Moreover, the depletion of glycogen stores in the body causes athletes to "hit the wall (HTW)"; the frequency of HTW among elite and non-elite runners was 51%, with the greatest proportion being found in non-elite runners. Thus, HTW also increases the risk of withdrawal as the distance of the competition increases [35].

Our data confirmed that a higher number of male finishers than females was also observed in a longer-distance event, which is similar to the "Marathon des Sables" (7-day competition) with a men-to-women ratio (MWR) of 6.76 [3], the "Western States 100-Mile Endurance Run" (161 km) with an MWR of 5.28 [36], or Double Iron Ultra-Triathlon

(MWR: 8.96) to Deca Iron Ultra-Triathlon (MWR: 6.94) [37]. However, over the past few years, an increase in women finishers was observed in half- and full-marathon events, as indicated by the decreased trend of MWR. A plausible explanation for the MWR variation by race distances/intensities might be the consideration of females as relatively "novice" runners compared to males. One study reported that the MWR was decreased from 10.2 in the 1970s to 1.5 in the 2010s in the "New York City Marathon" [38]. Women complete shorter-distance races first and then longer-distance races according to their ability and physiological features. The majority opted for the half marathon, resulting in a higher number of female finishers in the half marathon than in the full marathon. Regarding changes in finishers by gender and age group, similar trends were shown across all race distances, with older groups having a higher MWR than younger age groups.

The current findings showed faster running performance in males than in females and faster average running speed in shorter race distances. This may be attributable to the innate physiological advantage of male runners and gender differences in training habits, with males having greater body weights and lower body fat percentages in terms of physiology [3]. The research pointed out that men and women are born with different muscle fiber properties, and the advantage of men is that the circumference of muscle fibers is larger than that of women, so they are more powerful [39]. This is the difference between men and women in gene expression in human skeletal muscle [40]. Furthermore, male athletes exhibit higher maximal oxygen uptake (VO_2max) and anaerobic thresholds than females in long-distance running [41]; there is a positive correlation between VO_2max and thermoregulatory ability [42]. Some articles have pointed out that in the non-competition training phase, men have longer training distances than women and have more weekly training sessions, so the running experience of male runners is higher than that of women [43]; the same goes for training differences for a half marathon [3]. Some researchers have also found that the larger male-to-female ratio in the older group is due to the lower number of female finishers [44]. Our data also found that the average pace of women in half-marathon events increased with age. In previous research, the slowest pace occurred in the older age groups [22]. One of the reasons for this could be that most young female participants in the half marathon were attempting long-distance running for the first time, which makes the pace slower in younger age groups. At the same time, the running speeds of older Chinese women groups were better than Western women. Eastern women are morphologically thinner than Western women [38], thus saving more running economy in long-distance running and are, therefore, faster on average.

There were several limitations in the present study. First of all, the role of environmental conditions, such as detailed data on temperature, humidity, and wind, was not considered. It is reasonable to involve the effect of these environmental parameters on the endurance performance [45]. Secondly, the number of participants was higher than other studies, as four-year data were accessible. Long-term research should be conducted in future. Thirdly, other endurance events such as 10 km races should be included.

5. Conclusions

This study found that the number of female finishers in the half- and full-marathon races has increased, but, overall, there are still more males than females. A higher number of younger female finishers participated in both race distances. Moreover, the overall performance of male's running is better than female's running, but as the race distance and the age of participants increased, the difference in performance caused by gender gradually weakened. It should be emphasized that the analysis of performance trends is related to changes in MWR based on age group and race distance.

Author Contributions: Conceptualization, Y.-F.S., F.Y. and S.-J.Y.; methodology, F.Y. and S.-J.Y. and W.-K.L.; software, F.Y., Y.G. and S.-W.J.; validation, Y.G., S.-J.Y. and W.-K.L.; formal analysis, F.Y.; investigation, S.-J.Y., W.S. and Y.-F.S.; resources, S.-J.Y.; data curation, S.-W.J., S.-J.Y., Y.W. and W.S.; writing—original draft preparation, S.-J.Y.; writing—review and editing, W.-K.L. and F.Y.; visualization, S.-J.Y. and W.-K.L.; supervision, S.-J.Y. and Y.W.; project administration, F.Y.; funding acquisition, F.Y. and W.-K.L. All authors have read and agreed to the published version of the manuscript.

Funding: This research was funded by Beijing Technology and Innovation Service Development Research Fund, grant number 154218001.

Institutional Review Board Statement: Not applicable.

Informed Consent Statement: Informed consent was obtained from all subjects involved in the study.

Data Availability Statement: The data presented in this study are available on request from the corresponding author.

Conflicts of Interest: The authors declare no conflict of interest. The funders had no role in the design of the study; in the collection, analyses, or interpretation of data; in the writing of the manuscript, or in the decision to publish the results.

References

1. Ren, Z.; Zuo, Y.; Ma, Y.; Zhang, M.; Smith, L.; Yang, L.; Loprinzi, P.D.; Yu, Q.; Zou, L. The Natural Environmental Factors Influencing the Spatial Distribution of Marathon Event: A Case Study from China. *Int. J. Environ. Res. Public Health* **2020**, *17*, 2238. [CrossRef] [PubMed]
2. Guicciardi, M.; Carta, M.; Pau, M.; Cocco, E. The Relationships between Physical Activity, Self-Efficacy, and Quality of Life in People with Multiple Sclerosis. *Behav. Sci.* **2019**, *9*, 121. [CrossRef] [PubMed]
3. Knechtle, B.; Knechtle, P.; Rosemann, T.; Senn, O. Sex differences in association of race performance, skin-fold thicknesses, and training variables for recreational half-marathon runners. *Percept. Mot. Ski.* **2010**, *111*, 653–668. [CrossRef] [PubMed]
4. Hennig, E.M. Eighteen years of running shoe testing in Germany—A series of biomechanical studies. *Footwear Sci.* **2011**, *3*, 71–81. [CrossRef]
5. Statistics, R.M. Marathon Statistics 2019 Worldwide. Available online: https://runrepeat.com/research-marathon-performance-across-nations (accessed on 7 March 2020).
6. Zuo, Y.; Zou, L.; Zhang, M.; Smith, L.; Yang, L.; Loprinzi, P.D.; Ren, Z. The temporal and spatial evolution of marathons in China from 2010 to 2018. *Int. J. Environ. Res. Public Health* **2019**, *16*, 5046. [CrossRef]
7. Xing, X.; Zhang, R.; Taks, M. The effects of health, social, and consumption capital on running-related expenditures in China. *Eur. Sport Manag. Q.* **2020**, *22*, 1–21. [CrossRef]
8. Trudeau, M.B.; Willwacher, S.; Weir, G.; Rohr, E.; Ertel, C.; Bruggemann, G.-P.; Hamill, J. A novel method for estimating an individual's deviation from their habitual motion path when running. *Footwear Sci.* **2019**, *11*, 135–145. [CrossRef]
9. De Koning, J.J.; Foster, C.; Bakkum, A.; Kloppenburg, S.; Thiel, C.; Joseph, T.; Cohen, J.; Porcari, J.P. Regulation of pacing strategy during athletic competition. *PLoS ONE* **2011**, *6*, e15863. [CrossRef]
10. Cuk, I.; Nikolaidis, P.T.; Villiger, E.; Knechtle, B. Pacing in Long-Distance Running: Sex and Age Differences in 10-km Race and Marathon. *Medicina* **2021**, *57*, 389. [CrossRef]
11. Isherwood, J.; Wang, H.; Sterzing, T. Running biomechanics and running shoe perception of Chinese men and women. *Footwear Sci.* **2020**, *13*, 1–13. [CrossRef]
12. Lilley, K.; Dixon, S.; Stiles, V. A biomechanical comparison of the running gait of mature and young females. *Gait Posture* **2011**, *33*, 496–500. [CrossRef] [PubMed]
13. Sinclair, J.; Selfe, J. Sex differences in knee loading in recreational runners. *J. Biomech.* **2015**, *48*, 2171–2175. [CrossRef] [PubMed]
14. Davis, I.S.; Bowser, B.J.; Mullineaux, D.R. Greater vertical impact loading in female runners with medically diagnosed injuries: A prospective investigation. *Br. J. Sports Med.* **2016**, *50*, 887–892. [CrossRef] [PubMed]
15. Nikolaidis, P.T.; Rosemann, T.; Knechtle, B. Sex differences in the age of peak marathon race time. *Chin. J. Physiol.* **2018**, *61*, 85–91. [CrossRef] [PubMed]
16. Jokl, P.; Sethi, P.; Cooper, A. Master's performance in the New York City marathon 1983–1999. *Br. J. Sports Med.* **2004**, *38*, 408–412. [CrossRef] [PubMed]
17. Schneider, A.L.; Nikolaidis, P.T.; Knechtle, B. Improved performance in master runners competing in the european championships between 1978 and 2014. *J. Strength Cond. Res.* **2019**, *33*, 2559–2569. [CrossRef]
18. Cuk, I.; Nikolaidis, P.T.; Knechtle, B. Sex differences in pacing during half-marathon and marathon race. *Res. Sports Med.* **2020**, *28*, 111–120. [CrossRef]
19. Knechtle, B.; Barandun, U.; Knechtle, P.; Zingg, M.A.; Rosemann, T.; Rüst, C.A. Prediction of half-marathon race time in recreational female and male runners. *Springerplus* **2014**, *3*, 248. [CrossRef]

20. March, D.S.; Vanderburgh, P.M.; Titlebaum, P.J.; Hoops, M.L. Age, sex, and finish time as determinants of pacing in the marathon. *J. Strength Cond. Res.* **2011**, *25*, 386–391. [CrossRef]
21. Breen, D.; Norris, M.; Healy, R.; Anderson, R. Marathon pace control in masters athletes. *Int. J. Sports Physiol. Perform.* **2018**, *13*, 332–338. [CrossRef]
22. Nikolaidis, P.T.; Knechtle, B. Pacing in age group marathoners in the "New York City Marathon". *Res. Sports Med.* **2018**, *26*, 86–99. [CrossRef] [PubMed]
23. Nikolaidis, P.T.; Knechtle, B. Pacing strategies in the 'Athens classic marathon': Physiological and psychological aspects. *Front. Physiol.* **2018**, *9*, 1539. [CrossRef]
24. Hennig, E. Gender differences for running in athletic footwear. In Proceedings of the 5th Symposium on Footwear Biomechanics, Zurich, Switzerland, 5–7 July 2001.
25. Sinclair, J.; Greenhalgh, A.; Edmundson, C.J.; Brooks, D.; Hobbs, S.J. Gender differences in the kinetics and kinematics of distance running: Implications for footwear design. *Int. J. Sports Sci. Eng.* **2012**, *6*, 118–128.
26. Hangzhou Marathon Result Inquiry. Available online: http://en.hzim.org/p/hzim/match/queryresult.jsf (accessed on 4 May 2020).
27. Nikolaidis, P.T.; Cuk, I.; Rosemann, T.; Knechtle, B. Performance and Pacing of Age Groups in Half-Marathon and Marathon. *Int. J. Environ. Res. Public Health* **2019**, *16*, 1777. [CrossRef] [PubMed]
28. Nikolaidis, P.T.; Cuk, I.; Clemente-Suarez, V.J.; Villiger, E.; Knechtle, B. Number of finishers and performance of age group women and men in long-distance running: Comparison among 10 km, half-marathon and marathon races in Oslo. *Res. Sports Med.* **2021**, *29*, 56–66. [CrossRef] [PubMed]
29. Cuk, I.; Nikolaidis, P.T.; Markovic, S.; Knechtle, B. Age Differences in Pacing in Endurance Running: Comparison between Marathon and Half-MarathonMen and Women. *Medicina* **2019**, *55*, 479. [CrossRef] [PubMed]
30. Tian, H.B.; Qiu, Y.J.; Lin, Y.Q.; Zhou, W.T.; Fan, C.Y. The Role of Leisure Satisfaction in Serious Leisure and Subjective Well-Being: Evidence from Chinese Marathon Runners. *Front. Psychol.* **2020**, *11*, 581908. [CrossRef]
31. García-Naveira, A.; Barquín, R.R.; Pujals, C. Personality differences according to participation in or abstention from sport, competition level and age category in football players based on Costa and McCraes´ s Model. *Rev. De Psicol. Del Deporte* **2011**, *20*, 29–44.
32. Anthony, D.; Rüst, C.A.; Cribari, M.; Rosemann, T.; Lepers, R.; Knechtle, B. Differences in participation and performance trends in age group half and full marathoners. *Chin. J. Physiol.* **2014**, *57*, 209–219. [CrossRef]
33. Bairan, L. Research on Current Situation and Development Path of Marathon Events in Hubei Province. *J. Sports Sci.* **2019**, *7*, 65–70. [CrossRef]
34. Del Coso, J.; Fernández, D.; Abián-Vicen, J.; Salinero, J.J.; González-Millán, C.; Areces, F.; Ruiz, D.; Gallo, C.; Calleja-González, J.; Pérez-González, B. Running pace decrease during a marathon is positively related to blood markers of muscle damage. *PLoS ONE* **2013**, *8*, e57602. [CrossRef]
35. Buman, M.P.; Omli, J.W.; Giacobbi, P.R., Jr.; Brewer, B.W. Experiences and coping responses of "hitting the wall" for recreational marathon runners. *J. Appl. Sport Psychol.* **2008**, *20*, 282–300. [CrossRef]
36. Hoffman, M.D.; Wegelin, J.A. The Western States 100-mile endurance run: Participation and performance trends. *Med. Sci. Sports Exerc.* **2009**, *41*, 2191. [CrossRef] [PubMed]
37. Knechtle, B.; Knechtle, P.; Lepers, R. Participation and performance trends in ultra-triathlons from 1985 to 2009. *Scand. J. Med. Sci. Sports* **2011**, *21*, e82–e90. [CrossRef] [PubMed]
38. Vitti, A.; Nikolaidis, P.T.; Villiger, E.; Onywera, V.; Knechtle, B. The "New York City Marathon": Participation and performance trends of 1.2 M runners during half-century. *Res. Sports Med.* **2020**, *28*, 121–137. [CrossRef] [PubMed]
39. Miller, A.E.; MacDougall, J.D.; Tarnopolsky, M.A.; Sale, D.G. Gender diferences in strength and muscle fber characteristics. *Eur. J. Appl. Physiol. Occup. Physiol.* **1993**, *66*, 254–262. [CrossRef]
40. Welle, S.; Tawil, R.; Thornton, C.A. Sex-related diferences in gene expression in human skeletal muscle. *PLoS ONE* **2008**, *3*, e1385. [CrossRef]
41. Maldonado-Martin, S.; Mujika, I.; Padilla, S. Physiological variables to use in the gender comparison in highly trained runners. *J. Sports Med. Phys. Fit.* **2004**, *44*, 8–14.
42. Besson, T.; Macchi, R.; Rossi, J.; Morio, C.; Kunimasa, Y.; Nicol, C.; Vercruyssen, F.; Millet, G.Y. Sex Differences in Endurance Running. *Sports Med.* **2022**, *52*, 1235–1257. [CrossRef]
43. Leyk, D.; Erley, O.; Ridder, D.; Leurs, M.; Rüther, T.; Wunderlich, M.; Sievert, A.; Baum, K.; Essfeld, D. Age-related changes in marathon and half-marathon performances. *Int. J. Sports Med.* **2007**, *28*, 513–517. [CrossRef]
44. Hunter, S.K.; Stevens, A.A. Sex differences in marathon running with advanced age: Physiology or participation? *Med. Sci. Sports Exerc.* **2013**, *51*, 1–9. [CrossRef] [PubMed]
45. Knechtle, B.; Di Gangi, S.; Rüst, C.A.; Villiger, E.; Rosemann, T.; Nikolaidis, P.T. The role of weather conditions on running performance in the Boston Marathon from 1972 to 2018. *PLoS ONE* **2019**, *14*, e0212797. [CrossRef] [PubMed]

International Journal of
Environmental Research and Public Health

MDPI

Article

A Pilot Dance Intervention to Encourage Physical Activity Engagement for Adolescent Girls with Intellectual Disabilities

Aviva Must *, Linda G. Bandini, Carol Curtin, Katherine M. Rancaño, Misha Eliasziw, DJ Tybor and Heidi Stanish

Department of Public Health and Community Medicine, Tufts University School of Medicine, 136 Harrison Avenue, Boston, MA 02111, USA; linda.bandini@umassmed.edu (L.G.B.); carol.curtin@umassmed.edu (C.C.); katherine.rancano@tufts.edu (K.M.R.); misha.eliasziw@tufts.edu (M.E.); david.tybor@tufts.edu (D.J.T.); heidi.stanish@umassmed.edu (H.S.)

* Correspondence: aviva.must@tufts.edu

Abstract: Adolescent girls with intellectual disabilities (ID) are at risk for low physical activity (PA) participation due to their limited opportunities. Purpose: To evaluate the feasibility and preliminary efficacy of a 12-week dance intervention to promote engagement in moderate-to-vigorous PA (MVPA) and increase cardiorespiratory fitness. Methods: The 12-week intervention included two 75-min weekly dance sessions. Continuous heart-rate (HR) monitoring assessed time spent below/at/above each girl's target HR zone. Cardiorespiratory fitness was measured by the 6-min walk test (6MWT). Survey items assessed participant enjoyment and participant and parent satisfaction. Results: The mean (SD) age of 18 adolescent girls was 17.3 (2.7) years. Overall, girls attended 88% of sessions and spent 52.3% of each session in MVPA. Mean MVPA was unchanged across the 12 weeks, but the pattern differed across the three sites. We observed a non-significant pre-post increase of 74.6 feet on the 6MWT. Post-intervention surveys indicated that most girls liked the program, perceived improved fitness, and wished to continue dancing. The majority also reported a preference for a girls-only dance program exclusively for those with ID. Conclusion: Our findings suggest that dance is viable for promoting PA for girls with ID. More frequent exercise training is likely needed to improve cardiorespiratory fitness.

Keywords: dance; intellectual disabilities; physical activity; enjoyment; engagement; adolescent girls

1. Introduction

Intellectual disability (ID) is a developmental disability characterized by significant limitations in both intellectual functioning and adaptive behavior and is present before 22 years of age [1]. Intellectual functioning includes problem solving, learning, and reasoning (i.e., general mental capacity) and adaptive behavior refers to a collection of social, practical, and conceptual skills that are used in everyday life (e.g., language, occupational skills, number concepts, healthcare, self-esteem) [1]. Recent estimates indicate that ID affects approximately 3.2% of the global population of children and adolescents [2], with an estimated prevalence for children in the United States of 1.2% [3,4]. The five most common types of ID are autism spectrum disorder, Down syndrome, fragile X syndrome, and fetal alcohol syndrome [4]. ID is a lifelong disability and is associated with persistent functional limitations that often necessitate support in a variety of settings, contexts, and activities.

Participation in regular physical activity has many health benefits for children and adolescents, including increased cardiorespiratory fitness, healthy weight, increased bone mass, and fewer symptoms of anxiety and/or depression [5,6]. Yet, evidence indicates that youth with ID have low levels of physical activity [7–11]. Globally, adherence to physical activity guidelines among youth with ID is low, though the reported range is wide: from 0% of children with ID meeting guidelines [12,13] to 24% [14]. Consequentially, children and adolescents with ID have poor health-related fitness [15–18] and a high prevalence of obesity [19–22]; they also experience health inequities compared to youth with typical development (TD) [23]. The World Health Organization's (WHO) Global Action Plan on Physical Activity 2018–2030 [24] acknowledges the disparities in physical activity among individuals with disabilities. For the first time, the 2020 WHO guidelines on physical activity and sedentary behavior are inclusive of children and adolescents living with a disability and make specific recommendations for this population subgroup [25,26].

A multitude of individual/personal, family, social, and environmental factors hinder opportunities for youth with ID to be physically active. Examples of these include low skills, lack of accessible programming, and low motivation [27,28]. Limited evidence supports gender as a correlate of low physical activity participation in youth with ID, with girls being less active than boys [13,29]. Such gender-based disparities are well-documented in the general population [30,31]. In addition, physical activity levels decline from childhood through adolescence in both youth with ID [29,32] and youth with TD [6,33]. Children with ID—especially adolescent girls—need feasible and effective interventions to increase their physical activity engagement.

Dance is a form of physical activity that stands out as enjoyable and popular among adolescent girls [34–37]. Dance programs improve a host of mental and physical health outcomes in young people [38–42]. Dance increases social interaction, camaraderie, personal expression, intrinsic motivation, and creativity [43] in all youth, regardless of ability [44,45]. In our observational study of teenagers with ID, 75% of adolescent girls ranked dance (mostly at home) as the most common leisure time physical activity [10]. Dance has physical, social, and psychosocial benefits for children with various disabilities including ID [46]. Dance intervention studies have targeted subgroups of girls, such as racial/ethnic minorities [41,42,47] and low-income populations [48], but to our knowledge, none have determined the ability of dance programs to help adolescent girls with ID obtain the recommended 60 min of moderate to vigorous physical activity (MVPA) daily [49].

Despite the compelling reasons to believe that dance represents a suitable approach to increasing physical activity in community settings for girls with ID, there is a dearth of research in this area, perhaps due to the difficulty of developing programs that appeal to the interest, motivation, and learning styles of adolescent girls with ID. We postulated that a structured, supportive, and socially engaging dance program would promote MVPA among adolescent girls with ID and increase their cardiorespiratory fitness. Therefore, we aimed to determine the feasibility of a 12-week dance program for engaging adolescent girls with ID in MVPA and to assess the preliminary efficacy of the program to improve cardiorespiratory fitness. The overall goal of this line of research is to build evidence that supports intervention efforts to reduce the physical activity disparities experienced by individuals with ID.

2. Materials and Methods

2.1. Participants

We recruited girls with ID in the greater Boston area, who were 13 to 21 years of age, to participate in a 12-week dance program through public school special education programs, parent advisory councils, and local disability organizations. According to the US Individuals with Disabilities Education Act, youth with disabilities have access to educational services until their 22nd birthday, and so may remain in school until age 22 [50]. We determined eligibility and gave a study overview during parent/guardian telephone interviews. Eligible participants had an IQ score $\leq$75 as confirmed by parent report, were age 13–21 and were able to verbally communicate, follow simple instructions, and provide assent/consent in English. We excluded participants with untreated cardiac conditions, seizure disorder, psychiatric conditions (e.g., schizophrenia, bipolar disorder, or psychosis), heart disease, cancer, physical disabilities, orthopedic injury/impairment, disruptive behaviors (e.g., aggression, property destruction, or frequently running away from a program area) and any participants engaging in aerobic exercise outside of school for more than 60 min/day.

An in-person enrollment visit was scheduled for participants who met the screening criteria. At enrollment, eligibility was confirmed, the study protocol was thoroughly reviewed, parents provided informed written consent, and participants indicated their willingness to participate by signing an assent or consent form (depending on their age and guardianship status) that was read aloud to them. Written approval from a primary care physician was also required to participate. All procedures were approved by the university's review board for the protection of human subjects.

2.2. Settings

The 12-week intervention was conducted at three sites in eastern Massachusetts in order to recruit an adequate sample of girls with ID. Although each site varied by location/setting, number of participants and schedule (i.e., days/times), the components of the intervention were the same at all three sites, including the dance instructor and all study procedures. At Site A, the dance program was conducted during in-school hours at a fitness studio within a YMCA (an international community-based youth organization with branches across the US) located in an urban neighborhood of a small city. The special education program of the local public school transported the participating students to and from the YMCA so they could participate in the dance program during regular school hours. The Site B program was conducted during out-of-school time at a fitness studio within another YMCA fitness studio located in a suburban neighborhood in a second small city. Participants were transported to and from the facility by a parent, guardian, or other family members. At Site C, the dance program sessions were delivered during school hours in the gymnasium of a public high school located in a densely populated section of a large city. This school has a large special education program and participation in the dance program for Site C was restricted to female students with ID who were currently enrolled in the school. At Sites A and C, a teacher accompanied the girls to the facility/gymnasium, but they were not involved in the dance program and were not present during the dance sessions or testing. In-person contact with parents at these sites was limited to the screening and enrollment process, whereas at Site B there was ongoing in-person interaction with parents at drop-off and pick-up at the YMCA. All three sites completed the study within a single year.

2.3. Intervention

Study Design. The pilot intervention used a single-arm trial design for cardiorespiratory fitness. Engagement and satisfaction measures were assessed at baseline and then weekly post-intervention.

Group Dance Sessions. Group dance sessions were conducted twice weekly for 75 min over the 12-week intervention period. Sessions were led by a trained dance instructor with experience teaching children and youth in local dance programs. A student research assistant was present to assist the instructor and support participants. The first 10 min of each session was used to greet participants, provide an overview of the content for the class, and provide an opportunity for participants to socialize. The remainder of the session included: a 10-min warm-up period, 30–45 min of dance practice/choreography, and 5–10 min of cool-down activities.

Two dance styles were included in the 12-week program: 6 weeks of hip hop followed by 6 weeks of jazz. Dance sessions included simple choreography of each style (i.e., moves and routines) designed to be easy to learn and master by girls with ID without extended periods of instructional time when participants would be inactive. The dance moves and routines were also intended to be of moderate-to-vigorous intensity and the instructor-led activities were designed to keep participants moving at a level that would elicit their target HR. The target HR zone for participants during the dance was established as 60–79% of their age-predicted maximum HR (220 beats/min—age) [51]. Participants wore a Polar® HR monitor during each dance session to continuously monitor the intensity of their engagement and to provide them with feedback. Participants were taught to read the output on the HR watch and to recognize their own target HR zone. There were frequent HR checks throughout the dance sessions. During each session, participant engagement in MVPA by Polar® HR monitors (Polar Electro, Kempele, Finland) is reflected by the percentage of time spent in or above the participant's target HR zone.

At-home Dance Practice. Participants were instructed to dance at home at least twice each week for 45–60 min to increase their frequency of physical activity participation and to practice routines taught during the group sessions. Participants were encouraged to dance freely for the at-home practice or to use instructional videos that were provided and illustrated each dance style to support and motivate participants' engagement. The videos featured the dance instructor leading routines taught in class with demonstration, verbal instruction, and encouragement. The video format was similar to the group dance classes, with 10 min of warm-up, 30–45 min of dance practice, and 5 min of cool-down. In order to monitor the intensity of their activity during at-home dance and stay in their target HR zone, participants were asked to wear a Fitbit® Charge HR™ activity monitor (Fitbit, San Francisco, CA, USA) that was provided at the enrollment visit. Participants were encouraged to schedule consistent days/times to dance at home so that it became part of their weekly routine.

2.4. Feasibility Measures

Attendance and Retention. Attendance at each group dance session was recorded and the number of participants who withdrew from the study prior to week 12 was documented.

Engagement during Group Dance Sessions. Continuous HR monitoring was used to estimate the level of engagement in MVPA during each dance session using Polar® monitors. Participants put on a monitor (chest strap and output watch) at the start of each session and were asked to wear it for the full duration of the session. Assistance to put on the monitor and ensure proper placement was provided by a female member of the research team in a private space. HR data were stored and then downloaded using the Polar® software.

Participation in At-home Dance Practice. Participation in at-home dance practice sessions was estimated using the Fitbit® Charge HR™ activity monitor and an activity log. The device displays, records, and stores HR data and was synched wirelessly to a computer, tablet, or smartphone. Data were then retrieved from each participant's Fitbit® dashboard throughout the program. Participants, with help from a parent as needed, were instructed to manually record the date, start time, and end time of each at-home practice session on an activity log that was provided. The log was designed to assist in verifying the information collected from the Fitbit® Charge HR™, particularly the time period that the participant danced, and was a secondary source of documenting participation at home. Participants were instructed to bring the completed log to the group dance session each week.

Enjoyment and Satisfaction. A survey was used to assess participant enjoyment of and satisfaction with the dance program. The 5-item survey was administered following the second dance session each week for weeks 3–12. Four questions asked about the enjoyment of the weekly dance style, music, at-home practice, and dancing with other participants, and one question asked participants about their level of effort when dancing that week. The survey was administered verbally to participants and response choices were recorded by a member of the research team. Three response options (i.e., "liked it", "it was ok", and "did not like it") were presented and each option had a happy, neutral, or sad face to offer participants a visual cue when selecting a response. Few participants reported that they "did not like" components of the program; therefore, responses of "did not like" were combined with "just okay" and binary variables were created to indicate participants that "liked" components of the program. To examine participant enjoyment of at-home videos, a binary variable was created to indicate participants that tried and liked the at-home videos (i.e., 0 represents participants that did not try the at-home videos and participants that tried them but did not like them).

Surveys to assess participant satisfaction with the dance program overall were administered at the end of the session at weeks 6 and 12. The participant survey included 16 questions that asked about perceived benefits of the dance program (e.g., fitness, learned new dance routines), satisfaction with the instructor, the HR monitors, and videos for at-home practice, interest in continuing to dance, and preferences for including girls not in special education (i.e., those without ID) and boys in future dance programs. The survey was administered verbally to participants and response choices were recorded. The parent satisfaction survey, administered at weeks 6 and 12, included 20 questions about key program elements, such as intensity and difficulty of dance activities, appropriateness of routines, instructional strategies, and support for at-home sessions, perceived benefits of the program for their daughter (e.g., fitness, physical activity), satisfaction with program length and schedule, and barriers and facilitators of participation. Most questions were Yes/No or had up to five response options, the survey included one open-ended question on suggestions for improving the dance program. Paper copies of the parent surveys were distributed and returned by mail. At Site B, some parents returned their surveys directly to study staff when transporting their children to the YMCA.

2.5. Outcome Measure

Cardiorespiratory Fitness. The 6-min walk test (6MWT) was used to measure cardiorespiratory fitness at baseline and after the 12-week dance program (within 5 days of the last group dance session). The test, which is widely used in research involving people with ID [52,53], was administered at the site of the dance sessions (i.e., YMCA or school gymnasium). Following a demonstration and simple verbal instructions, participants were instructed to walk as quickly as possible between two cones on a flat indoor surface for 6 min. To assist with pacing and motivation during the 6MWT, a research assistant walked slightly ahead of each participant and provided verbal encouragement.

2.6. Statistical Analyses

Participant characteristics were summarized using means for continuous and percentages for categorical variables. The average rates of session time spent in or above the participants' target HR zone over the 12-week intervention were estimated from Poisson regression models with a compound symmetry covariance structure to account for participants' repeated measures of HR over time. In the models, total time spent in or above the target HR zone was the outcome variable and total session time was the offset variable. Results are summarized as the percentage of session time spent in or above the target HR zone with corresponding 95% confidence intervals (CI) for all sites and each site separately.

Changes in the average distance walked in the 6MWT between pre- and post-intervention were assessed using linear mixed models. The models included a random intercept to account for the within-subject correlation. The fixed effects included site, timepoint (i.e., pre- and post-intervention), and a site-by-timepoint cross-product term. Results are summarized as the mean difference in distance walked with corresponding 95% CIs for all sites and each site separately. Despite four participants having missing data for the 6MWT at pre- or post-intervention, and not being included in this analysis, the baseline characteristics were similar between the analyzed sample and participants with complete 6MWT.

Participant attendance, satisfaction with program components, and activity logs returned for at-home use of the Fitbit® Charge HR™ from week 3 to week 12 were estimated with logistic regression models using a generalized estimating equation (GEE) approach. A compound symmetry covariance structure was used in the models to account for the repeated measures from each participant. The results are summarized as average percentages with corresponding 95% CIs.

Participants' satisfaction with the program post-intervention is summarized in terms of percentages. One participant from site B was missing post-intervention assessments and was excluded from this analysis. Parent satisfaction and parent perceptions of at-home videos post-intervention are summarized in terms of percentages and are limited to site

B parents. Parents from site A and site C were not included because they had limited knowledge of the intervention's content and delivery, given that the intervention at these sites was carried out during the school day. SAS version 9.4 was used for all statistical analyses and results with p-values less than 0.05 are considered to be statistically significant.

3. Results

Eighteen adolescent girls with ID participated in the intervention at the three sites of the 12-week dance program. Table 1 displays demographic characteristics overall and by study site. Overall, the mean (SD) age of the sample was 17.3 (2.7) years. The sample was diverse, with the greatest diversity in Site C. On average, slightly fewer than half of the girls' parents had earned less than a bachelor's degree, with striking differences by site: all of the Site B participants had at least one parent with a college education or more, whereas those participating in Site A had no parents with a college education or more.

Table 1. Characteristics of the study sample.

	All Sites (n = 18)	Site A (n = 6)	Site B (n = 7)	Site C (n = 5)
Age in years, mean (SD)	17.3 (2.7)	18.4 (2.5)	16.0 (2.8)	17.7 (2.3)
Race/ethnicity, n (%)				
Non-Hispanic White	8 (44.4)	3 (50.0)	4 (57.1)	1 (20.0)
Non-Hispanic Black	1 (5.6)	0 (0.0)	0 (0.0)	1 (20.0)
Hispanic	1 (5.6)	0 (0.0)	0 (0.0)	1 (20.0)
Asian	4 (22.2)	2 (33.3)	1 (14.3)	1 (20.0)
More than one race	4 (22.2)	1 (16.7)	2 (28.6)	1 (20.0)
Max parental education, n (%)				
Less than a bachelor's degree	8 (44.4)	6 (100.0)	0 (0.0)	2 (40.0)
Bachelor's degree or higher	10 (55.6)	0 (0.0)	7 (100.0)	3 (60.0)

Attendance at the sessions was high. On average, participants attended 88% of sessions and was similar across sites; at the session level, attendance ranged from 69% to 100%. Two participants withdrew from the study: one moved out of the area and the other lost interest and withdrew. Overall, girls spent 52.3% (95% CI: 39.3% to 65.3%) of each session engaged in MVPA; defined as the time in or above their individual target HR zone. Interestingly, the pattern of engagement also varied substantially between and within sites (Figure 1, $p < 0.001$). The pattern across the 12 weeks differed significantly by the site ($p < 0.001$); site A decreased, site B increased, and site C remained constant. As observed in Figure 2, the highest mean percentage of session time participants spent in or above their target HR zone was observed at Site C (71.6%, 95%CI: 52.5% to 90.7%) and the lowest in Site B (36.7%, 95%CI: 20.4% to 53.0%). MVPA engagement levels varied among participants; one girl averaged 4% of the dance session in her target HR zone and another averaged 94%.

Overall, we observed a non-significant mean increase of 73.4 feet in distance walked on the 6MWT from baseline to post-test for the 14 participants with data at both time points (p = 0.22, Table 2). There were similar increases in distance walked at each site, which ranged from an increase of 55.7 to 82.9 feet; however, none of these differences were statistically significant (Table 2).

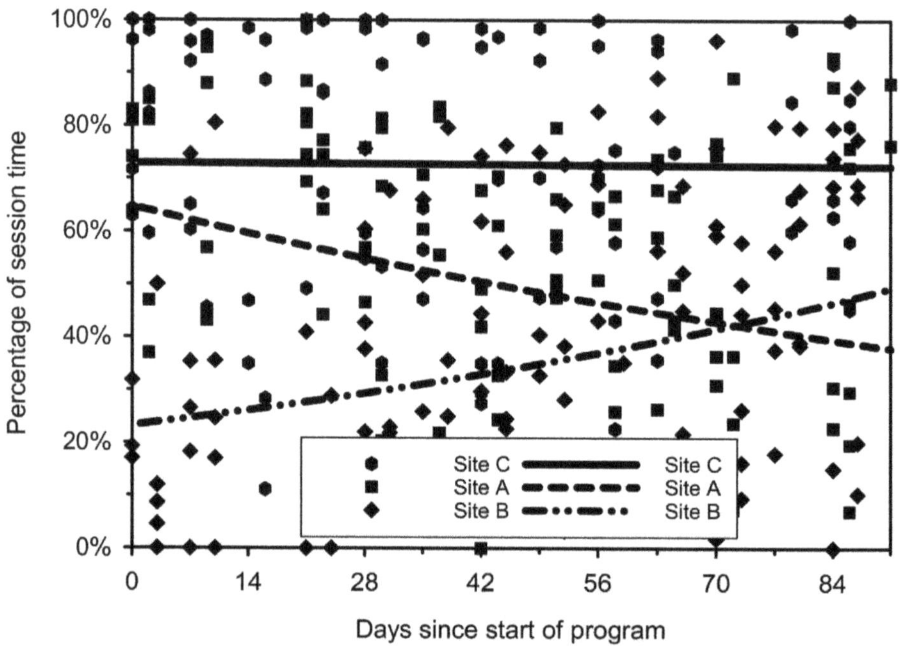

Figure 1. Scattergram of percentage of session time spent in or above participant target heart rate zone across time by site. The fitted regression lines are derived from a multivariable Poisson model.

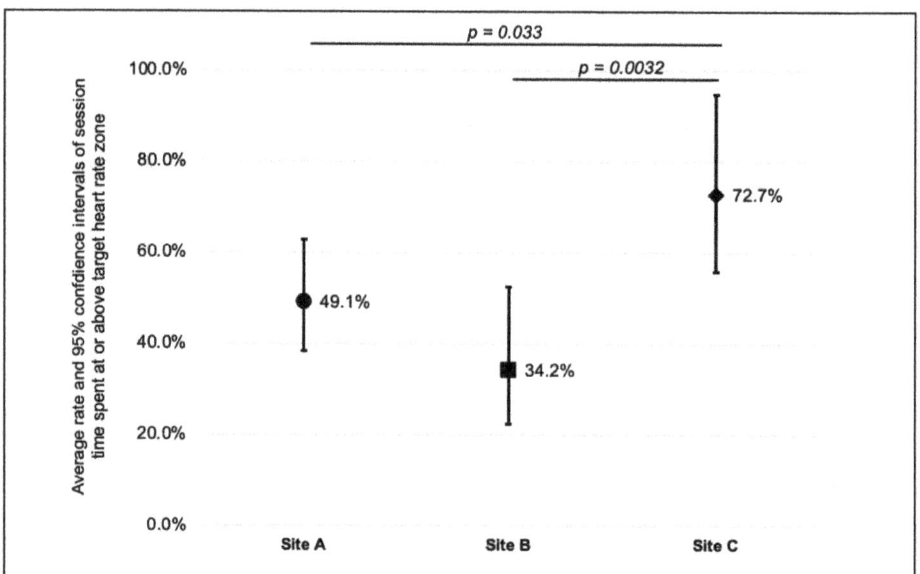

Figure 2. Average percentage and 95% confidence intervals of session time spent in or above participant target heart rate zone, by site.

Table 2. Six-minute walk test results pre- and post-intervention.

Distance in Meters	All Sites (n = 14) [1]	Site A (n = 5)	Site B (n = 5)	Site C (n = 4)
Pre-Intervention, mean (SD)	469.7 (75.2)	464.9 (120.0)	472.7 (36.8)	475.0 (57/5)
Post-intervention, mean (SD)	492.5 (38.9)	486.7 (36.3)	497.7 (36.9)	492.8 (53.7)
Change between Pre- and Post-Intervention, mean (95% CI)	22.4 (−15.9 to 60.6)	24.9 (−38.8 to 87.6)	25.3 (−38.4 to 89.0)	17.0 (−17.0 to 88.2)
p-value	0.22	0.41	0.40	0.61

[1] Three participants were missing data for the walk test (pre-intervention, n = 1; post-intervention, n = 2) and one participant was missing data for both pre- and post-intervention.

Participants reported enjoying the dance sessions. On average, over the 10-week period that participant enjoyment was assessed (weekly for weeks 3 through 12), 83.7% (95% CI: 74.2% to 95.2%) of participants indicated they liked the type of dance, 80.3% (95% CI: 63.1% to 97.5%) liked the music played, and 85.0% (95% CI: 74.0% to 96.0%) liked dancing with other girls. There were only small differences in participants' enjoyment across sites. With respect to perceived physical activity intensity, the majority (72.8%, 95% CI: 53.4% to 92.2%) reported that they worked "really hard" during sessions. Notably, Site A had the lowest prevalence of participants that worked "really hard" (48.4%, 95% CI: 20.9% to 76.9%) and 100% of Site B participants reported working "really hard" (Table 3).

Table 3. Assessment of participants' enjoyment of the dance program over the 12-week dance program.

	All Sites (n = 18) % (95% CI)	Site A (n = 6) % (95% CI)	Site B (n = 7) % (95% CI)	Site C (n = 5) % (95% CI)
Attendance	87.8 (84.2 to 91.6)	89.2 (80.9 to 94.1)	88.5 (81.4 to 93.1)	85.5 (81.1 to 88.9)
Liked dance style	83.7 (74.2 to 95.2)	79.3 (55.9 to 92.1)	86.6 (63.4 to 96.0)	84.0 (58.6 to 95.2)
Liked music played	80.3 (63.1 to 97.5)	74.7 (43.3 to 92.0)	83.8 (43.3 to 97.2)	87.5 (64.0 to 96.5)
Liked dancing with other girls	85.0 (74.0 to 96.0)	72.3 (51.8 to 86.4)	100.0 — [1]	82.0 (62.1 to 92.7)
Worked really hard	72.8 (53.4 to 92.2)	48.4 (20.9 to 76.9)	100.0 — [1]	71.2 (43.7 to 88.7)
Tried and liked the at-home videos	49.0 (31.3 to 66.6)	55.4 (36.5 to 72.8)	100.0 — [1]	32.0 (12.7 to 60.3)

Satisfaction surveys were administered once per week starting with Week 3 of the intervention 12-week intervention. A total of ten surveys were administered. [1] 95% confidence intervals are not provided because all participants reported that they "liked" dancing with other girls, worked "really hard," and tried and reported liking the at-home videos.

Surveys with participants at week 12 reflected a high level of satisfaction with the program overall (Table 4). The assessment at week 6 found a similarly high and consistent level of satisfaction as the week 12 assessment. At both time points, 82.4% of the girls reported that they "liked" the dance program overall, and none reported disliking it. By the end of the program, most girls (76.5%) found the level of difficulty just right and none found it too hard. Almost all participants perceived improved fitness (88.2%), and almost all wished to continue dancing after the program ended (88.2%) and wanted to come back to the program (88.2%). Interestingly, most girls also indicated a preference for a girls-only dance program (87.5%) and for a program exclusively for those enrolled in special education (64.7%).

Table 4. Assessment of participant satisfaction with the dance intervention program post-intervention.

	Post-Intervention (n = 17) [1] n (%)
Overall satisfaction with the program	
Did not like it	0 (0.0)
It was okay	3 (17.7)
Liked it	14 (82.4)
How difficult were the dance steps	
Too hard	0 (0.0)
Too easy	4 (23.5)
Just right	13 (76.5)
How much work	
Didn't work at all	0 (0.0)
Worked a little	4 (23.5)
Worked a lot	13 (76.5)
Learned new dance steps	
No	0 (0.0)
Yes	100.0
Got more fit	
No	2 (11.8)
Yes	15 (88.2)
Want to come back to program	
No	2 (11.8)
Yes	15 (88.2)
Want to keep dancing after program	
No	2 (11.8)
Yes	15 (88.2)
Include other girls not in special education	
Girls in special education only	11 (64.7)
Other girls	6 (35.3)
Want to include boys	
Include girls only	14 (87.5)
Include boys	2 (12.5)

[1] One participant did not complete the post-intervention satisfaction survey.

Parents of the participants in Site B (only) also reported their daughters had high levels of satisfaction with the program (Table 5). At the end of the intervention, 100% of those reporting agreed or strongly agreed that their daughter enjoyed the dance program, 100% agreed or strongly agreed that the program was taught at an appropriate level, and 90% thought dancing with one's peers was important. All of those reporting indicated that their daughter learned new dance steps and routines. Fitness improvements were less consistently perceived: 67% of parents agreed or strongly agreed with the statement that their daughter's fitness had improved over the course of the program, 83% reported that their daughter had shown new interest or motivation for participation in dance and that their daughter's physical activity level had increased from before the program. All parents at Site B were interested in re-enrolling their daughter in the program.

Table 5. Parent satisfaction with the dance program at post-intervention at site B only.

	Post-Intervention (n = 6) [1] n (%)
Daughter enjoyed the program	
Neutral/Disagree/Strongly Disagree	0 (0.0)
Strongly Agree/Agree	6 (100.0)
Program was at an appropriate level for their daughter to understand	
Neutral/Disagree/Strongly Disagree	0 (0.0)
Strongly Agree/Agree	6 (100.0)
Dancing with peers was important for their daughter's participation	
Neutral/Disagree/Strongly Disagree	0 (0.0)
Strongly Agree/Agree	6 (100.0)
Daughter's fitness improved	
Neutral/Disagree/Strongly Disagree	2 (33.3)
Strongly Agree/Agree	4 (66.6)
Daughter learned new dance steps and routines	
Neutral/Disagree/Strongly Disagree	0 (0.0)
Strongly Agree/Agree	6 (100.0)
Daughter's physical activity level increased from before the program	
Neutral/Disagree/Strongly Disagree	1 (16.7)
Strongly Agree/Agree	5 (83.3)
Daughter gave a good effort during classes and at home	
Neutral/Disagree/Strongly Disagree	1 (16.7)
Strongly Agree/Agree	5 (83.3)
Daughter has shown new interest/motivation in participating in dance	
No	1 (16.7)
Yes	5 (83.3)
Noted positive changes in their daughter attributed to the program	
No	0 (0.0)
Yes	6 (100.0)
Interested in re-enrolling your daughter in the program	
No	0 (0.0)
Yes	6 (100.0)

[1] Six parents completed satisfaction surveys post-intervention.

The study protocol included directions for at-home practice with monitoring using a dance log and a Fitbit® Charge HR™. On average, 54% of participants completed the Fitbit® dance logs. There was substantial variation across the sites: 20% of logs were completed by participants at Site A and 40% at Site C. In contrast, more than 95% of logs were completed by participants at Site B. Table 6 summarizes the parent survey for Site B. Of the six parents who completed the post-intervention survey, three parents indicated that their child had practiced at home less than once per week; their data are tabulated in Table 6. Based on the parent report, two girls practiced 1–2 times per week: one girl danced every day. Barriers to the at-home practice varied and included practical considerations. The most frequently cited facilitating factor was having someone else dance with the participant. Parents varied regarding the difficulty of using the Fitbit® Charge HR™ when their daughter danced at home.

Table 6. Parent perceptions of the at-home dance videos and Fitbit monitors post- intervention at site B only.

	Post-Intervention (n = 6) n (%)
Average number of times daughter practiced dance at home using the video	
<1 time/week	3 (50.0)
1 to 2 times/week	2 (33.3)
3 to 4 times/week	0 (0.0)
5 to 6 times/week	0 (0.0)
Everyday	1 (16.6)
Barriers for daughter's participation in at-home dance	
Did not enjoy dancing at home	1 (16.7)
Difficult to follow along to the video	0 (0.0)
Did not have an appropriate space	0 (0.0)
Daughter's schedule was too busy	1 (16.6)
Daughter was too tired	1 (16.6)
Did not have the time to remind/encourage daughter	1 (16.6)
Factors that helped daughter's participation in at-home dance	
Daughter has always danced a lot at home	2 (33.3)
Daughter enjoyed the video	1 (16.7)
Scheduled day/time	1 (16.7)
Reminded/encouraged daughter	2 (33.3)
Someone else would dance with daughter/motivate her	0 (0.0)
Gave daughter a reward	6 (100.0)
Level of difficulty using Fitbit when daughter danced at-home [1]	
Not difficult at all	2 (40.0)
A bit difficult	0 (0.0)
Difficult	3 (60.0)
Really difficult	0 (0.0)

[1] One participant was missing data for this item (n = 5).

4. Discussion

Our pilot dance intervention was successfully implemented in three distinct venues, reflecting a successful partnership among our research team, local community organizations, and a large public school. Overall, our results suggest that dance represents a promising approach to increasing time spent in MVPA in adolescent girls with ID and thereby could help girls with ID meet current physical activity recommendations. Girls enrolled in the study spent more than half of the 75-min session at an intensity level considered moderate to vigorous, based on heart rate monitoring. This intensity level was confirmed by participants; most participants reported they worked "really hard" during sessions. Engagement during the sessions varied substantially, based on time in or above their target heart rate zone. We did not observe increases in cardiorespiratory fitness as measured by the 6MWT, although a modest non-significant increase in distance walked between pre- and post- fitness testing was observed.

Our pilot effort adds to the small number of dance interventions for children, adolescents, and young adults with ID [54–58]. The five previously published dance interventions conducted with adolescents with ID examined outcomes that included balance, coordination, and locomotor skills; none measured MVPA by heart rate or cardiorespiratory fitness by 6MWT as we did in the present study. Only one previous investigation employed a randomized controlled trial study design, [54] and, like our study, the remaining four studies employed pre-post designs [55–58] and lacked a control group. Additionally, like ours, these studies were typically small, enrolling 10 to 36 participants. Prior work focused on younger children, ages 4 to 16.9 years. Participant diagnoses also varied, enrolling participants with Down syndrome [54,56] and autism spectrum disorder [58]. A trial of 36 Indian children aged 6–10 years with Down syndrome randomized to either traditional Indian dance or neuromuscular coordination exercises demonstrated that those who were randomized to dance experienced greater improvements in locomotor skills, but showed similar improvements in balance after the 6-week intervention period [54]. The four other smaller intervention studies with pre-post trial designs reported significant improvements in coordination, balance, vertical jump, flexibility, and sprint [55–58]. It is noteworthy that all published intervention studies in this population have demonstrated positive fitness outcomes, though mostly in skill-related fitness [54–58]. Our study adds to this research base in our positive, albeit variable, MVPA findings using heart rate monitoring.

We found very high levels of satisfaction with the program by participants overall. None of the previous dance intervention studies have reported participant satisfaction. Parents of participants in an adapted dance intervention for youth with Down syndrome reported high levels of satisfaction on a 10-point scale for almost all participants [56]. Interestingly, most participants in our study did not favor including boys in the program, nor did they favor including girls with typical development who were not receiving special education. There have been numerous calls to increase the capacity and accessibility of existing physical activity programs to meet the needs of youth with disabilities, rather than focusing efforts on developing specialized, separate programs that promote exclusion [59–61]. The preference for exclusive programming in our study may reflect past negative experiences in inclusive activities or their general overall satisfaction with the current program [62–64].

The at-home practice component was not well-received, as evidenced by both low reported compliance and barriers identified by parents who responded to the post-survey. Participants were encouraged to dance outside of the group sessions by the instructor and were verbally commended when they reported dancing at home. More deliberate strategies are clearly needed to stimulate this change in behavior, however. The videos may not have been sufficiently motivating to engage the girls, nor was wearing the Fitbit® while dancing. With a growing array of dance-focused activities online, in apps, and streamed through social media (e.g., TikTok), getting adolescent girls with ID to dance outside of group programs may now be far easier.

Our study had several notable limitations in addition to its strengths. As a pilot, we focused on assessing the feasibility and acceptability of the intervention and did not include a control group. Despite having three implementation venues, our sample size was small. We did not collect data on other relevant fitness outcomes, such as dynamic or static balance or coordination. Notwithstanding these limitations, our study also had numerous strengths. Our design allowed us to demonstrate intervention feasibility in three distinct settings. Despite the multiplicity of venues, the intervention content, which featured two popular dance forms, was the same across all sites and delivered by the same instructor. In addition to gathering cardiorespiratory fitness data at multiple time points, satisfaction and preference information was obtained from the girls themselves, which represents an essential and overdue advance over prior studies [65]. We also were successful in partnering with community-based organizations, which may support program sustainability by building capacity for uptake in programming beyond a discreet research project. Finally, we were able to recruit a very diverse sample of adolescent girls with ID, who represent a woefully underrepresented and underserved population along several dimensions.

5. Conclusions

Our intervention was successful in that it resulted in participants engaging in dance at an MVPA intensity level for more than half of the 75-min dance sessions. Satisfaction with the dance program was high: the girls themselves expressed their enjoyment of the program and wanted it to continue. Together, this suggests that dance represents a viable approach to help adolescent girls with ID meet current physical activity guidelines. Further, partnering with community-level organizations holds promise for fostering inclusion in community and other settings (46).

Given the success of this pilot study for increasing engagement in physical activity, several directions for future study emerge. Establishing feasibility and preliminary efficacy in children with other developmental disabilities such as autism and among boys would increase the potential for including this program in school settings. A properly powered cluster-randomized controlled trial that includes an attention comparison group is needed to demonstrate efficacy. Additionally, to achieve an impact on cardiorespiratory fitness, more frequent training would be necessary; the at-home component of the intervention would also require additional development and implementation in a pilot context.

Author Contributions: Conceptualization, H.S., A.M., L.G.B., C.C.; Methodology, H.S., A.M., L.G.B., C.C.; Investigation, H.S.; Formal Analysis, K.M.R., M.E., A.M., D.J.T.; Resources, H.S., A.M.; Data Curation, D.J.T., M.E., K.M.R., A.M.; Writing—Original Draft Preparation, A.M., H.S.; Writing—Review & Editing, C.C., K.M.R., M.E., D.J.T., L.G.B.; Visualization M.E., K.M.R.; Project Administration, H.S.; and Funding Acquisition, H.S. All authors have read and agreed to the published version of the manuscript.

Funding: Funding for this work was provided by the Healthy Weight Research Network, Health Resources and Services Administration, and Maternal and Child Health Bureau (UA3MC25735), and the Joseph P. Healey Research Fund at the University of Massachusetts Boston.

Institutional Review Board Statement: The study was conducted in accordance with the Declaration of Helsinki, and approved by the Institutional Review Board of the University of Massachusetts Boston (12 August 2015, Assurance #: FWA00004634).

Informed Consent Statement: Informed consent was obtained from all parents. Participants indicated their willingness to participate by signing an assent or consent form (depending on their age and guardianship status).

Data Availability Statement: The data presented in this study are available upon request from the corresponding author.

Acknowledgments: The authors would like to thank Uma Rajiyah for her assistance with the literature review, the team who helped with the study, and the girls and their families for their enthusiastic participation.

Conflicts of Interest: The authors declare no conflict of interest.

References

1. Schalock, R.L.; Luckasson, R.; Tassé, M.J. An Overview of Intellectual Disability: Definition, Diagnosis, Classification, and Systems of Supports. *Am. J. Intellect. Dev. Disabil.* **2021**, *126*, 439–442. [CrossRef] [PubMed]
2. Olusanya, B.O.; Wright, S.M.; Nair, M.; Boo, N.-Y.; Halpern, R.; Kuper, H.; Abubakar, A.A.; Almasri, N.A.; Arabloo, J.; Arora, N.K. Global burden of childhood epilepsy, intellectual disability, and sensory impairments. *Pediatrics* **2020**, *146*, e20192623. [CrossRef] [PubMed]
3. Zablotsky, B.; Black, L.I.; Blumberg, S.J. Estimated Prevalence of Children With Diagnosed Developmental Disabilities in the United States, 2014–2016. *NCHS Data Brief* **2017**, *291*, 1–8.
4. Patrick, M.E.; Shaw, K.A.; Dietz, P.M.; Baio, J.; Yeargin-Allsopp, M.; Bilder, D.A.; Kirby, R.S.; Hall-Lande, J.A.; Harrington, R.A.; Lee, L.-C. Prevalence of intellectual disability among eight-year-old children from selected communities in the United States, 2014. *Disabil. Health J.* **2021**, *14*, 101023. [CrossRef] [PubMed]
5. Kumar, B.; Robinson, R.; Till, S. Physical activity and health in adolescence. *Clin. Med.* **2015**, *15*, 267. [CrossRef]
6. Katzmarzyk, P.T.; Denstel, K.D.; Beals, K.; Carlson, J.; Crouter, S.E.; McKenzie, T.L.; Pate, R.R.; Sisson, S.B.; Staiano, A.E.; Stanish, H. Results from the United States 2018 report card on physical activity for children and youth. *J. Phys. Act. Health* **2018**, *15*, S422–S424. [CrossRef]
7. Einarsson, I.; Johannsson, E.; Daly, D.; Arngrimsson, S.A. Physical activity during school and after school among youth with and without intellectual disability. *Res. Dev. Disabil.* **2016**, *56*, 60–70. [CrossRef]
8. Hinckson, E.A.; Curtis, A. Measuring physical activity in children and youth living with intellectual disabilities: A systematic review. *Res. Dev. Disabil.* **2013**, *34*, 72–86. [CrossRef]

9. Frey, G.C.; Stanish, H.I.; Temple, V.A. Physical activity of youth with intellectual disability: Review and research agenda. *Adapt. Phys. Act. Q.* **2008**, *25*, 95–117. [CrossRef]
10. Stanish, H.I.; Curtin, C.; Must, A.; Phillips, S.; Maslin, M.; Bandini, L.G. Does physical activity differ between youth with and without intellectual disabilities? *Disabil. Health J.* **2019**, *12*, 503–508. [CrossRef]
11. Wouters, M.; Evenhuis, H.M.; Hilgenkamp, T.I. Physical activity levels of children and adolescents with moderate-to-severe intellectual disability. *J. Appl. Res. Intellect. Disabil.* **2019**, *32*, 131–142. [CrossRef] [PubMed]
12. Einarsson, I.Ó.; Ólafsson, Á.; Hinriksdóttir, G.; Jóhannsson, E.; Daly, D.; Arngrímsson, S.A. Differences in physical activity among youth with and without intellectual disability. *Med. Sci. Sports Exerc.* **2015**, *47*, 411–418. [CrossRef] [PubMed]
13. Phillips, A.C.; Holland, A.J. Assessment of objectively measured physical activity levels in individuals with intellectual disabilities with and without Down's syndrome. *PLoS ONE* **2011**, *6*, e28618. [CrossRef] [PubMed]
14. Downs, S.J.; Fairclough, S.J.; Knowles, Z.R.; Boddy, L.M. Physical activity patterns in youth with intellectual disabilities. *Adapt. Phys. Act. Q.* **2016**, *33*, 374–390. [CrossRef] [PubMed]
15. Onyewadume, I.U. Fitness of black African early adolescents with and without mild mental retardation. *Adapt. Phys. Act. Q.* **2006**, *23*, 277–292. [CrossRef]
16. Skowroński, W.; Horvat, M.; Nocera, J.; Roswal, G.; Croce, R. Eurofit special: European fitness battery score variation among individuals with intellectual disabilities. *Adapt. Phys. Act. Q.* **2009**, *26*, 54–67. [CrossRef]
17. Gillespie, M. Cardiovascular fitness of young Canadian children with and without mental retardation. *Educ. Train. Dev. Disabil.* **2003**, *38*, 296–301.
18. Oppewal, A.; Hilgenkamp, T.I.; Van Wijck, R.; Evenhuis, H.M. Cardiorespiratory fitness in individuals with intellectual disabilities—A review. *Res. Dev. Disabil.* **2013**, *34*, 3301–3316. [CrossRef]
19. González-Agüero, A.; Vicente-Rodríguez, G.; Moreno, L.; Guerra-Balic, M.; Ara, I.; Casajus, J. Health-related physical fitness in children and adolescents with Down syndrome and response to training. *Scand. J. Med. Sci. Sports* **2010**, *20*, 716–724. [CrossRef]
20. Wallen, E.F.; Müllersdorf, M.; Christensson, K.; Malm, G.; Ekblom, Ö.; Marcus, C. High prevalence of cardio-metabolic risk factors among adolescents with intellectual disability. *Acta Paediatr.* **2009**, *98*, 853–859. [CrossRef]
21. Rimmer, J.H.; Yamaki, K.; Lowry, B.M.; Wang, E.; Vogel, L.C. Obesity and obesity-related secondary conditions in adolescents with intellectual/developmental disabilities. *J. Intellect. Disabil. Res.* **2010**, *54*, 787–794. [CrossRef] [PubMed]
22. Maiano, C. Prevalence and risk factors of overweight and obesity among children and adolescents with intellectual disabilities. *Obes. Rev.* **2010**, *12*, 189–197. [CrossRef] [PubMed]
23. Allerton, L.A.; Welch, V.; Emerson, E. Health inequalities experienced by children and young people with intellectual disabilities: A review of literature from the United Kingdom. *J. Intellect. Disabil.* **2011**, *15*, 269–278. [CrossRef] [PubMed]
24. World Health Organization. *Global Action Plan on Physical Activity 2018–2030: More Active People for a Healthier World*; World Health Organization: Geneva, Switzerland, 2019.
25. Bull, F.C.; Al-Ansari, S.S.; Biddle, S.; Borodulin, K.; Buman, M.P.; Cardon, G.; Carty, C.; Chaput, J.-P.; Chastin, S.; Chou, R. World Health Organization 2020 guidelines on physical activity and sedentary behaviour. *Br. J. Sports Med.* **2020**, *54*, 1451–1462. [CrossRef] [PubMed]
26. Carty, C.; van der Ploeg, H.P.; Biddle, S.J.H.; Bull, F.; Willumsen, J.; Lee, L.; Kamenov, K.; Milton, K. The First Global Physical Activity and Sedentary Behavior Guidelines for People Living With Disability. *J. Phys. Act. Health* **2021**, *18*, 86–93. [CrossRef] [PubMed]
27. Barr, M.; Shields, N. Identifying the barriers and facilitators to participation in physical activity for children with Down syndrome. *J. Intellect. Disabil. Res.* **2011**, *55*, 1020–1033. [CrossRef] [PubMed]
28. McGarty, A.M.; Melville, C.A. Parental perceptions of facilitators and barriers to physical activity for children with intellectual disabilities: A mixed methods systematic review. *Res. Dev. Disabil.* **2018**, *73*, 40–57. [CrossRef]
29. Izquierdo-Gomez, R.; Martínez-Gómez, D.; Acha, A.; Veiga, O.L.; Villagra, A.; Diaz-Cueto, M.; UP&DOWN Study Group. Objective assessment of sedentary time and physical activity throughout the week in adolescents with Down syndrome. The UP&DOWN study. *Res. Dev. Disabil.* **2014**, *35*, 482–489.
30. Guthold, R.; Stevens, G.A.; Riley, L.M.; Bull, F.C. Global trends in insufficient physical activity among adolescents: A pooled analysis of 298 population-based surveys with 1· 6 million participants. *Lancet Child Adolesc. Health* **2020**, *4*, 23–35. [CrossRef]
31. Camacho-Miñano, M.J.; LaVoi, N.M.; Barr-Anderson, D.J. Interventions to promote physical activity among young and adolescent girls: A systematic review. *Health Educ. Res.* **2011**, *26*, 1025–1049. [CrossRef]
32. Esposito, P.E.; MacDonald, M.; Hornyak, J.E.; Ulrich, D.A. Physical activity patterns of youth with Down syndrome. *Intellect. Dev. Disabil.* **2012**, *50*, 109–119. [CrossRef] [PubMed]
33. Kahn, J.A.; Huang, B.; Gillman, M.W.; Field, A.E.; Austin, S.B.; Colditz, G.A.; Frazier, A.L. Patterns and determinants of physical activity in US adolescents. *J. Adolesc. Health* **2008**, *42*, 369–377. [CrossRef] [PubMed]
34. Grieser, M.; Vu, M.B.; Bedimo-Rung, A.L.; Neumark-Sztainer, D.; Moody, J.; Young, D.R.; Moe, S.G. Physical activity attitudes, preferences, and practices in African American, Hispanic, and Caucasian girls. *Health Educ. Behav.* **2006**, *33*, 40–51. [CrossRef] [PubMed]
35. Jago, R.; Davis, L.; McNeill, J.; Sebire, S.J.; Haase, A.; Powell, J.; Cooper, A.R. Adolescent girls' and parents' views on recruiting and retaining girls into an after-school dance intervention: Implications for extra-curricular physical activity provision. *Int. J. Behav. Nutr. Phys. Act.* **2011**, *8*, 91. [CrossRef]

36. Richards, R.; Reeder, A.; Darling, H. Interest and participation in selected sports among New Zealand adolescents. *J. N. Z. Med. Assoc.* **2004**, *117*, 1–3.
37. O'Neill, J.R.; Pate, R.R.; Beets, M.W. Physical activity levels of adolescent girls during dance classes. *J. Phys. Act. Health* **2012**, *9*, 382–388. [CrossRef]
38. O'Neill, J.R.; Pate, R.R.; Hooker, S.P. The contribution of dance to daily physical activity among adolescent girls. *Int. J. Behav. Nutr. Phys. Act.* **2011**, *8*, 87. [CrossRef]
39. Burkhardt, J.; Brennan, C. The effects of recreational dance interventions on the health and well-being of children and young people: A systematic review. *Arts Health* **2012**, *4*, 148–161. [CrossRef]
40. May, T.; Chan, E.S.; Lindor, E.; McGinley, J.; Skouteris, H.; Austin, D.; McGillivray, J.; Rinehart, N.J. Physical, cognitive, psychological and social effects of dance in children with disabilities: Systematic review and meta-analysis. *Disabil. Rehabil.* **2021**, *43*, 13–26. [CrossRef]
41. Flores, R. Dance for health: Improving fitness in African American and Hispanic adolescents. *Public Health Rep.* **1995**, *110*, 189–193.
42. Romero, A.J. A pilot test of the Latin Active Hip Hop Intervention to increase physical activity among low-income Mexican-American adolescents. *Am. J. Health Promot.* **2012**, *26*, 208–211. [CrossRef] [PubMed]
43. Olvera, A.E. Cultural dance and health: A review of the literature. *Am. J. Health Educ.* **2008**, *39*, 353–359. [CrossRef]
44. Woodmansee, C.; Hahne, A.; Imms, C.; Shields, N. Comparing participation in physical recreation activities between children with disability and children with typical development: A secondary analysis of matched data. *Res. Dev. Disabil.* **2016**, *49*, 268–276. [CrossRef] [PubMed]
45. Zitomer, M.R. 'Dance Makes Me Happy': Experiences of children with disabilities in elementary school dance education. *Res. Danc. Educ.* **2016**, *17*, 218–234. [CrossRef]
46. Prieto, L.A.; Haegele, J.A.; Columna, L. Dance programs for school-age individuals with disabilities: A systematic review. *Adapt. Phys. Act. Q.* **2020**, *37*, 349–376. [CrossRef]
47. Robinson, T.N.; Killen, J.D.; Kraemer, H.C.; Wilson, D.M.; Matheson, D.M.; Haskell, W.L.; Pruitt, L.A.; Powell, T.M.; Owens, A.S.; Thompson, N.S. Dance and reducing television viewing to prevent weight gain in African-American girls: The Stanford GEMS pilot study. *Ethn. Dis.* **2003**, *13* (Suppl. 1), S1–S65.
48. Beaulac, J.; Kristjansson, E.; Calhoun, M. 'Bigger than hip-hop?'Impact of a community-based physical activity program on youth living in a disadvantaged neighborhood in Canada. *J. Youth Stud.* **2011**, *14*, 961–974. [CrossRef]
49. Piercy, K.L.; Troiano, R.P.; Ballard, R.M.; Carlson, S.A.; Fulton, J.E.; Galuska, D.A.; George, S.M.; Olson, R.D. The physical activity guidelines for Americans. *JAMA* **2018**, *320*, 2020–2028. [CrossRef]
50. Turnbull, H.; Turnbull, A. *Re Appropriate Public Education: The Law and Children with Disabilities*, 5th ed.; Love Publishing Company: Denver, CO, USA, 1998.
51. American College of Sports Medicine. *ACSM's Exercise Management for Persons with Chronic Diseases and Disabilities*, 3rd ed.; Human Kinetics: Champaign, IL, USA, 2009.
52. Nasuti, G. The Six-Minute Walk Test in adults with intellectual disability: A study of validity and reliability. *J. Intellect. Dev. Disabil.* **2010**, *38*, 31–38. [CrossRef]
53. Elmahgoub, S.S.; Van de Velde, A.; Peersman, W.; Cambier, D.; Calders, P. Reproducibility, validity and predictors of six-minute walk test in overweight and obese adolescents with intellectual disability. *Disabil. Rehabil.* **2012**, *34*, 846–851. [CrossRef]
54. Raghupathy, M.K.; Divya, M.; Karthikbabu, S. Effects of traditional Indian dance on motor skills and balance in children with Down syndrome. *J. Mot. Behav.* **2021**, *54*, 212–221. [CrossRef] [PubMed]
55. Dorsan, A.; Gözde, K.; Elif, K.; Emine, B.; ÇALIŞKAN, E. The effect of 12 weeks dance education on physical fitness values at mentally retarded children. *Int. J. Sport Cult. Sci.* **2014**, *2*, 283–286. [CrossRef]
56. McGuire, M.; Long, J.; Esbensen, A.J.; Bailes, A.F. Adapted dance improves motor abilities and participation in children with Down syndrome: A pilot study. *Pediatric Phys. Ther.* **2019**, *31*, 76–82. [CrossRef] [PubMed]
57. Ito, Y.; Hiramoto, I.; Kodama, H. Factors affecting dance exercise performance in students at a special needs school. *Pediatrics Int.* **2017**, *59*, 967–972. [CrossRef] [PubMed]
58. Arzoglou, D.; Tsimaras, V.; Kotsikas, G.; Fotiadou, E.; Sidiropoulou, M.; Proios, M.; Bassa, E. The effect of [alpha] tradinional dance training program on neuromuscular coordination of individuals with autism. *J. Phys. Educ. Sport* **2013**, *13*, 563.
59. Rimmer, J.H. Promoting inclusive community-based obesity prevention programs for children and adolescents with disabilities: The why and how. *Child. Obes.* **2011**, *7*, 177–184. [CrossRef]
60. Rimmer, J.H. Physical activity for people with disabilities: How do we reach those with the greatest need? *NAM Perspect.* **2015**. [CrossRef]
61. Rimmer, J.H.; Rowland, J.L. Health promotion for people with disabilities: Implications for empowering the person and promoting disability-friendly environments. *Am. J. Lifestyle Med.* **2008**, *2*, 409–420. [CrossRef]
62. Brewster, S.; Coleyshaw, L. Participation or exclusion? Perspectives of pupils with autistic spectrum disorders on their participation in leisure activities. *Br. J. Learn. Disabil.* **2010**, *39*, 284–291. [CrossRef]

63. Schleien, S.J.; Miller, K.D.; Walton, G.; Pruett, S. Parent perspectives of barriers to child participation in recreational activities. *Ther. Recreat. J.* **2014**, *48*, 61–73.
64. Thompson, D.; Emira, M. 'They say every child matters, but they don't': An investigation into parental and carer perceptions of access to leisure facilities and respite care for children and young people with Autistic Spectrum Disorder (ASD) or Attention Deficit, Hyperactivity Disorder (ADHD). *Disabil. Soc.* **2011**, *26*, 65–78.
65. Curtin, C.; Bandini, L.G.; Must, A.; Phillips, S.; Maslin, M.C.T.; Lo, C.; Gleason, J.M.; Fleming, R.K.; Stanish, H.I. Including youth with intellectual disabilities in health promotion research: Development and reliability of a structured interview to assess the correlates of physical activity among youth. *J. Appl. Res. Intellect. Disabil. JARID* **2016**, *29*, 378–386. [CrossRef] [PubMed]

International Journal of
Environmental Research and Public Health

MDPI

Review

A Systematic Review of the Influence of Overweight and Obesity across the Lifespan on Obstacle Crossing during Walking

Matthias Chardon [1,2,*], Fabio A. Barbieri [2], Tiago Penedo [1,2], Paulo C. R. Santos [1,3] and Nicolas Vuillerme [1,4,*]

1 Autonomie, Gérontologie, E-santé, Imagerie et Société (AGEIS), Université Grenoble Alpes, 38400 Grenoble, France
2 Human Movement Research Laboratory (MOVI-LAB), Department of Physical Education, School of Sciences, São Paulo State University (Unesp), Bauru 15782, Brazil
3 Department of Computer Science and Applied Mathematics, Weizmann Institute of Science, Rehovot 7632706, Israel
4 Institut Universitaire de France, 75005 Paris, France
* Correspondence: matthias.chardon@univ-grenoble-alpes.fr (M.C.); nicolas.vuillerme@univ-grenoble-alpes.fr (N.V.)

Abstract: This study aimed to systematically review and summarize the available data regarding the influence of overweight and obesity across the lifespan on obstacle crossing during walking. Four databases were systematically searched with no limitation on publication date following the Cochrane Handbook for Systematic Reviews and PRISMA guidelines. Only full-text English-language articles published in a peer-reviewed journal were eligible. They had to compare obstacle crossing during walking by overweight or obese individuals with individuals of normal body weight. Five studies were considered eligible. All the studies assessed kinematics; only one assessed kinetics, but none investigated muscle activity or obstacle contact. Compared to normal individuals crossing obstacles, overweight or obese individuals exhibited lower velocity, shorter step length, lower cadence, and less time spent in single-limb support. They also exhibited increased step width, more time spent in double support, and greater trailing leg ground force reaction and centre of mass acceleration. Overall, the small number of included studies did not allow us to draw any conclusions. However, being overweight or obese seems to have a potentially negative influence on the kinematics of gait parameters due to a tendency to trip, fall, and suffer severe fall-related injuries when negotiating obstacles on foot in real-life environments.

Keywords: obesity; overweight; obstacle crossing; gait; systematic review

1. Introduction

The World Health Organization defines overweight (OW) and obesity (OB) as "abnormal or excessive fat accumulation that may impair health" [1]. OW and OB have become major health issues worldwide, and the prevalence of obesity continues to increase [2]. A 2016 World Health Organization report [1] estimated that 39% of the world population was considered OW and 13% was OB. Specific data for children and adolescents indicated that ~340 million 5–19-year-olds were OW or OB [1]. OW and OB are commonly characterised based on body mass index (BMI). For adults, a BMI of 25.0–29.9 kg/m^2 is defined as OW, and a BMI of 30 kg/m^2 or greater is defined as OB [3]. One emerging public health concern is that OW and OB are associated with several comorbidities that accentuate the risks of hospitalisation [4], sudden death [5] and functional impairments [6]. Among these functional impairments, static and dynamic balance and gait behaviours are particularly affected [7–9].

Molina-Garcia et al. [9] recently reported that OW and OB children and adolescents exhibited different gait behaviours than their normal-weight peers, including greater pelvis transversal plane motion, internal rotation/flexion, extension and abduction moments, power generation and absorption, knee abduction and adduction motion, and knee abduction and adduction moments. These biomechanical alterations are likely to increase the risk of injuries during the activities of daily living [10], musculoskeletal disorders [7,11], and fall risk [12] among individuals with OW and OB. However, although much has been reported about the influence of OW and OB on gait during unobstructed walking [13–18], little is known about how these conditions might impact gait under more challenging conditions, such as environments with obstacles [18–22].

Indeed, tripping during obstacle crossing represents one of the main causes (up to 53%) of falls among healthy older adults [23]. Over the past 25 years, obstacle crossing has been reported to reflect a greater risk of imbalance and trips and could lead to falls [24–29]. A possible explanation for the increased risk of tripping during obstacle crossing could be the increased neuromuscular demands during this activity compared to unobstructed walking [26,30,31]. Accordingly, given the functional limitations that OW and OB impose on the musculoskeletal system (see [9,10,32] for recent reviews), it seemed particularly interesting to evaluate whether and how OW and OB might impact obstacle crossing during walking. The present study aimed to systematically review and summarize the available data regarding the influence of overweight and obesity across the lifespan on obstacle crossing during walking.

2. Methods

2.1. Protocol and Registration

This systematic review's protocol was registered with the International Prospective Register of Systematic Reviews (PROSPERO) (CRD#42021269949) and published in May 2022 [33]; it follows the recommendations of the Preferred Reporting Items for Systematic Reviews and Meta-Analyses (PRISMA) statement [34] (checklist available in the Supplementary Materials: Supplementary File S1) and the guidelines of the Cochrane Handbook for Systematic Reviews [35]. As this review was limited to publicly available materials, it did not require any ethical approval. Note that there was no deviation from the recently published protocol for systematic review [33].

2.2. Eligibility, Inclusion, and Exclusion Criteria

A population, intervention, comparison, outcome and study design (PICOS) tool was used to select the eligibility, inclusion and exclusion criteria for the studies reviewed. Two reviewers (MC and TP) independently included studies based on samples of OW or OB individuals (together defined as having a BMI $\geq$ 25 kg/m^2 for adult studies or being at or above the 85th percentile of the Centers for Disease Control and Prevention's Weight-for-recumbent-length Growth Charts for child studies [36]), excluding studies that selected participants with acute or overuse injuries or with neurological, musculoskeletal, or systemic diseases unrelated to OB comorbidities (population). We included studies addressing the influence of an obstacle-crossing task (intervention: obstacle-crossing while walking). Included articles must have compared obstacle-crossing during walking by OW or OB individuals to individuals of normal weight (NW) (BMI 18–24.9 kg/m^2). No other walking tasks were considered (comparison). We included studies reporting kinematic, kinetic, or electromyographic parameters, and the following outcomes were also extracted (outcomes): gait spatial and temporal stride parameters (e.g., stride length and duration; and horizontal and vertical foot–obstacle clearance distances), kinetics (e.g., force outcomes such as momentum, work, power, and ground reaction force), muscle activation outcomes (e.g., amplitude, muscle onset, muscle activation duration, muscle synergy, mean frequency, and power density) and obstacle contact. Randomised controlled trials, non-randomised controlled trials, and non-randomised, non-controlled trials (study design) were all included. Accordingly, study design inclusion criteria required original articles to have been published in English in a peer-reviewed scientific journal. Finally, we excluded case reports, abstracts, editorials, letters to the editor, case studies, reviews, meta-analyses, theses, grey literature (annual, research, technical, or project reports), working papers, and government documents. The inclusion and exclusion criteria using the PICOS tool are described in Table 1.

Table 1. Eligibility criteria of the included studies using PICOS.

	Inclusion Criteria	Exclusion Criteria
Population	Overweight or obese individuals	Acute or overuse injuries or with neurological, musculoskeletal or systemic diseases unrelated to OB comorbidities
Intervention	Obstacle-crossing task during walking	Obstacle avoidance during a non-walking task Walking task without obstacle crossing
Comparator	Healthy normal-weight individuals	Non-healthy normal-weight individuals
Outcomes	Kinematic, kinetic, and electromyographic	None
Study design	Randomised controlled trials, non-randomised controlled trials, and non-randomised, non-controlled trials. Published in English in a peer-reviewed journal	Case reports, abstracts, editorials, letters to the editor, case studies, reviews, meta-analyses, theses, grey literature (annual, research, technical, or project reports), working papers, and government documents

2.3. Data Sources and Search Strategy

Team members developed and agreed upon the search strategy and selection criteria in line with the review questions. Following the recommendations in the PRISMA statement [34] and the guidelines in the Cochrane Handbook for Systematic Reviews [35], two reviewers (MC and TP) independently performed a systematic computerised literature search of PubMed, Web of Science, Scopus, and SportDiscus from their dates of inception to April 2022, and the search was repeated on February 2023. The search strategy targeted articles containing information relating to overweight or obesity and gait during obstacle-crossing tasks and all subsets of these terms. No filters were used, and the full combination of keywords for all the databases was:

(obes* OR overweight OR over-weight OR adipos* OR "body mass index" OR BMI) AND ("obstacle crossing" or "obstacle negotiation" or "obstacle avoidance" or "obstructed walking"). The references of included studies were not checked for potential citations. No experts in the field were contacted.

2.4. Study Selection

The same two reviewers (MC and TP) independently selected the studies, screened the titles, abstracts, and keywords identified via the search strategy, and applied the eligibility criteria. After this initial selection, full-length texts were subjected to the same procedure. In cases of disagreement, and if subsequent discussions between the two reviewers were inconclusive, a third reviewer (NV) was contacted to arbitrate until a consensus was found.

2.5. Data Extraction

In line with the PRISMA guidelines [34], the number of citations reviewed at each stage of the review was summarised in a flow diagram. The same two reviewers (MC and TP) independently completed the data extraction process using a standardised data extraction form. The following four datasets were extracted from each article retrieved:

(1) Study characteristics: first author, title, year of publication, journal name, country, study design, mention of any adverse events occurring during the study, and funding;
(2) Sample description: sample size, age, sex, body weight, body height, body mass index, lower limb length, health status, fall status, and limb preference;
(3) Obstacle-crossing protocol: task requirement, instrumentation, data acquisition methodology, and gait parameters assessed;
(4) Main results obtained from gait measurement: spatial-temporal parameters, muscle activity, joint angle and moment, ground reaction force, and obstacle contacts.

2.6. Quality Assessment

The same two reviewers (MC and TP) independently performed a qualitative analysis of the selected studies [34]. To do this, they used a grid specifically developed by Galna and colleagues to assess the quality of the evidence contained within a systematic review investigating obstacle crossing by older adults [37]. Quality issues and risks of bias in the present systematic review centred on the internal validity, external validity, and reproducibility of the methods used in the articles retained. However, Galna's grid [37] contains no items related to the study participants' anthropometric characteristics. We thus modified the grid to allow us to address our review question: "How do overweight and obesity influence gait parameters during obstacle crossing across the lifespan?" (CRD#42021269949). The items of body mass and body mass index were added to the grid. The scoring system developed by Galna and colleagues [37] was used to quantify the quality of each of the studies retained and to assess the methodological strengths and weaknesses of those reviewed. Each question in our modified quality assessment [37] was scored as follows: 1 = assessment criterion met, 0 = assessment criterion not met, and 0.5 = lack of information or clarity on that criterion. Any discrepancies between the two reviewers' findings were resolved by consensus. If disagreements persisted, a third reviewer (NV) was consulted to arbitrate a final decision.

2.7. Data Synthesis

Given the small number of included studies, the wide range of age of the participants included in these studies, and the variety of experimental protocols and reported outcomes, we were unable to conduct meta-analyses of the extracted data. As an alternative, we provided a narrative synthesis of the available data regarding the influence of overweight and obesity on kinematic (Section 3.6.1) and kinetic parameters (Section 3.6.2) related to executing the obstacle-crossing task.

3. Results

3.1. Study Selection

The study selection process is presented in Figure 1.

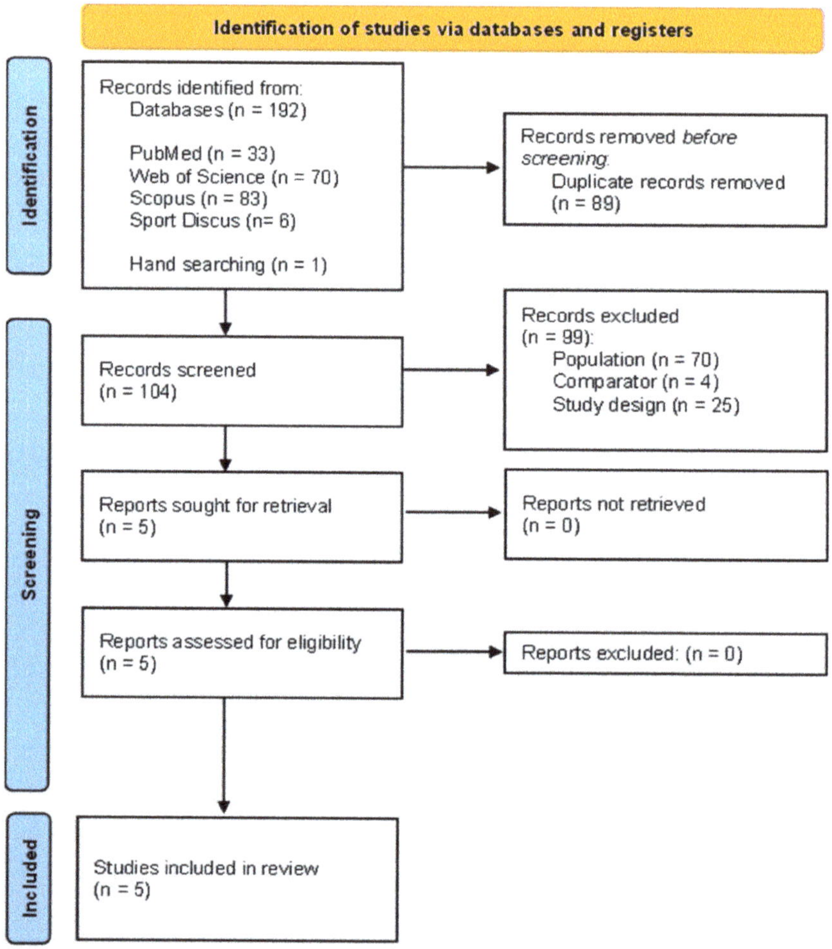

Figure 1. Flow diagram of the articles included in the review. The number of original articles is indicated at each stage of the search.

Our searches of PubMed, Web of Science, Scopus, and SportDiscus resulted in 33, 70, 83 and 6 records, respectively. One article was found via hand searching [21]. After duplicate removal (n = 89), 104 records remained. After screening titles, abstracts and keywords, five full texts were read to verify and confirm their eligibility [18–22]. All five met our eligibility criteria and were retained for review [18–22].

3.2. *General Information about the Studies Included in the Systematic Review*

Table 2 shows the basic information about the studies included in the systematic review.

Table 2. Studies included in the review in order of publication.

Author	Gill and Hung [19]	Gill and Hung [20]	Silva et al. [21]	Gill [22]	Desrochers et al. [18]
Publication year	2012	2014	2018	2019	2021
Country	USA	USA	Portugal	USA	USA
Title	Influence of weight classification on children stepping over obstacles	Effects of overweight and obese body mass on motor planning and motor skills during obstacle crossing in children	Foot rollover temporal parameters during walking straight ahead and stepping over obstacles: obese and non-obese post-menopausal women	Effects of obesity class on flat ground walking and obstacle negotiation	Association between the Functional Gait Assessment and spatiotemporal gait parameters in individuals with obesity compared to normal-weight controls: A proof-of-concept study
Journal	*American Journal of Physical Medicine and Rehabilitation*	*Research in Developmental Disabilities*	*Journal of Aging and Physical Activity*	*Journal of Musculoskeletal Neuronal Interactions*	*Journal of Musculoskeletal Neuronal Interactions*
Study design	Observational cross-sectional	Observational cross-sectional	Observational cross-sectional	Observational cross-sectional	Observational cross-sectional, proof-of-concept
Main objective	To examine how weight classification relates to children's ability to meet a task constraint: crossing obstacles of various heights.	To examine whether body mass index would influence the ability of 4- to 13-year-olds to plan and coordinate their movements to cross obstacles of various heights.	To explore the potential differences between walking straight ahead and walking stepping over obstacles for OB and NOB post-menopausal women.	To investigate how increasing obesity classes affected gait and gait variability in adults.	To determine how to capture gait and balance impairments in adults with obesity using an inexpensive method as a proof-of-concept for possible future validation.
Main Findings	During obstacle crossing, children who were overweight or obese took longer to cross obstacles and had a dorsiflexed ankle position when landing. We also found that children demonstrated high variability in ankle position when crossing medium obstacles and during the final baseline trials.	Differences in motor planning and motor skills between normal weight and overweight/obese children during obstacle crossing may reflect movement patterns evident during early skill acquisition in which children attempt to freeze degrees of freedom, exhibit difficulty planning and controlling their movements with excess adiposity, or use unknown mechanisms responsible for motor planning and motor skill abilities	Significant differences were found in temporal characteristics of foot rollover during walking straight ahead and stepping over obstacles in both groups, with most of these differences being common for both OB and NOB subjects.	Increases in classes of obesity are associated with more difficulties with spatiotemporal gait and gait variability. Most importantly, there were few differences between Class II and Class III obesity.	Poorer FGA scores in the obese group were associated with slowing of gait when encountering obstacles but not during flat over-ground walking. Further, the presence of obstacles during gait tasks may be helpful in revealing meaningful gait impairments in obesity and other populations.

Table 2. *Cont.*

Author	Gill and Hung [19]	Gill and Hung [20]	Silva et al. [21]	Gill [22]	Desrochers et al. [18]
Funding	No funding information reported.	Boston University start-up funds.	European Investment Funds via FEDER/COMPETE/POCI—Operational Competitiveness and Internationalisation Programme, under project POCI-01-0145-FEDER-006958 and National Funds via FCT—Portuguese Foundation for Science and Technology, under project UID/AGR/04033/2013	R03 AR066344-01 A1 (Gill, PI).	NIH R03 AR066344-01A1 (Gill, PI).

Note: FGA: Functional Gait Assessment; NOB: non-obese; OB: obese.

3.3. Study Characteristics

Table 2 summarises the characteristics of the studies included in the review in order of publication.

The studies retained were published from 2012 to 2021, with one study each published in 2012 [19], 2014 [20], 2018 [21], 2019 [22] and 2021 [18].

The articles were published in four different journals: two in the *Journal of Musculoskeletal Neuronal Interactions* [18,22], and one each in the *Journal of Aging and Physical Activity* [21], *Research in Developmental Disabilities* [20] and the *American Journal of Physical Medicine and Rehabilitation* [19].

The studies originated from just two countries: four from the USA [18–20,22] and one from Portugal [21].

3.4. Quality Assessment

Table 3 summarises our quality assessment for each article retained [18–22].

Table 3. Methodological quality appraisal results adapted from the grid developed by Galna et al. [36].

Question	Scoring Criteria	Gill and Hung [19]	Gill and Hung [20]	Silva et al. [21]	Gill [22]	Desrochers et al. [18]	Average
1. Research aims or questions stated clearly	Y = 1; L = 0.5; N = 0	1	1	1	1	1	1
2. Participants detailed	Number	1	1	1	1	1	1
	Age	1	1	1	1	1	1
	Sex	1	1	1	1	1	1
	Height	0	0	1	0	1	0.4
	Body mass	0	0	1	0	1	0.4
	Body mass index	1	1	1	1	1	1
	Subtotal	0.67	0.67	1	0.67	1	0.8
3. Recruitment and sampling methods described	Y = 1; L = 0.5; N = 0	1	1	1	1	1	1
4. Inclusion and exclusion criteria detailed	Y = 1; L = 0.5; N = 0	1	1	1	1	0.5	0.9
5. Covariates controlled for	Age	1	1	1	1	1	1
	Sex	0	0	1	1	0	0.4
	Height	0	0.5	1	0	0	0.3
	Body mass	0	0	0	0	0	0
	Body mass index	1	1	1	1	1	1
	Limb asymmetries	0	0	1	0	1	0.4
	Strength	0	0	0	0	0	0
	Stride/step Speed	1	1	1	1	0	0.8
	Subtotal	0.38	0.44	0.88	0.5	0.38	0.52
6. Key outcome variables clearly described	Y = 1; L = 0.5; N = 0	1	1	1	1	1	1
7. Adequate methodology ables study replication	Participants	0.5	0.5	1	0.5	1	0.7
	Equipment	1	1	1	1	1	1
	Procedure	1	1	1	1	1	1
	Processing	1	1	1	1	1	1
	Statistics	1	1	1	1	1	1
	Subtotal	0.9	0.9	1	0.9	1	0.94

Table 3. *Cont.*

Question	Scoring Criteria	Gill and Hung [19]	Gill and Hung [20]	Silva et al. [21]	Gill [22]	Desrochers et al. [18]	Average
8. Methodology able to answer the research question	Participants	1	1	1	1	1	1
	Equipment	1	1	1	1	1	1
	Procedure	1	1	1	1	1	1
	Processing	1	1	1	1	1	1
	Statistics	1	1	1	1	1	1
	Subtotal	1	1	1	1	1	1
9. Reliability of the methodology is stated	Y = 1, N = 0	0	0	0	0	0	0
10. Internal validity of the methodology was stated	Y = 1, N = 0	0	0	0	0	0	0
11 Research questions were answered adequately in the discussion	Y = 1, N = 0	1	1	1	1	1	1
12. Key findings were supported by the results	Y = 1, N = 0	1	1	1	1	1	1
13. Key findings were interpreted logically, supported by references	Y = 1, N = 0	1	1	1	1	1	1
14. Clinical implications were stated	Y = 1; L = 0.5; N = 0	0	0.5	0	0	0	0.1
Study average		0.69	0.71	0.85	0.72	0.75	0.74

Y = yes; L = lacking detail or clarity; N = no. A score of 1 indicated high-quality research, and 0 indicated lower quality.

The articles included adequately stated their objectives, provided an appropriate description of their participants (although three studies reported participants' BMI but not their height or body mass [19,20,22]), described their inclusion and exclusion criteria, detailed their main findings, used appropriate methodologies to answer their research questions, and appropriately discussed their study results. The details provided were adequate to replicate their study. All five studies lacked detail and clarity on the clinical implications of their research [18–22].

Sample Characteristics

The basic demographic and anthropometric characteristics of each study's participants are presented in Table 4.

Table 4. Basic demographic and anthropometric characteristics of the participants in each study.

Author	Gill and Hung [19]	Gill and Hung [20]	Silva et al. [21]	Gill [22]	Desrochers et al. [18]
Number of groups (n)	2:	2:	2:	4:	2:
	Normal BMI (between 5th and 85th percentile). [C]	Normal weight (between 5th and 85th percentile). [C]	Non-OB (<27 kg/m^2).	Normal BMI (≥18.5 kg/m^2 and <25 kg/m^2).	Normal BMI (≥19 kg/m^2 and ≤25 kg/m^2).
	High BMI (children at or above 85th percentile and below 95th percentile were classified as OW; those above 95th percentile were classified as OB). (C)	OW/OB (children at or above 85th percentile and below 95th percentile were classified as OW; those above 95th percentile were classified as OB). (C)	OB (Z) (>27 kg/m^2).	OW/Class I OB (C) (≥25 kg/m^2 and <35 kg/m^2).	OB BMI (≥30 kg/m^2). (C)
				Class II OB (C) (≥35 kg/m^2 and <40 kg/m^2).	
				Class III OB (C) (>40 kg/m^2).	
Number of participants (n)	Non-OB: 10	Non-OB: 10	Non-OB: 27	Normal BMI: 13	Non-OB: 20
				OW/Class I OB: 18	
	OW/OB: 12	OW/OB: 12	OB: 40	Class II OB: 16	OB: 14
				Class III OB: 20	
Sex (F: female; M: male) (n)	Non-OB: F:6; M: 6	All participants: F: 9; M: 13	Non-OB: F: 27	Normal BMI: F: 13	Non-OB: F: 14; M: 6
				OW/Class I OB: F: 18	
	OW/OB: F:5; M: 7		OB: F: 40	Class II OB: F: 16	OB: F: 12; M: 2
				Class III OB: F: 20	
Exclusion criteria	Not reported.	Not reported.	(1) Diabetes and/or signs associated with neuropathy, (2) acute foot pain and deformities, (3) severe lower extremity trauma, and (4) coordination problems resulting from eye disorders. Scheduled to undergo knee surgery, having no significant cardiovascular, musculoskeletal, vestibular or other neurological disorders. These criteria were confirmed via participant reports and investigators' observations.	Scheduled to undergo knee surgery, having no significant cardiovascular, musculoskeletal, vestibular or other neurological disorders. These criteria were confirmed via participant reports and investigators' observations.	Not reported.

Table 4. *Cont.*

Author	Gill and Hung [19]	Gill and Hung [20]	Silva et al. [21]	Gill [22]	Desrochers et al. [18]
Inclusion criteria	Being free of intellectual impairment or physical conditions that precluded independent walking based on parents' reports and investigators' observations and being 4–13 years old.	Having normal cognitive abilities, no known physical conditions that would preclude independent walking, and being 4–13 years old.	Not reported.	All participants could walk without the aid of an assistive device.	All participants were free of neurological difficulties, had normal or corrected-to-normal vision, and could walk without assistive devices.
Age, mean (SD) (Range), years	Non-OB: 8.42 (1.00) (4.5–13). OW/OB: 8.58 (0.73) (6–13).	All participants: 8.62 (0.93) (not reported).	Non-OB: 58.2 (4.8) (not reported). OB: 57.1 (4.7) (not reported).	Normal BMI: 33.2 (7.04) (not reported). OW/Class I OB: 36.16 (12.76) (not reported). Class II OB: 41.17 (5.89) (not reported) Class III OB: 42.72 (11.43) (not reported).	Non-OB: 45.55 (8.77) (35–64). OB: 50.36 (10.97) (35–66).
Height, mean (SD) (Range), cm	Not reported.	Not reported.	Non-OB: 155.8 (5.2) (not reported). OB: 156.3 (4.5) (not reported).	Not reported.	Non-OB: 170.15 (8) (150–180). (X) OB: 168.83 (8.69) (155–184). (X)
Body mass, mean (SD) (Range), kg	Not reported.	Not reported.	Non-OB: 58.4 (7.1) (not reported). OB: 73.1 (7.3) (not reported).	Not reported.	Non-OB: 69.36 (12.17) (47.20–86.20). (X) OB: 120.58 (20.13) (99.20–173.01). (X)
BMI, mean (SD) (Range), kg/m^2	Non-OB: 15.85 (0.68) (11.65–18.35). (C) OW/OB: 21.41 (1.31) (16.67–31.23). (C)	Non-OB: 15.85 (0.68) (not reported). (C) OW/OB: 21.85 (0.50) (not reported). (C)	Non-OB: 24.0 (2.0) (not reported). OW/OB: 29.9 (2.5) (not reported).	Normal BMI: 22.56 (1.61) (not reported). OW/Class I OB: 29.36 (3.19) (not reported). (C) Class II OB: 37.78 (1.42) (not reported). (C) Class III OB: 44.31 (4.24) (not reported). (C)	Non-OB: 23.77 (2.53) (18.59–27.55). (C) OB: 40.95 (5.46) (35.3–52.64). (C)

BMI: body mass index. Class I obesity: $30\ kg/m^2 \leq BMI < 35\ kg/m^2$; Class II obesity: $35\ kg/m^2 \leq BMI < 40\ kg/m^2$; Class III obesity: $BMI > 40\ kg/m^2$). (C) indicates an OW and OB classification according to the Centers for Disease Control and Prevention [38]; (Z) indicates that OB levels were determined using the cut-off value of $27\ kg/m^2$: Brochu et al., 2008. "Contribution of the Lean Body Mass to Insulin Resistance in Postmenopausal Women with Visceral Obesity: A Monet Study" [39]; (X) indicates that the value was calculated by the reviewers. Non-OB: non-overweight/obese individuals; OW: overweight individuals.

Regarding sample size, a total of 132 OW/OB individuals and 82 NW individuals were included. Sample sizes ranged from 12 [19,20] to 54 [22] for OW/OB individuals and from 10 [20] to 27 [21] for NW individuals.

Regarding sex, two studies only included female participants [21,22], with 134 female participants in total (94 OW/OB; 40 NW). Three studies included male and female participants [18–20], totalling 34 males and 46 females. Two of these studies also reported the number of male and female participants in each BMI group, namely 9 OW/OB males and 17 OW/OB females vs. 12 NW males and 20 NW females [18,19]. No sex comparisons were made.

Regarding age, two studies only included children [19,20], with a total of 46 children (24 OW/OB individuals and 22 NW individuals). Children ranged from 4 to 13 years old across both studies [19,20].

Gill and Hung in 2012 reported their mean participant age as 8.58 ± 0.73 years for OW/OB individuals and 8.42 ± 1.00 years for NW individuals [19]. The mean participant age in the other study (including NW and OW/OB children) was 8.62 ± 0.93 years [20]. Three studies included adults [18,21,22], with a total of 168 participants (108 OW/OB; 60 NW), with mean ages ranging from 36.2 ± 12.8 [22] to 57.1 ± 4.7 [21] years for OW/OB individuals and from 33.2 ± 7.0 [22] to 58.2 ± 4.8 [21] years old for NW individuals. None of these three studies reported age inclusion criteria [18,21,22].

Considering anthropometry, two studies reported the heights and weights of their adult participants [18,21]. Heights ranged from 156.3 ± 4.5 cm [21] to 168.83 ± 8.69 cm [18] for OW/OB individuals and from 155.8 ± 5.2 cm [21] to 170.15 ± 8 cm [18] for NW individuals. Weights ranged from 73.1 ± 7.3 kg [21] to 120.58 ± 20.13 kg [18] for OW/OB individuals and from 58.4 ± 7.1 kg [21] to 69.36 ± 12.17 kg [18] for NW individuals. For the two studies involving children [19,20], BMIs were 21.41 ± 1.31 kg/m^2 [19] and 21.85 ± 0.50 kg/m^2 [20] for OW/OB individuals and 15.85 ± 0.68 kg/m^2 for NW individuals [19,20]. For the three studies involving adults [18,21,22], BMIs ranged from 29.9 ± 2.5 kg/m^2 [21] to 43.31 ± 4.24 kg/m^2 [22] for OW/OB individuals and from 22.56 ± 1.61 kg/m^2 [22] to 24.0 ± 2.0 kg/m^2 [21] for NW individuals. Only Desrochers et al. (2021) reported participants' heights and weights using fixed obstacle height [18].

Regarding obesity classification, four studies [18–20,22] used the Centers for Disease Control and Prevention classification [36,38], and the fifth [21] used a classification developed for Brochu et al.'s study [39] of post-menopausal women, where participants were considered OB above a BMI cut-off value of 27 kg/m^2. In Desrochers et al.'s 2021 study involving adults [18], OB individuals had a BMI above 30 kg/m^2. In another study, three OW/OB groups were established according to their BMI: OW/Class I OB (25 kg/m^2 $\leq$ BMI < 35 kg/m^2); Class II OB (35 kg/m^2 $\leq$ BMI < 40 kg/m^2); and Class III OB: (BMI < 40 kg/m^2) [22].

In the two studies involving children aged 4–13 years old [19,20], participants at or above the 85th percentile and below the 95th percentile were classified as OW (approximately 17–25.2 kg/m^2 and 17.2–26.2 kg/m^2 for boys and girls, respectively), and those above the 95th percentile were classified as OB (approximately 17.8 to more than 25.2 kg/m^2 and from 18 to more than 26.2 kg/m^2 for boys and girls, respectively) [36].

3.5. Obstacle-Crossing Task

The obstacle-crossing tasks used in the retained studies are described in Table 5.

Table 5. Description of the obstacle-crossing tasks used in the retained studies.

Author	Gill & Hung [19]	Gill & Hung [20]	Silva et al. [21]	Gill [22]	Desrochers et al. [18]
Task	Participants first walked once along a 406-cm-long walkway. In balance order, they walked and stepped over low, medium, and high obstacles.	Children walked along a 406-cm-long walkway and crossed low, medium, and high obstacles.	Walking straight ahead with or without stepping over an obstacle whose height was 30% of the leg length in a two-step protocol.	Participants walked down a 1600 cm walkway with a gait carpet (610 cm long × 89 cm wide) in the centre and crossed 3 obstacles of low, medium, and high height placed halfway down the path.	Participants walked along the GAITRite (488 cm long × 61 cm wide) walkway under five conditions.
Obstacle	A wooden dowel inserted into two 25-cm-high wooden towers at 4 cm (low obstacle), 11 cm (medium obstacle), and 16 cm (high obstacle).	A wooden dowel inserted into two 25-cm-high wooden towers at 4 cm (low obstacle), 11 cm (medium obstacle), and 16 cm (high obstacle).	Not reported.	The obstacles were created using a wooden dowel (121 cm long) and two rectangular towers (9 cm × 10 cm × 22 cm) with holes drilled at 4 cm, 8 cm, and 16 cm (low, medium, and high).	The obstacle was a wooden dowel suspended across the walkway that was inserted into holes in two wooden towers. Participants encountered small (4 cm), medium (8 cm), or large (16 cm) obstacles.
Expected/ Unexpected	Expected.	Expected.	Expected.	Expected.	Expected.
Starting point	Not reported.	203 cm from the obstacle.	Two-step protocol with the left leg as the leading limb during obstacle crossing.	800 cm from the obstacle.	244 cm from the obstacle.
Number of sessions	1.	1.	1.	1.	1.
Number of conditions	5: No obstacle = flat surface without obstacle (baseline initial and final trials). Low obstacle height (4 cm). Medium obstacle height (11 cm). High obstacle height (16 cm).	5: No obstacle = flat surface without obstacle (baseline initial and final trial). Low obstacle height (4 cm). Medium obstacle height (11 cm). High obstacle height (16 cm).	2: Straight ahead walking without obstacle = flat ground surface without obstacle. Straight ahead walking and stepping over an obstacle height of 30% of leg length.	5: No obstacle = flat ground surface without obstacles (baseline initial and final trials). Low obstacle height (4 cm). Medium obstacle height (8 cm). High obstacle height (16 cm).	5: No obstacle = flat ground surface without obstacles (baseline initial and final trials). Low obstacle height (4 cm). Medium obstacle height (8 cm). High obstacle height (16 cm).
Obstacle condition order	Initial and final overground trials. Obstacle conditions were counterbalanced.	Not reported.	Two-step protocol without obstacle. Two-step protocol with obstacle.	Initial and final overground trials Obstacle conditions were randomised.	Initial and final overground trials Obstacle conditions were counterbalanced.

Table 5. *Cont.*

Author	Gill & Hung [19]	Gill & Hung [20]	Silva et al. [21]	Gill [22]	Desrochers et al. [18]
Number of trials per condition	5 for obstacle-crossing trials. 1 for baseline and final trials (no obstacle condition).	5.	5 valid trials. [y]	5.	5.
Walking speed	Self-selected pace.	Self-selected pace.	Self-selected pace.	Self-selected pace.	Self-selected pace.
Experimental condition	Single task.	Single task.	Single task.	Single task.	Single task.
Practice	Not reported.	3 practice trials.	10 min familiarisation period.	Not reported.	Not reported.

[y]: Whenever a participant trod on the pressure platform, if foot contact was incomplete or the coefficient of variation of the duration of contact was greater than 4%, the trial was discarded. Note that all studies included single-task conditions and self-selected walking speed instruction and had the same number of experimental session and trials per obstacle crossing conditions.

Regarding the walkway, four studies [18–20,22] reported fixed walkway lengths between 406 cm [19,20] and 1600 cm [22], and one [21] used a two-step protocol (left leg as the leading limb during obstacle crossing). Three studies placed their obstacles in the middle of their walkway [18,20,22], and one [19] did not report the obstacle's location.

Concerning the starting point, studies' starting points and walking distances before arriving at their obstacles ranged from 203 cm [20] to 800 cm [22] or two steps before the obstacle [21]. Gill and Hung's 2012 study did not report the starting point's distance from the obstacle [19].

For the obstacle conditions and experimental conditions, all five studies performed an overground gait task and obstacle-crossing tasks [18–22]. Four studies used baseline and final overground walking trials [18–20,22]; three studies executed five consecutive overground walking trials before and after their obstacle-crossing tasks [18,20,22] Desrochers et al., 2021 used a single overground walking trial before and after the obstacle-crossing task [19]. In the last study, participants performed five trials using the two-step protocol without the presence of the obstacle [21].

Regarding obstacle height and shape, Silva et al., 2018 [21] used an obstacle height that varied according to the participant's leg length (30% of leg length), with obstacle heights of 22.2 ± 0.9 cm for non-OB participants and 22.1 ± 1 cm for OB participants. The obstacle's shape was not described, however. Four studies [18–20,22] used three fixed obstacle heights: two [19,20] used small (4 cm), medium (11 cm), and high (16 cm) obstacles; two [18,22] used different respective small (4 cm), medium (8 cm), and high (16 cm) obstacles. All four [18–20,22] used a wooden dowel suspended across the walkway and inserted into holes in two wooden towers as their obstacle.

As concerns instructions, in all five studies, participants were instructed to walk at a self-selected speed and cross an obstacle. In the study by Gill (2019) [22], participants walked barefoot; in the other four studies [18–20,22], footwear was not specified. The obstacle's presence on the walkway was expected in all five studies. Participants executed 5 consecutive trials for each obstacle condition [18–22]. The mean [18–22] or mean and SD were used to calculate coefficients of variation using the following equation: the mean/SD [22] of the 5 trials was used for data analysis. Three studies reported that the obstacle condition order was counterbalanced [18,19] or randomised [22] across individuals; Gill and Hun, 2014 did not mention any obstacle condition order [20].

Regarding practice and familiarisation, two studies [20,21] reported that the participants were allowed to practice before the experimental trials, with one permitting three practice trials [20] and the other allotting a 10 min familiarisation period [21].

Table 6 reports the categories of parameters related to the performance of the obstacle-crossing tasks assessed in each of the retained studies, including the parameters measured during obstacle crossing, and the data acquisition methods for kinematic and kinetic gait parameters related to the performance of the obstacle-crossing tasks.

Table 6. Gait parameters measured and data acquisition methods.

Author	Gill and Hung [19]	Gill and Hung [20]	Silva et al. [21]	Gill [22]	Desrochers et al. [18]
Parameters measured	Kinematics: Time from foot lift to maximum knee height, time from maximum knee height to foot contact, and maximum knee height. Ankle angles at foot contact to determine neutral (angles near 90 degrees) or dorsiflexed ankle positions (angles < 90 degrees) and sagittal knee and ankle angles at maximum knee height. Estimated variability of ankle positions at foot contact by calculating the coefficient of variation.	Kinematics: Maximum toe height for each leg during obstacle crossing; hip and knee angles in sagittal and frontal planes; vertical, anterior/posterior, and medial/lateral acceleration of centre of mass. Kinetics: Ground reaction force: normalised vertical, anterior/posterior, and medial/lateral ground reaction forces of both legs.	Kinematics: Plantar pressure parameters: relative foot temporal data for the initial contact, final contact, and duration of contact.	Kinematics: Velocity, percentage of gait cycle spent in swing and in stance, and coefficient of variation for each variable to obtain a measure of variability.	Kinematics: Gait velocity, step length and width, cadence, and single- and double-limb support during leading leg step across the obstacle.
Acquisition system	Vicon Nexus Model 1.4 motion capture system (120 Hz) and 41 reflective markers.	Whole-body plug-in-gait model of Vicon Nexus 1.51 (120 Hz) with 7 infrared cameras and 41 reflective markers. Two AMTI OR6-6 force platforms (46 × 50 cm; 1200 Hz).	Two Footscan platforms (100 × 40 cm, 8192 sensors; RSscan International, Olen, Belgium; 250 Hz).	Gait carpet (Protokinetics, LLC; Peekskill, NY, USA; 610 cm long × 89 cm wide; 120 Hz).	-GAITRite software and custom Matlab scripts (Mathworks, Inc., Natick, MA, USA) (488 cm long × 61 cm wide; 120 Hz).

All five studies assessed kinematic parameters [18–22], but only one assessed both the kinematic and kinetic parameters related to executing the obstacle-crossing task [20]. None of the studies assessed muscular activity or obstacle contacts.

Regarding kinematic parameters, the kinematic measurement tools used were Protokinetics LLC's 610 cm long × 89 cm wide gait carpet [22], GAITRite's 488 cm long × 61 cm wide carpet [18] and two Footscan platforms (100 × 40 cm) [21]. Two studies used the Vicon Nexus Model motion capture system [19,20].

The only kinematic parameter investigated by two studies was gait velocity during obstacle crossing [18,22]. The following 63 kinematic parameters were only assessed in one study each:

- Step length, width, cadence, and single- and double-limb support phases [18];
- Stance and swing time and their coefficients of variation, and the coefficient of variation of velocity [22];
- Time from foot lift to maximum knee height and from maximum knee height to foot contact, maximum knee height (plus sagittal knee and ankle angles at maximum knee height), and ankle angle at foot contact [19];
- Leading- and trailing-leg toe clearance, hip and knee angles at maximum knee height in the sagittal and frontal planes, COM (centre of mass) anterior and posterior, and medial, lateral and vertical acceleration at the leading and trailing legs' maximum knee height during crossing [20];
- Relative foot temporal data at initial and final foot contact and duration of contact of the HL (lateral heel), HM (medial heel), MF (midfoot), M1-5 (metatarsal areas), T2-5 (toes), and T1 (hallux) areas of the leading and trailing legs [21].

Regarding kinetic parameters, Gill and Hung, 2014 [20] assessed six kinetic parameters using two AMTI OR6-6 force platforms (46 cm × 50 cm): leading and trailing leg normalised anterior and posterior; and medial, lateral, and vertical ground reaction force at maximum knee height of the contralateral leg during obstacle crossing [20].

3.6. *Influence of Overweight/Obesity on Obstacle Crossing during Walking*

3.6.1. Kinematic Parameters

Table 7 reports the influence of OW/OB on kinematic parameters during obstacle crossing.

Table 7. The influence of overweight/obesity on gait parameters during obstacle crossing.

Gait Parameters	Number of Studies	Study	Between-Group Differences	Results (Mean ± SD or Median (IQR)) and Direction of Difference (↑↓)
Kinematics outcomes				
Velocity (cm/s)	2	Gill, 2019	**NW vs. OBI: $p = 0.03$** **NW vs. OBII: $p = 0.000002$** **NW vs. OBIII: $p = 0.000000058$** **OBI vs. OBII: $p = 0.018$** **OBI vs. OBIII: $p = 0.001$**	**NW = 125.08 ± 1.98** **OBI = 105.72 ± 3.08 (↓ 15.5% vs. NW)** **OBII = 91.46 ± 3.06 (↓ 26.9% vs. NW; ↓ 13.5% vs. OBI)** **OBIII = 85.46 ± 2.43 (↓ 31.7% vs. NW; ↓ 19.2% vs. OBI).**
		Desrochers et al., 2021	**$p = 0.0001$ (OB vs. C)**	**NW = 97.49 ± 6.14** **OB = 67.53 ± 5.83 (↓ 30.7% vs. NW)**
Leading-leg step length (cm)	1	Desrochers et al., 2021	**NW vs. OB: $p = 0.01$**	**NW = 60.40 ± 0.37** **OB = 51.94 ± 0.18 (↓ 14.0% vs. NW)**
Leading-leg step width (cm)	1	Desrochers et al., 2021	**NW vs. OB: $p = 0.01$**	**NW = 8.40 ± 0.21** **OB = 11.54 ± 0.70 (↑ 37.4% vs. NW)**
Leading-leg single-limb support (% of gait cycle)	1	Desrochers et al., 2021	**NW vs. OB: $p = 0.001$**	**NW = 41.38 ± 1.16** **OB = 38.87 ± 1.03 (↓ 6.1% vs. NW)**
Double-limb support (% of gait cycle)	1	Desrochers et al., 2021	**NW vs. OB: $p = 0.001$**	**NW = 8.90 ± 0.85** **OB = 11.09 ± 0.96 (↑ 24.5% vs. NW)**
Cadence (steps/min)	1	Desrochers et al., 2021	**NW vs. OB: $p = 0.001$**	**NW = 104.46 ± 2.33** **OB = 90.24 ± 3.07 (↓ 13.6% vs. NW)**
Stance time (% of gait cycle)	1	Gill, 2019	**NW vs. OBI: $p = 0.012$** **OBI vs. OBII: $p = 0.029$** **NW vs. OBI, low obstacle: $p = 0.004$** **NW vs. OBI, medium obstacle: $p = 0.007$**	**NW = 61.64 ± 1.71** **OBI = 65.13 ± 0.35 (↑ 5.7% vs. NW; ↑ 4.6% vs. OBII)** **OBII = 62.83 ± 0.02** **Low obstacle (4 cm):** **NW = 60.79 ± 6.97** **OBI = 64.85 ± 2.31 (↑ 6.7% vs. NW)** **Medium obstacle (8 cm):** **NW = 60.52 ± 8.04** **OBI = 65.01 ± 3.71 (↑ 7.4% vs. NW)**
Swing time (% of gait cycle)	1	Gill, 2019	**NW vs. OBI: $p = 0.003$** **NW vs. OBII: $p = 0.001$** **NW vs. OBIII: $p = 0.00024$**	**C = 42.55 ± 0.85** **OBI = 38.42 ± 0.85 (↓ 9.7% vs. NW)** **OBII = 37.72 ± 0.02 (↓ 11.4% vs. NW)** **OBIII = 37.14 ± 0.21 (↓ 12.7% vs. NW)**
CV velocity	1	Gill, 2019	**NW vs. OBII: $p = 0.00042$** **OBI vs. OBII: $p = 0.00015$** **NW vs. OBIII: $p = 0.000023$** **OBI vs. OBIII: $p = 0.000006$**	**NW = 0.03 ± 0.01** **OBI = 0.03 ± 0.01** **OBII = 0.06 ± 0 (↑ 80% vs. NW and OBI)** **OBIII = 0.07 ± 0.01 (↑ 100% vs. NW and OBI)**

Table 7. *Cont.*

Gait Parameters	Number of Studies	Study	Between-Group Differences	Results (Mean ± SD or Median (IQR)) and Direction of Difference (↑↓)
CV stance time	1	Gill, 2019	NS	
CV swing time	1	Gill, 2019	NS	
Time from foot lift to maximum knee height (s)	1	Gill and Hung, 2012	**NW vs. OB, high obstacle: $p = 0.04$** NW vs. OB, low obstacle: $p = 0.41$ NW vs. OB, medium obstacle: $p = 0.31$	**High obstacle (16 cm):** **NW = 0.08 ± 0.01** **OB = 0.11 ± 0.01 (↑ 37.5% vs. NW)**
Time from maximum knee height to foot contact (s)	1	Gill and Hung, 2012	**NW vs. OB, high obstacle: $p = 0.04$** NW vs. OB, low obstacle: $p = 0.13$ NW vs. OB, medium obstacle: $p = 0.96$	**High obstacle (16 cm):** **NW = 0.0011 ± 0.001** **OB = 0.0006 ± 0.0005 (↓ 45.5% vs. NW)**
Maximum knee height	1	Gill and Hung, 2012	C vs. OB: $p = 0.57$	
Ankle angle at foot contact (°)	1	Gill and Hung, 2012	**C vs. OB, low obstacle: $p = 0.04$** NW vs. OB, medium obstacle: $p = 0.07$ NW vs. OB, high obstacle: $p = 0.89$	**Low obstacle (4 cm):** **NW = 99.24 ± 6.18** **OB = 79.90 ± 6.18 (↓ 19.5% vs. NW)**
Sagittal ankle angle at maximum knee height (°)	1	Gill and Hung, 2012	NW vs. OB: $p = 0.65$	
Sagittal knee angle at maximum knee height (°)	1	Gill and Hung, 2012	NW vs. OB: $p = 0.18$	
Leading-leg toe clearance (cm)	1	Gill and Hung, 2014	NS	
Trailing-leg toe clearance (cm)	1	Gill and Hung, 2014	**NW, high low obstacle: $p = 0.02$** **OB, low vs. high obstacle: $p = 0.01$**	**Low obstacle (4 cm):** **NW = 13.73 ± 1.47** **O = 23.13 ± 1.53 (↑ 38% vs. high obstacle)** **High obstacle (16 cm):** **NW = 18.38 ± 1.53 (↑ 33.9% vs. low obstacle)** **OB = 16.76 ± 1.59**
Leading-leg hip angles at maximum knee height in frontal plane (°)	1	Gill and Hung, 2014	**OB, high vs. medium and low obstacles: $p = 0.02$** No other effects were observed	**Low obstacle (4 cm):** **OB = 47.28 ± 0.47** **Medium obstacle (11 cm):** **OB = 50.28 ± 0.52** **High obstacle (16 cm):** **OB = 66.75 ± 0.57 (↑ 32.8% and 41.18% vs. medium and low obstacles, respectively)**
Trailing-leg hip angles at maximum knee height in frontal plane (°)	1	Gill and Hung, 2014	No BMI or BMI*condition effects were observed ($p > 0.05$).	
Hip angles at maximum knee height in sagittal plane (°)	1	Gill and Hung, 2014	No BMI or BMI*condition effects were observed for both legs ($p > 0.05$).	

Table 7. *Cont.*

Gait Parameters	Number of Studies	Study	Between-Group Differences	Results (Mean ± SD or Median (IQR)) and Direction of Difference (↑↓)
Trailing-leg knee angles at maximum knee height in sagittal plane (°)	1	Gill and Hung, 2014	**NW vs. OB, high obstacle: $p = 0.04$** **NW vs. OB, low obstacle: $p = 0.04$** No other effects were observed.	**Low obstacle (4 cm):** **NW = 6.99 ± 0.66** **OB = 11.09 ± 1.16 (↑ 58.7% vs. NW)** **High obstacle (16 cm):** **NW = 4.64 ± 0.64** **OB = 12.02 ± 1.05 (↑ 159.1% vs. NW)**
COM acceleration in anterior/posterior direction at maximum knee height of leading leg during crossing	1	Gill and Hung, 2014	**NW vs. OB, low obstacle: $p = 0.006$** No other effects were observed.	**Low obstacle (4 cm):** **C = 0.63 ± 0.08** **OB = 1.05 ± 0.05 (↑ 66.7% vs. NW)**
COM acceleration in anterior/posterior direction at maximum knee height of trailing leg during crossing	1	Gill and Hung, 2014	**NW vs. OB, low obstacle: $p = 0.01$** **OB, low vs. medium and high obstacles: $p = 0.01$**	**Low obstacle (4 cm):** **NW = 0.66 ± 0.12** **OB = 1.02 ± 0.12 (↑ 54.5% vs. NW; ↑ 45.7% and 82.1% vs. medium and high obstacles, respectively)** **Medium obstacle (11 cm):** **NW = 0.83 ± 0.06** **OB = 0.70 ± 0.06** High obstacle (16 cm): NW = 0.73 ± 0.09 OB = 0.56 ± 0.09
COM acceleration in medial/lateral direction at maximum knee height	1	Gill and Hung, 2014	No BMI or BMI*condition effects were observed for both legs ($p > 0.05$).	
COM acceleration in vertical direction at maximum knee height	1	Gill and Hung, 2014	No BMI or BMI*condition effects were observed for both legs ($p > 0.05$).	
Duration of contact of HL, HM, MF, M5, M4, M3, M2, M1, T2-5, T1 of leading and trailing leg (ms)	1	Silva et al., 2018	No difference between OB and C for any area for both legs.	

Table 7. *Cont.*

Gait Parameters	Number of Studies	Study	Between-Group Differences	Results (Mean ± SD or Median (IQR)) and Direction of Difference (↑↓)
			Kinetics outcomes	
Trailing-leg normalised, anterior/posterior ground reaction forces at maximum knee height of leading leg during crossing (N/kg)	1	Gill and Hung, 2014	**OB, low vs. medium and high obstacles: $p = 0.001$** **NW, high vs. medium and low obstacles: $p = 0.001$** No other effects were observed.	**Low obstacle (4 cm):** **NW = 0.17 ± 0.06** **OB = 0.66 ± 0.02 (↑266.7%, and 100% vs. medium and high obstacles, respectively)** **Medium obstacle (11 cm):** **NW = 0.29 ± 0.03** **OB = 0.18 ± 0.08** **High obstacle (16 cm):** **NW = 0.33 ± 0.04 (↑ 94,1%, and 13.8% vs. low and medium obstacles, respectively)** **OB = 0.33 ± 0.12**
Leading-leg normalised, anterior/posterior ground reaction forces at maximum knee height of trailing leg during crossing (N/kg)	1	Gill and Hung, 2014	No BMI or BMI*condition effects were observed ($p > 0.05$).	
Trailing-leg normalised, medial/lateral ground reaction forces at maximum knee height of leading leg during crossing (N/kg)	1	Gill and Hung, 2014	**OB, high vs. medium obstacle: $p = 0.01$** No other effects were observed.	**Medium obstacle (11 cm):** **NW = 0.19 ± 0.06** **OB = 0.04 ± 0.02** **High obstacle (16 cm):** **NW = 0.12 ± 0.07** **OB = 0.19 ± 0.05 (↑ 375% vs. medium obstacle)**
Leading-leg normalised, medial/lateral ground reaction forces at maximum knee height of trailing leg during crossing (N/kg)	1	Gill and Hung, 2014	No BMI or BMI*condition effects were observed ($p > 0.05$).	

Table 7. *Cont.*

Gait Parameters	Number of Studies	Study	Between-Group Differences	Results (Mean ± SD or Median (IQR)) and Direction of Difference (↑↓)
Trailing-leg normalised, vertical ground reaction forces at maximum knee height of leading leg during crossing (N/kg)	1	Gill and Hung, 2014	**OB, high vs. medium obstacle: p = 0.05** **NW, medium vs. low obstacle: p = 0.05** No other effects were observed.	**Low obstacle (4 cm):** **NW = 1.38 ± 0.27** **OB = 1.99 ± 0.19** **Medium obstacle (11 cm):** **NW = 2.14 ± 0.22 (↑ 55.1% vs. low obstacle)** **OB = 1.58 ± 0.29** **High obstacle (16 cm):** **NW = 1.92 ± 0.26** **OB = 2.23 ± 0.24 (↑ 41.1% vs. medium obstacle)**
Leading-leg normalised, vertical ground reaction forces at maximum knee height of leading leg during crossing (N/kg)	1	Gill and Hung, 2014	No BMI or BMI*condition effects were observed (p > 0.05).	

CV: coefficient of variation; COM: centre of mass; HM: medial heel; HL: lateral heel; M1-M5: metatarsal areas, MF: midfoot; NS: non-significant differences; NW: normal-weight group; OB: overweight/obese group; OBI: Class I obesity group; OBII: Class II obesity group; OBIII: Class III obesity group; T1: hallux; T2-5: toes.* No BMI effect nor interaction between BMI and condition were observed. All five studies investigated kinematic parameters during obstacle crossing [18–22].

Regarding gait velocity, both studies that investigated gait velocity [18,22] reported that the OB (>30 BMI), [18] OW/Class I OB (25 kg/m^2 $\leq$ BMI < 35 kg/m^2), Class II OB (35 kg/m^2 $\leq$ BMI < 40 kg/m^2), and Class III OB (BMI > 40 kg/m^2) [22] groups' step-crossing velocities were slower than those of the NOB (non-OW/OB) group ($\geq$18.5 kg/m^2 and <25 kg/m^2) [18,22]. Results also showed that Class II OB and Class III OB participants had a slower step-crossing velocity than Class I OB participants [22].

Being OB led to a significantly lower crossing step length [18].
The OB group showed a significantly lower cadence [18].
OB individuals spent less time in single limb support [18].
The OB group had a greater step width [18].
OB individuals spent more time in the double-limb support phase [18].
The OW/Class I OB group spent more time in stance than the NOB and Class II OB groups [22].
The OW/Class I OB, Class II OB, and Class III OB groups had lower swing times during crossing [22].

OB individuals showed faster COM anterior/posterior (A/P) acceleration when crossing the low obstacle (4 cm) during both-leg crossing [20]. Additionally, when the trailing leg crossed the obstacle, COM A/P acceleration was faster on low obstacles than on medium and high obstacles, but only for the OB group [20].

Regarding leg motion during crossing, OB individuals took longer from foot lift to maximum knee height and less time from maximum knee height to foot contact in the high obstacle (16 cm) condition, with obstacle conditions having no effects on maximum knee height [19].

The OB group had a smaller ankle angle at foot contact during the low obstacle (4 cm) condition [19].

Regarding vertical clearance, OB individuals showed greater trailing-leg toe clearance in the low (4 cm) obstacle condition than in the high one (16 cm), whereas the NOB group showed greater trailing-toe clearance in the high obstacle condition than in the low one. No influence of OB was observed for leading-leg toe clearance [19].

The OB group's leading-leg frontal hip angle at maximum knee height was greater in high (16 cm) obstacle conditions than in medium (11 cm) and low (4 cm) ones. No effects were observed for the NOB group [20].

The OB group showed a greater trailing leg sagittal knee angle at maximum knee height than the NOB group for the low and high obstacle conditions, but no effect was observed for the medium obstacle condition [20].

Regarding temporal foot data, there were no differences between the OB and NOB groups regarding their relative temporal data at initial and final contact or the contact duration of the plantar areas assessed (HL; HM; MF; M1; M2; M3; M4; M5; T2-5; T1) [21].

Regarding the coefficient of variation of gait velocity, no differences were found between the OW/Class I OB and NOB groups [22]. The Class II OB and Class IIB OB groups had a greater coefficient of variation of velocity than the NOB and OW/Class I OB groups [22].

3.6.2. Kinetic Parameters

Table 7 reports the influence of OW/OB on kinetic parameters during obstacle crossing. Gill and Hung, 2014 investigated kinetic parameters during obstacle crossing [20].

Regarding trailing-leg normalised ground reaction forces (GRF), the OB group showed a greater trailing-leg normalised A/P GRF during the low obstacle condition (4 cm) than in the medium (11 cm) and high conditions (16 cm) [20]. The NOB group showed greater trailing-leg normalised A/P GRF in high obstacle conditions than in medium and low ones [20]. Trailing-leg normalised medial/lateral (M/L) GRF was only greater in the high obstacle condition than in the medium one for the OB group [20]. In the OB group, trailing-leg normalised vertical GRF was greater in the high obstacle condition than in the medium one, whereas for the NOB group, trailing-leg normalised vertical GRF was greater during the medium obstacle condition than during the low one.

For leading-leg normalised GRF, no effects on the OB group were observed for any GRF [20].

3.7. Synthesis

Five studies were considered eligible and were retained [18–22]. Overall, these studies were evaluated as "good" despite their lack ofs detail and clarity on the clinical implications of their research. Among these 5 studies, 2 included children [19,20], and 3 included adults [18,21,22]. One study used an obstacle height that varied according to the participant's leg length (30% of leg length) [21], while four studies used three fixed obstacle heights [18–20,22]. All the studies [18–22] included single-task conditions, used self-selected walking speed instruction, and had the same number of experimental sessions (n = 1) and trials per obstacle crossing conditions (n = 5). Finally, all the studies assessed kinematics [18–22], one assessed kinetics [20], and none investigated muscle activity or obstacle contact. Compared to normal individuals crossing obstacles, overweight or obese individuals exhibited lower velocity [18,22], shorter step length [18], lower cadence [18] and less time spent in single limb support [18]. They also exhibited increased step width [18], more time spent in double support [18], and greater trailing leg ground force reaction [20] and center of mass acceleration [20]. Furthermore, these observed between-group differences were also dependent on obstacle height [19,20].

4. Discussion

This work aimed to systematically review and summarize all the available biomechanical-parameter data regarding the influence of OW and OB across the lifespan on obstacle-crossing tasks during walking tests. Our broad search and selection retained five studies for evaluation. Two studies involved children [19,20], and three involved adults [18,21,22], for a total of 82 NW individuals and 132 OW/OB individuals. Their performances in the different obstacle-crossing tasks were assessed using a wide variety of kinematic and kinetic parameters. Overall, results suggested that compared to NW individuals, OW and OB individuals walked more slowly and with a lower cadence, shorter step length, shorter single-limb support duration, shorter swing time, longer leg-raising and shorter leg-dropping times, and a smaller ankle angle at foot contact.

4.1. Influence of Overweight/Obesity on Kinematic Parameters during Obstacle Crossing

The most consistent between-group difference (NW vs. OB) in obstacle-crossing performance was the lower gait velocity in OB adults reported in two studies comparing them to NW adults [18,22]. One of those two studies [22] reported that adults in the OW/Class I OB ($\geq$25 kg/m^2 and <35 kg/m^2) group had faster gait velocities and less variable velocities than those in the Class II OB ($\geq$35 kg/m^2 and <40 kg/m^2) or Class III OB (>40 kg/m^2) groups. In addition to slower velocity, Desrochers et al. (2021) [18] reported that OB adults had a greater step width and double-limb support duration and shorter step length, single-limb support duration, and cadence than NW individuals. This study's authors [18] proposed the following interpretation for their results: "These gait changes likely represent adaptive behaviors in the face of unstable postural control, where individuals with obesity increase their base of support for a greater amount of time relative to a single gait cycle" [18]. It is noteworthy that these authors [18] further speculated that the shorter single-limb support duration measured in OB adults might increase the likelihood of tripping as they cross the obstacle more quickly and with less clearance.

All five studies assessed spatial outcome measures of gait [18–22]. Ankle angle at landing after obstacle crossing differed significantly between NW and OB children in the low obstacle condition (4 cm) [19]. NW children tended to land in a neutral ankle-angle position (around 90°, corresponding to a flat-foot landing strategy), whereas OB children were more dorsiflexed (<90°, corresponding to a heel–toe landing strategy) [19]. The study authors [19] suggested that NW children may have used a flat-foot strategy during obstacle crossing because it was the most useful for increasing landing stability, as a heel–toe strategy was less stable. Walking impairments could lead to falls and injuries in OB children [40]. Note that the heel–toe landing strategy reported in OW/OB children was not observed in OB post-menopausal women, who exhibited similar relative initial, final, and duration of contact for all ten-foot areas and foot total-contact duration to NW post-menopausal women [21]. NW and OB children had different trailing-vertical-toe clearances depending on the obstacle condition [20]. Interestingly, OB children had a higher clearance over low obstacles than over high ones, whereas NW children had a higher clearance over high obstacles than over low ones. This study's authors [20] suggested that: "overweight/obese children's difficulty with motor planning may have contributed to the use of a less effective strategy when crossing high obstacles. (...) differences in motor skills and strategies used during obstacle crossing can increase the risk of injury; less toe clearance on high obstacles increases the chance of tripping and falling" ([20], p. 51).

All five studies assessed temporal outcome measures of gait [18–22]. Compared with NW children, OB children took longer to reach maximum knee height and less time to move from maximum knee height to foot contact in the high (16 cm) obstacle condition [19]. These authors suggested that this behaviour could stem from OB children's relatively limited capacity to accelerate lower-leg segments due to the relatively higher effort and energy they expend compared to NW children [19]. They also suggested that the longer time OB children required to lift their knees (with no difference in knee height) compared to NW children may be due to musculoskeletal difficulties [19], especially due to OB children's heavier lower limbs [41]. This interpretation is supported by overground level-walking data showing that even when over-activating ankle muscles, obesity-typical spatiotemporal changes in gait were observed [42]. However, it is important to mention that this interpretation remains speculative since no studies have directly measured muscle activation during obstacle crossing to compare OB and/or OW individuals to NW ones. This point reinforces the relevance and necessity of future studies investigating physiological and mechanical mechanisms related to impaired gait control in OW/OB individuals. Interestingly, significant differences in COM anterior/posterior acceleration between NW and OB children were only observed in the low obstacle condition (4 cm), where COM acceleration at the maximum knee height of both legs during crossing was higher among OB children [20]. The authors suggested that this observation could reflect the difficulties OB children had in controlling forward acceleration [20] when crossing a low obstacle.

4.2. *Influence of Overweight/Obesity on Kinetic Parameters during Obstacle Crossing*

The impaired gait control and stability observed during obstacle crossing due to OW/OB were reiterated in the kinetics results. NW and OB children exhibited significant differences in trailing-leg ground force reactions. Compared to the NW group, in the anterior/posterior direction, OB children had a higher normalised ground reaction force in low obstacle conditions than in medium or high obstacle conditions, and in the vertical and medial/lateral directions, their ground forces were significantly higher in the high obstacle condition than in the medium one (Table 7, [20]). Among NW children, differences in obstacle conditions were only observed in the anterior/posterior direction (a higher value on the high obstacle condition than on the medium or low ones) and the vertical direction (a higher value on the medium obstacle condition than on the low one) [20]. This study's authors [20] suggested that OB children's balance issues [43] and musculoskeletal disorders [41] could have been exacerbated by their larger hip abduction angles and higher vertical and medial/lateral ground reaction forces, especially on high obstacles. They also suggested that OB children's efforts to maintain stability could have been more difficult due to changes in hip abduction angles and the vertical and medial/lateral ground reaction forces on high obstacles [44].

4.3. Limitations and Strengths

The present systematic review had some limitations, most notable of which was the low number of studies (n = 5) [18–22] meeting our selection criteria and their heterogeneity, including differences in the sample populations, experimental procedures, and gait outcomes. Indeed, participants' age groups differed widely between the 5 included studies; two included children aged 4–13 years old [19,20], while three included adults [18,21,22] aged 36.16 ± 12.76 [22] and 57.1 ± 4.7 years old [21], resulting in small sample sizes within each age category (with a total of 24 OW/OB child participants vs. 22 NW child participants [19,20] and 108 OW/OB adult participants vs. 60 NW adult participants) [18,21,22]. However, the large age range of the individuals can also be regarded as a strength of the present review that allowed us to summarize the available data regarding the influence of overweight and obesity across the lifespan on obstacle crossing during walking. Another limitation is that none of the studies that included both male and female participants [18–20] evaluated the influence of sex on gait outcomes, although previous studies have reported sex differences in gait patterns during unobstructed level walking [45]. It is also noteworthy that although all the studies included had assessed BMI-group-related differences in gait outcomes during obstacle crossing [18–22], none had specifically reported the possible influence of body mass and body height, i.e., the two constitutive anthropometric parameters of BMI. This observation is all the more important given that 4 of the 5 included studies [18–20,22] used three fixed obstacle heights (low, medium and high obstacles, measuring from 4 cm to 16 cm), i.e., not personalised to each participant's bodily dimensions. Note that, in an effort to scale the difficulty of an obstacle crossing task to each participant's bodily dimensions, one of the five included studies [21] used an obstacle height that reflected a percentage of each individual's leg length (i.e., 30%, representing approximately 22 cm for NW and OW/OB individuals) [21]. In addition to the above-mentioned differences in sample populations and experimental procedures, the present systematic review also revealed the heterogeneity in gait outcomes in each of the included articles, which further hampered the comparison of published results. Interestingly, although it is likely that greater toe–obstacle clearance may help decrease the risk of tripping over an obstacle (e.g., [31,46–49]), this parameter (namely leading-leg toe clearance and trailing-leg toe clearance) was reported in only one of the five included studies [20]. Furthermore, participants' obstacle contacts (errors) during the execution of the obstacle-crossing task were not reported in any of the 5 included studies.

4.4. Practical Implications and Future Directions

Given the results, limitations, and strengths of the present review, several practical implications can be considered. It is presumable that the performance of an obstacle-crossing task depends on the participant's height (and/or their lower limb length) and the height of the obstacle [31]. Accordingly, a description of the participant's height and leg length should be reported in a systematic way. As above-mentioned, in addition, or in combination with the influence of anthropometric parameters, future studies should investigate how sex could affect the performance of obstacle-crossing tasks in normal weight and OW/OB individuals. Finally, we believe that obstacle contacts and foot clearances should be assessed and reported in a systematic way. We believe, indeed, that these parameters could be used to identify OW/OB individuals at risk of falling and to evaluate the outcomes of interventions aimed at fall prevention.

5. Conclusions

Despite the small number of studies included, the present findings suggest that overweight and obesity do indeed affect kinematic and kinetic gait parameters during obstacle-crossing tasks executed by both children [19,20] and adults [18,21,22]. At this point, however, the kinematic parameters assessed in each study were diverse; only one of these five studies investigated kinetics, and none assessed muscular parameters or obstacle contacts. These could be appropriate research elements for future studies, as could investigating the influence of specific anthropometric parameters. Finally, these findings should be interpreted with caution as no overarching or generalizable conclusions could be drawn regarding the influence of overweight and obesity across the lifespan on obstacle crossing during walking.

Supplementary Materials: The following supporting information can be downloaded at: https://www.mdpi.com/article/10.3390/ijerph20115931/s1, File S1: PRISMA checklist. Ref [50] is cited in the Supplementary Materials.

Author Contributions: F.A.B., M.C. and N.V. conceived and designed this study. M.C. and T.P. extracted the data. F.A.B., M.C., N.V., P.C.R.S. and T.P. interpreted the data. M.C. wrote the manuscript's first draft. F.A.B., M.C., N.V., P.C.R.S. and T.P. contributed to the manuscript's revision, read and approved the final version, and approved its submission for publication. They have agreed to be personally accountable for the first author's contributions, and they assure that questions related to the accuracy or integrity of any part of the work, even ones in which they were not personally involved, were appropriately investigated, resolved, and documented in the literature. All authors have read and agreed to the published version of the manuscript.

Funding: This work was supported by the French National Research Agency (ANR) in the framework of the Investissements d'avenir program (ANR-10-AIRT-05 and ANR-15-IDEX-02), the MIAI @ Grenoble Alpes (ANR-19-P3IA-0003), the Coordination for the Improvement of Higher Education Personnel Brazil (grant 001), and the Estate of Naomi K. Shapiro (grant 721926).

Institutional Review Board Statement: Not applicable.

Informed Consent Statement: Not applicable.

Data Availability Statement: No new data was created.

Acknowledgments: This work is part of the Ph.D. thesis of the first author (M.C.) at Université Grenoble Alpes, France, and São Paulo State University, Bauru, Brazil. The sponsors were not involved in the review or approval of the manuscript for publication. This work also forms part of a broader translational and interdisciplinary research programme—GaitAlps (NV).

Conflicts of Interest: The authors declare that they have no proprietary, financial, professional, or other competing or conflicting interest regarding this study and the publication of this paper.

References

1. Obesity and Overweight. Available online: https://www.who.int/news-room/fact-sheets/detail/obesity-and-overweight (accessed on 4 October 2022).
2. Akram, D.S.; Astrup, A.V.; Atinmo, T.; Boissin, J.L.; Bray, G.A.; Caroll, K.K.; Chitson, P.; Chunming, C.; Dietz, W.H.; Hill, J.O.; et al. *Obesity: Preventing and Managing the Global Epidemic. Report of a WHO Consultation*; World Health Organization Technical Repport Series: Geneva, Switzerland, 2000; Volume 894, pp. 1–253.
3. Apovian, C. Obesity: Definition, Comorbidities, Causes, and Burden. *Am. J. Manag. Care* **2016**, *22*, s176–s185. [PubMed]
4. Han, E.; Truesdale, K.P.; Taber, D.R.; Cai, J.; Juhaeri, J.; Stevens, J. Impact of Overweight and Obesity on Hospitalization: Race and Gender Differences. *Int. J. Obes.* **2009**, *33*, 249–256. [CrossRef] [PubMed]
5. di Angelantonio, E.; Bhupathiraju, S.N.; Wormser, D.; Gao, P.; Kaptoge, S.; de Gonzalez, A.B.; Cairns, B.J.; Huxley, R.; Jackson, C.L.; Joshy, G.; et al. Body-Mass Index and All-Cause Mortality: Individual-Participant-Data Meta-Analysis of 239 Prospective Studies in Four Continents. *Lancet* **2016**, *388*, 776–786. [CrossRef]
6. Heo, M.; Pietrobelli, A.; Wang, D.; Heymsfield, S.B.; Faith, M.S. Obesity and Functional Impairment: Influence of Comorbidity, Joint Pain, and Mental Health. *Obesity* **2010**, *18*, 2030–2038. [CrossRef] [PubMed]
7. Steinberg, N.; Nemet, D.; Pantanowitz, M.; Eliakim, A. Gait Pattern, Impact to the Skeleton and Postural Balance in Overweight and Obese Children: A Review. *Sports* **2018**, *6*, 75. [CrossRef]
8. del Porto, H.; Pechak, C.; Smith, D.; Reed-Jones, R. Biomechanical Effects of Obesity on Balance. *Int. J. Exerc. Sci.* **2012**, *5*, 301–320.
9. Molina-Garcia, P.; Migueles, J.H.; Cadenas-Sanchez, C.; Esteban-Cornejo, I.; Mora-Gonzalez, J.; Rodriguez-Ayllon, M.; Plaza-Florido, A.; Vanrenterghem, J.; Ortega, F.B. A Systematic Review on Biomechanical Characteristics of Walking in Children and Adolescents with Overweight/Obesity: Possible Implications for the Development of Musculoskeletal Disorders. *Obes. Rev.* **2019**, *20*, 1033–1044. [CrossRef]
10. Backholer, K.; Wong, E.; Freak-Poli, R.; Walls, H.L.; Peeters, A. Increasing Body Weight and Risk of Limitations in Activities of Daily Living: A Systematic Review and Meta-Analysis. *Obes. Rev.* **2012**, *13*, 456–468. [CrossRef]

11. Wearing, S.C.; Hennig, E.M.; Byrne, N.M.; Steele, J.R.; Hills, A.P. The Biomechanics of Restricted Movement in Adult Obesity. *Obes. Rev.* **2006**, *7*, 13–24. [CrossRef]
12. Neri, S.G.R.; Oliveira, J.S.; Dario, A.B.; Lima, R.M.; Tiedemann, A. Does Obesity Increase the Risk and Severity of Falls in People Aged 60 Years and Older? A Systematic Review and Meta-Analysis of Observational Studies. *J. Gerontol. A Biol. Sci. Med. Sci.* **2020**, *75*, 952–960. [CrossRef]
13. Capodaglio, P.; Gobbi, M.; Donno, L.; Fumagalli, A.; Buratto, C.; Galli, M.; Cimolin, V. Effect of Obesity on Knee and Ankle Biomechanics during Walking. *Sensors* **2021**, *21*, 7114. [CrossRef] [PubMed]
14. de Oliveira Máximo, R.; de Oliveira, D.C.; Ramírez, P.C.; Luiz, M.M.; de Souza, A.F.; Delinocente, M.L.B.; Steptoe, A.; de Oliveira, C.; da Silva Alexandre, T. Dynapenia, Abdominal Obesity or Both: Which Accelerates the Gait Speed Decline Most? *Age Ageing* **2021**, *50*, 1616–1625. [CrossRef]
15. Kim, D.; Lewis, C.L.; Gill, S.V. Effects of Obesity and Foot Arch Height on Gait Mechanics: A Cross-Sectional Study. *PLoS ONE* **2021**, *16*, e0260398. [CrossRef] [PubMed]
16. Pau, M.; Capodaglio, P.; Leban, B.; Porta, M.; Galli, M.; Cimolin, V. Kinematics Adaptation and Inter-Limb Symmetry during Gait in Obese Adults. *Sensors* **2021**, *21*, 5980. [CrossRef] [PubMed]
17. Choi, H.; Lim, J.; Lee, S. Body Fat-Related Differences in Gait Parameters and Physical Fitness Level in Weight-Matched Male Adults. *Clin. Biomech.* **2021**, *81*, 105243. [CrossRef] [PubMed]
18. Desrochers, P.C.; Kim, D.; Keegan, L.; Gill, S.V. Association between the Functional Gait Assessment and Spatiotemporal Gait Parameters in Individuals with Obesity Compared to Normal Weight Controls: A Proof-of-Concept Study. *J. Musculoskelet. Neuronal Interact.* **2021**, *21*, 335–342.
19. Gill, S.V.; Hung, Y.C. Influence of Weight Classification on Children Stepping over Obstacles. *Am. J. Phys. Med. Rehabil.* **2012**, *91*, 625–630. [CrossRef]
20. Gill, S.V.; Hung, Y.C. Effects of Overweight and Obese Body Mass on Motor Planning and Motor Skills during Obstacle Crossing in Children. *Res. Dev. Disabil.* **2014**, *35*, 46–53. [CrossRef]
21. Silva, D.; Gabriel, R.; Moreira, H.; Abrantes, J.; Faria, A. Foot Rollover Temporal Parameters During Walking Straight Ahead and Stepping Over Obstacles: Obese and Non-Obese Postmenopausal Women. *J. Aging Phys. Act.* **2018**, *26*, 227–234. [CrossRef]
22. Gill, S.V. Effects of Obesity Class on Flat Ground Walking and Obstacle Negotiation. *J. Musculoskelet. Neuronal Interact.* **2019**, *19*, 448–454.
23. Pavol, M.J.; Owings, T.M.; Foley, K.T.; Grabiner, M.D. Mechanisms Leading to a Fall from an Induced Trip in Healthy Older Adults. *J. Gerontol. A Biol. Sci. Med. Sci.* **2001**, *56*, 428–437. [CrossRef] [PubMed]
24. Berg, W.P.; Alessio, H.M.; Mills, E.M.; Tong, C. Circumstances and Consequences of Falls in Independent Community-Dwelling Older Adults. *Age Ageing* **1997**, *26*, 261–268. [CrossRef]
25. Brown, L.A.; McKenzie, N.C.; Doan, J. Age-Dependent Differences in the Attentional Demands of Obstacle Negotiation. *J. Gerontol. A Biol. Sci. Med. Sci.* **2005**, *60*, 924–927. [CrossRef] [PubMed]
26. Hahn, M.E.; Lee, H.-J.; Chou, L.-S. Increased Muscular Challenge in Older Adults during Obstructed Gait. *Gait Posture* **2005**, *22*, 356–361. [CrossRef] [PubMed]
27. Kannus, P.; Sievänen, H.; Palvanen, M.; Järvinen, T.; Parkkari, J. Prevention of Falls and Consequent Injuries in Elderly People. *Lancet* **2005**, *366*, 1885–1893. [CrossRef]
28. Uemura, K.; Yamada, M.; Nagai, K.; Ichihashi, N. Older Adults At High Risk of Falling Need More Time for Anticipatory Postural Adjustment in the Precrossing Phase of Obstacle Negotiation. *J. Gerontol. A Biol. Sci. Med. Sci.* **2011**, *66*, 904–909. [CrossRef]
29. Pieruccini-Faria, F.; Montero-Odasso, M.; Newman, A. Obstacle Negotiation, Gait Variability, and Risk of Falling: Results From the "Gait and Brain Study". *J. Gerontol. A Biol. Sci. Med. Sci.* **2019**, *74*, 1422–1428. [CrossRef]
30. Patla, A.E.; Prentice, S.D.; Robinson, C.; Neufeld, J. Visual Control of Locomotion: Strategies for Changing Direction and for Going Over Obstacles. *J. Exp. Psychol. Hum. Percept. Perform.* **1991**, *17*, 603–634. [CrossRef]
31. Patla, A.; Rietdyk, S. Visual Control of Limb Trajectory over Obstacles during Locomotion: Effect of Obstacle Height and Width. *Gait Posture* **1993**, *1*, 45–60. [CrossRef]
32. Walsh, T.P.; Arnold, J.B.; Evans, A.M.; Yaxley, A.; Damarell, R.A.; Shanahan, E.M. The Association between Body Fat and Musculoskeletal Pain: A Systematic Review and Meta-Analysis. *BMC Musculoskelet. Disord.* **2018**, *19*, 233. [CrossRef]
33. Chardon, M.; Barbieri, F.A.; Penedo, T.; Santos, P.C.R.; Vuillerme, N. The Effects of Overweight and Obesity on Obstacle Crossing During Walking: Protocol for a Systematic Review. *JMIR Res. Protoc.* **2022**, *11*, e36234. [CrossRef] [PubMed]
34. Page, M.J.; McKenzie, J.E.; Bossuyt, P.M.; Boutron, I.; Hoffmann, T.C.; Mulrow, C.D.; Shamseer, L.; Tetzlaff, J.M.; Akl, E.A.; Brennan, S.E.; et al. The PRISMA 2020 Statement: An Updated Guideline for Reporting Systematic Reviews. *BMJ* **2021**, *372*, n71. [CrossRef]
35. Higgins, J.P.T.; Thomas, J.; Chandler, J.; Cumpston, M.; Li, T.; Page, M.J.; Welch, V.A. *Cochrane Handbook for Systematic Reviews of Interventions*, 2nd ed.; John Wiley & Sons: Hoboken, NJ, USA, 2019.
36. Kuczmarski, R.J.; National Center for Health Statistics (U.S.); National Health and Nutrition Examination Survey (U.S.). *2000 CDC Growth Charts for the United States: Methods and Development*; Department of Health and Human Services: Washington, DC, USA; Centers for Disease Control and Prevention: Atlanta, GA, USA; National Center for Health Statistics: Hyattsville, MD, USA, 2002.

37. Galna, B.; Peters, A.; Murphy, A.T.; Morris, M.E. Obstacle Crossing Deficits in Older Adults: A Systematic Review. *Gait Posture* **2009**, *30*, 270–275. [CrossRef] [PubMed]
38. Overweight & Obesity | CDC. Available online: https://www.cdc.gov/obesity/index.html (accessed on 14 December 2021).
39. Brochu, M.; Mathieu, M.E.; Karelis, A.D.; Doucet, É.; Lavoie, M.E.; Garrel, D.; Rabasa-Lhoret, R. Contribution of the Lean Body Mass to Insulin Resistance in Postmenopausal Women with Visceral Obesity: A Monet Study. *Obesity* **2008**, *16*, 1085–1093. [CrossRef] [PubMed]
40. Gill, S.V. Optimising Motor Adaptation in Childhood Obesity. *Aust. Occup. Ther. J.* **2011**, *58*, 386–389. [CrossRef]
41. Wearing, S.C.; Hennig, E.M.; Byrne, N.M.; Steele, J.R.; Hills, A.P. The Impact of Childhood Obesity on Musculoskeletal Form. *Obes. Rev.* **2006**, *7*, 209–218. [CrossRef]
42. Maktouf, W.; Durand, S.; Boyas, S.; Pouliquen, C.; Beaune, B. Interactions among Obesity and Age-Related Effects on the Gait Pattern and Muscle Activity across the Ankle Joint. *Exp. Gerontol.* **2020**, *140*, 111054. [CrossRef] [PubMed]
43. Singh, D.; Park, W.; Levy, M.S.; Jung, E.E. The Effects of Obesity and Standing Time on Postural Sway during Prolonged Quiet Standing. *Ergonomics* **2009**, *52*, 977–986. [CrossRef] [PubMed]
44. Deforche, B.I.; Hills, A.P.; Worringham, C.J.; Davies, P.S.W.; Murphy, A.J.; Bouckaert, J.J.; de Bourdeaudhuij, I.M. Balance and Postural Skills in Normal-Weight and Overweight Prepubertal Boys. *Int. J. Pediatr. Obes.* **2009**, *4*, 175–182. [CrossRef]
45. Smith, L.; Johansson, J.; Kerrigan, D. Gender Differences in Pelvic Motions and Center of Mass Displacement during Walking: Stereotypes Quantified. *J. Womens Health Gend. Based Med.* **2002**, *11*, 453–458. [CrossRef]
46. Chardon, M.; Barbieri, F.A.; Penedo, T.; Santos, P.C.R.; Vuillerme, N. The Effects of Experimentally-Induced Fatigue on Gait Parameters during Obstacle Crossing: A Systematic Review. *Neurosci. Biobehav. Rev.* **2022**, *142*, 104854. [CrossRef] [PubMed]
47. Chou, L.S.; Draganich, L.F. Stepping over an Obstacle Increases the Motions and Moments of the Joints of the Trailing Limb in Young Adults. *J. Biomech.* **1997**, *30*, 331–337. [CrossRef] [PubMed]
48. Chen, H.L.; Lu, T.W. Comparisons of the Joint Moments between Leading and Trailing Limb in Young Adults When Stepping over Obstacles. *Gait Posture* **2006**, *23*, 69–77. [CrossRef] [PubMed]
49. Chen, H.-C.; Ashton-Miller, J.; Alexander, N.; Schultz, A. Stepping Over Obstacles: Gait Patterns of Healthy Young and Old Adults. *J. Gerontol.* **1991**, *46*, M196–M203. [CrossRef]
50. Moher, D.; Shamseer, L.; Clarke, M.; Ghersi, D.; Liberati, A.; Petticrew, M.; Shekelle, P.; Stewart, L.A.; PRISMA-P Group. Preferred reporting items for systematic review and meta-analysis protocols (PRISMA-P) 2015 statement. *Syst. Rev.* **2015**, *4*, 1. [CrossRef]

International Journal of
Environmental Research and Public Health

MDPI

Review

Adherence to eHealth-Delivered Exercise in Adults with no Specific Health Conditions: A Scoping Review on a Conceptual Challenge

Andrea Fuente-Vidal [1,2,*], Myriam Guerra-Balic [1], Oriol Roda-Noguera [3], Javier Jerez-Roig [2] and Joel Montane [1,4]

1 Research Group on Health, Physical Activity and Sport (SAFE), Blanquerna School of Psychology, Education and Sport Sciences, Universitat Ramon Llull, 08022 Barcelona, Spain
2 Research Group on Methodology, Methods, Models and Outcomes of Health and Social Sciences (M_3O), Faculty of Health Sciences and Welfare, Centre for Health and Social Care Research (CESS), University of Vic—Central University of Catalonia (UVic-UCC), 08500 Vic, Spain
3 Fundació Naccari-Ravà, 08036 Barcelona, Spain
4 Blanquerna School of Health Science, Universitat Ramon Llull, 08025 Barcelona, Spain
* Correspondence: andreafv@blanquerna.url.edu

Abstract: Adherence has emerged as a focal point and critical determinant of success for physical activity interventions. The term is used for both traditional and digital interventions, and for prescribed and nonprescribed activities. Many other terms for adherence are being used interchangeably, as there is no consensus on its precise conceptualization. This scoping review aimed to advance the definition of adherence to eHealth programs, specifically for the adult population with no specific health conditions. A total of 2983 papers, published between 1 January 2016 and 13 March 2022, were retrieved from different databases (including grey literature). Of those, 13 studies met the eligibility criteria and were included for review. The selected studies used a wide array of technologies and consisted mainly of exercise interventions. Most of the reviewed publications contemplated exercise adherence as a percentage of expected dose. Most (8 out of 13) studies neither assessed nor specified an expected use of the involved technology. Results suggest a need for homogeneity in the conceptualization of adherence to physical activity and exercise, including those interventions delivered digitally.

Keywords: eHealth; mHealth; smartphone; physical activity; exercise; adherence; engagement; attrition; apps; digital health; treatment adherence and compliance

1. Introduction

The beneficial effects of active living and regular physical exercise have a solid evidence base [1]. The World Health Organization (WHO) has consequently made it a worldwide public health priority to increase physical activity and to concurrently decrease sedentary behavior [2]. In spite of this, Guthold et al. established a global age-standardized prevalence of insufficient physical activity of 27.5% in 2016, with a difference between sexes of more than 8 percentage points (23.4%, 21.1–30.7, in men vs. 31.7%, 28.6–39.0, in women) [1].

Research and innovation funding programs such as Horizon Europe have established tools, technologies and digital solutions for health and care as their main areas of intervention [3]. In an ever more digitalized world, robust monitoring and evaluation plans for digital interventions have been specifically identified as essential to support potential intervention scale-up [4]. In both digital and nondigital physical activity research, adherence has been emerging as a focal point and relevant variable [5–8]. Adherence to eHealth technology is an underdeveloped and often improperly used concept in the existing body of literature [7]. One of the most persistent issues in the consistent operationalization of the term adherence is the lack of a clear definition of this concept [5–8], especially when a medical prescription or otherwise preset exercise calendar is not involved. However, even for the most structured therapeutic exercise interventions, an agreed communicable definition of adherence is lacking [5]. The latter constitutes a problem, since it prevents patients and healthcare providers from working toward a shared goal while hindering measurement and the ability to monitor its variability [5]. All of these barriers become considerably more relevant when the term adherence is applied to voluntary (nonprescribed) activity, when recommendations or assessments lack specificity (e.g., exercise volume), and when technology is involved—which often leads to a duplication of adherences (i.e., adherence to the expected behavior vs. adherence to the technology usage). In terms of comparability between studies, an additional barrier is the fact that compliance is often defined as a binary variable, using a combination of two outcomes (e.g., 10 h a day for 3 out of 7 days) [9].

In summary, as long as a valid, reliable and acceptable measure of adherence to different physical activity or exercise interventions is not agreed upon, interventions or methods for improving adherence may be questioned [5].

1.1. Adherence to Physical Activity (PA)

Research has commonly focused on the assessment of adherence to PA, as per the physical activity guidelines by the WHO, both for people with and without pathological conditions. The WHO's 2020 PA guidelines recommend that adults undertake at least 150 min of moderate-intensity (or an equivalent combination) of physical activity per week, plus 2 or more days of muscle strengthening activities for additional health benefits [10]. When using the WHO—or any other recognized institution—as a reference, adherence can be easily categorized as a binary variable (i.e., user is either adherent or not adherent to the recommended levels of PA).

In those cases where the study design specified particular PA goals (different to those in guidelines), authors commonly categorized adherence as good when objective behavior equaled 80% or more of the planned behavior [5]. Several studies were in line with this approach [11], most of which involved individuals with health conditions. When PA was programmed, attainment (as opposed to adherence) was generally high. According to Sperandei et al., this could have been keeping the proportion of active people stable while at the same time failing to ensure individuals participate long enough to achieve their objectives [12].

1.2. Adherence to Exercise

Whereas PA includes all skeletal body movements and energy expenditure, it can only be categorized as exercise when it is "planned, structured, repetitive and purposefully focused on improvement or maintenance of one or more components of physical fitness" [13].

Adherence to exercise is a widely used term, subject to a range of interpretations. It has been estimated that 60% of research studies on therapeutic exercise do not provide a clearly identifiable definition of adherence [5]. Additionally, even when they do, it is often constructed ad hoc [5], a fact that has led authors to recommend that a more consistent and standard validated measure of exercise adherence be developed [14].

A systematic review, by Bailey et al., on exercise adherence for musculoskeletal pain disorders pointed out that most of the reviewed studies defined adherence as a function of the parameters used for its assessment, with frequency being the most commonly measured parameter [5]. In this regard, frequency can be interpreted as a predetermined cut-off or as a distribution method, which explained why adherence levels ranged from 15% to 100% completion of the prescribed exercises [5]. While frequency is certainly a useful parameter, the authors highlighted that other parameters, such as intensity, time, accuracy or behavioral components, could also contribute to adherence and would be worth considering [5].

In clinical settings, adequate adherence to physician instructions has generally been reported to be low, with values ranging from 30% to 60%, depending on the complexity of the behavior changes required [15,16]. Most research on exercise has been conducted while focusing on structured exercise programs, often supervised and commonly performed within clinical settings [14]. When it comes to the temporal dynamics of adherence in unsupervised/unstructured settings, there is an evident gap in the literature [12].

In the context of fitness centers, for instance, the probability of an individual maintaining their membership uninterrupted for more than 12 months has been estimated at around 5% [12].

1.3. Adherence to eHealth

A 2021 systematic review on digital health usage associations concluded that a small but significant positive relationship existed between engagement with a digital health intervention and PA outcomes in healthy adults [17]. The WHO itself recommended that digital health interventions (DHI) be used to promote and support participation in PA [2]. Accordingly, an increase of 26% in article publications on DHI to improve PA was documented between 2000 and 2018 [18].

In contrast, evidence up until 2017 highlighted the fact that many eHealth evaluations lacked or did not report positive effects [7]. The same systematic review established that the interventions were often not used or were abandoned after a period, which, in either case, resulted in the available technological elements not being used as intended by their developers [7]. Within a broader spectrum—and considering digital behavior change interventions as a whole usage—levels have been found to be typically low [4,19]. Informal data suggest that 26% of apps are used only once after downloading and only 26% of users access the app more than ten times [20]. Our own results, from the evaluation of a popular commercial fitness app, showed that only 17% of subscribers actually completed their first workout and as few as 2% of initial enrollments reached practical session number eight [21].

When it comes to electronic interventions, the traditional definition of adherence—based on completion of the prescribed intervention—seems to fall short. Several research papers, including a series of systematic reviews, have drawn attention to the heterogeneity of definitions and the need to unify criteria [6–8]. Variables most often used to measure adherence to eHealth interventions include number of logins, number of days of technology use, time spent on the platform, number of lessons or modules accessed or finished, and number of elements accessed or used [7,17].

To our knowledge, three authors, in particular, have attempted to categorize adherence to health interventions delivered through electronic means. In 2017, Sieverink et al., determined that there were three requisites for measuring adherence to eHealth interventions. Those included: 1) that the design provides a justification (empirical, theoretical or rational) of the intended use; 2) that operationalization of intended use is provided; and 3) the ability to measure actual usage [7]. Consequently, the authors operationalized the definition of adherence in three different categories: Category A was assigned when an intended use of a technology was not specified and adherence was operationalized in terms of "the more usage, the better". Category B was assigned when intended use of a technology was specified but not justified (for example: "a user is adherent when logging in at least once a week for three subsequent weeks"). Category C was assigned when the intended use of the technology was provided, together with some form or rationale [7]. A year later, Payne et al. conducted a narrative review on adherence to dietary self-monitoring using a mobile app [6]. Their results indicated that adherence was operationally defined in two ways: as either adherent or nonadherent, or by frequency (of dietary intake recording, interaction with apps, timing of recording), with some studies simultaneously using both definitions [6]. Finally, data published by Yang et al., in 2020 provided similar insights in regard to PA app adherence [8]. Further detail is provided in the Adherence to eHealth for General PA and Exercise, below.

1.4. Adherence to eHealth for General PA and Exercise

Increased engagement in DHI has been suggested to have a weak but positive relationship with PA outcomes, in terms of both objective and subjective experiences in adults [17]. Augmenting PA levels in all populations has been set as a priority [2] and eHealth has the potential to address this matter, potentially with high effectiveness and at a low cost [22]. A recent systematic review revealed that interventions using eHealth could strongly increase PA levels and reduce sedentary time among inactive participants [23]. Among the many appealing features of DHI, an important factor is their capacity to be scaled for larger populations [8,24].

It is widely accepted that motivation is a determinant of behavior change. It has been pointed out that continuous use of eHealth could make this feasible and cost-effective [23]. In a fitness facility in Brazil, weight loss was found to be the most prevalent motivation to start an exercise program [12]. However, it was also found to be significantly related to higher chances of an early drop out [12]. Exploring baseline motivation has been common practice, but Sperandei's results indicated that the potential changes in motivation during intervention could be highly significant, and that looking at motivation alone does not seem sufficient to promote adherence [12]. As far as technology is concerned, we now know that app glitches are able to profoundly influence app adherence in a negative manner [8], yet researchers seem to be lacking a consensus of conceptualization for adherence [7,8,12,25] and other related terms.

Research participants have traditionally self-reported their activity by using logs [5]. More recently, fitness trackers, pedometers and accelerometers have become popular instruments for obtaining reliable estimates of PA [26]. Some of these technologies, alone or in combination with others, allow researchers to measure not only wear duration and step count, but also other relevant factors related to exercise, such as activity intensity and energy expenditure [25]. Even for activity tracking publications, heterogeneity in the analyses and reporting of data has been observed—and authors have recommended that minimum reporting thresholds be determined in the future [25].

It has been suggested that whenever PA/exercise practice is linked to the use of eHealth, it is not sufficient to promote the effects of the technologies without an accompanying assessment of its influence on the intervention [27]. This should be borne in mind, as it has been shown that more complex behavioral recommendations tend to lead to higher nonadherence rates [16]. In an attempt to tackle this, researchers focused on assessing adherence to the prompts delivered via health technologies and found that it tended to diminish over time [28].

In a 2020 scoping literature review on PA app adherence, Yang et al. were able to establish a total of four possible category dimensions for adherence to PA apps: (1) frequency of PA app usage, (2) intention/motivation to sustain use of the PA app, (3) degree of function use within the PA app, and (4) the duration of PA app usage [8].

The explanations above on the particularities of eHealth intervention design point to the existing split between traditional adherence to exercise and adherence to eHealth-delivered exercise, where the technology itself can be a determining factor in intervention effects. A standard, validated measure of exercise adherence that can be consistently used in future studies is required [14]. This review aimed to offer insight into how adherence to eHealth-delivered exercise has been utilized in recent scientific literature. Being aware of past conceptualizations could constitute a first, necessary step toward increased homogeneity in research—and could allow clinicians and researchers to analyze and report in a more standardized and replicable manner.

2. The Goal of the Review

The primary goal of this scoping review was to analyze and report how researchers have approached the definition and operationalization of adherence to physical activity interventions via eHealth for the adult population with no specific health conditions. This subsample of the population constitutes a particularly challenging group, since their access to interventions is often voluntary, lacks the urge of a health-specific need and, most importantly, lacks a formal medical prescription. These characteristics, together with the fact that the interventions were delivered via technology, meant that these scenarios do not fit as easily into the traditional definition of adherence—the percentage of actual compliance over the prescribed dose.

The broad directive in this review was to determine whether the inclusion of e-Health technologies in physical activity/exercise interventions required a new conceptualization of the term adherence. The research question was: how has eHealth exercise adherence for the healthy adult population been defined and operationalized in the literature over the last six years? These questions directed the subsequent search and selection of relevant e-Health publications presented in this review. This paper include the review findings and accompanying analysis, which together provide insight into how adherence to exercise has been operationalized in the past, both for in-person and electronic exercise plans.

3. Methods

This scoping review followed the stages as outlined by Levac et al. [29] in their update to the work of Arksey and O'Malley in 2005 [27]. Six steps to the review process were followed: (1) identifying the research question, (2) identifying the relevant studies, (3) study selection, (4) charting the data, (5) collating, summarizing and reporting results, and (6) optional consultation [29]. This framework recommended that scoping reviews employ both a broad and a more focused questions for step one [29].

3.1. Protocol and Registration

This review was not previously registered, as it is not customary to do so with scoping reviews. PROSPERO, an open access online database of systematic review protocols and registry for systematic review protocols, was nevertheless consulted (with the search terms "adherence", "physical activity", and "exercise") in order to determine whether any similar reviews were ongoing. Sixty-one related publications were found, of which eleven were initially perceived as relevant to our study. After a thorough reading of their designs, it was determined that none of them matched or were otherwise relevant to our study. Five were disregarded for not involving technologies and the remaining six were found not relevant for involving patients with pathologies.

3.2. Search Strategy

A preliminary search strategy was used during step two to determine the medical subject headings (MeSH) and keywords. The portal-related search terms were separated into four categories: "telemedicine", "exercise", "physical fitness", and "treatment adherence and compliance". A combination of the constructs and related keywords was used for a comprehensive literature search using the Cochrane Library, Science Direct, Scielo, PubMed, Sport Discus, and Greynet International databases. The exact search terms used can be found in Figure 1. An additional manual search was performed to complete the review, and spontaneous findings were not systematically disregarded. Papers were searched regardless of their study design, language, and publication status.

The literature search was conducted at two different points in time, using the same search queries on both occasions. The first search was carried out during February 2021 and encompassed published articles from 1 January 2016 to 31 December 2020. The second search was carried out in March 2022 and was restricted to publications from 1 January 2021 until 13 March 2022, in order to better reflect the impact of the COVID-19 pandemic.

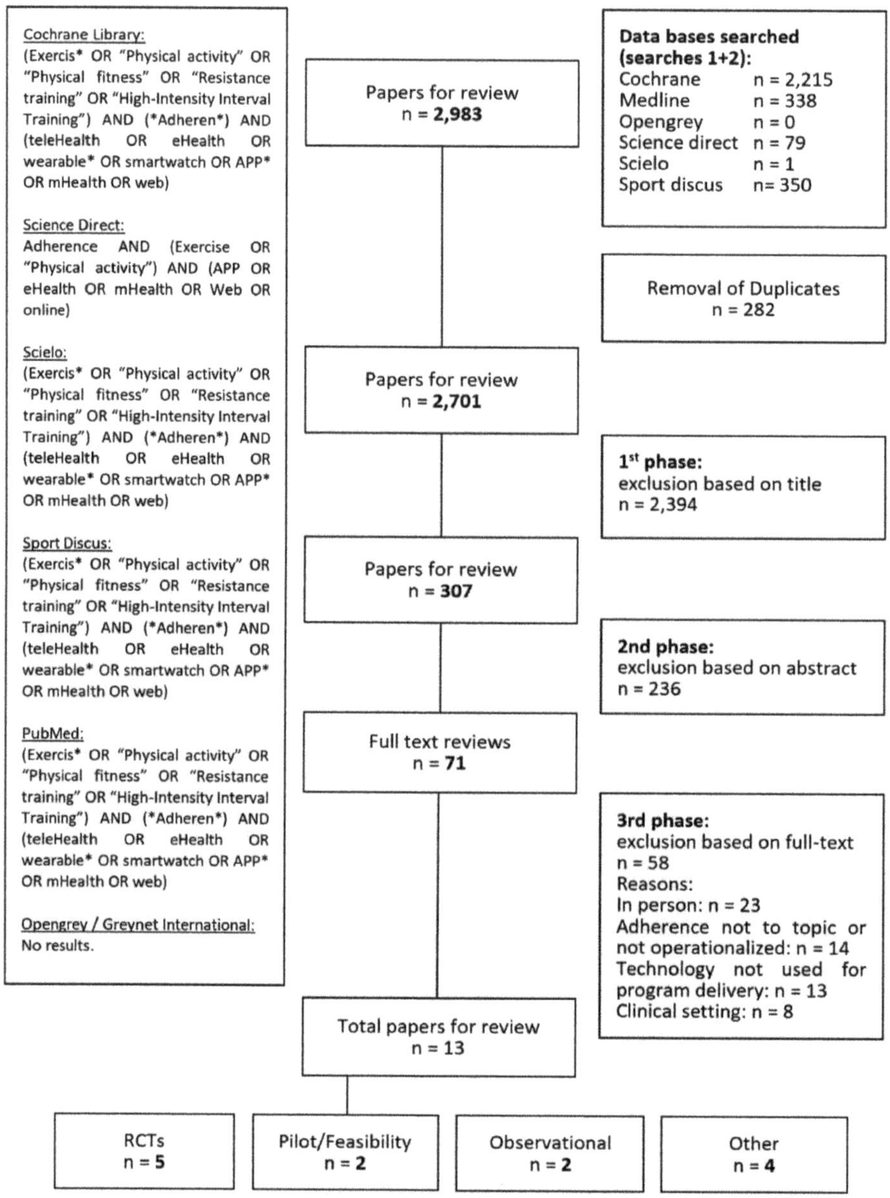

Figure 1. Scoping review strategy and results.

A detailed description of keywords and search queries for each database is provided in the Multimedia Appendix A.

3.3. Eligibility Criteria

In the third step of the review process, inclusion and exclusion criteria were used. All articles that met or seemed to meet the following criteria were included in the review: (1) involved humans, with no specific health conditions; (2) subjects were 18 years of age or above; (3) intervention consisted of physical activity or exercise, delivered or supported remotely; (4) the article specifically mentioned adherence, referring to exercise, physical activity, sedentary behavior, or app use. Articles which did not fulfill the inclusion criteria were excluded, as well as those in the following situations: (1) if the article dealt with pathology or related problems (e.g., referring to pathology, therapeutic, rehabilitation, chronic conditions, painful conditions, disability, frail, fragility, clinical, hypertension, prescription, critical, disorders, primary care, doctor, nurse, practitioner); (2) adherence was not conceptualized, defined, or measured; (3) adherence referred to variables other than physical activity, sedentary behavior, exercise, or app use (e.g., diet, combined interventions, activity tracker wear time); (4) studies relating to pregnancy or performance sports.

3.4. Data Extraction

The studies (n = 13) selected for review were screened for data, and key points were extracted and registered in a Microsoft Excel sheet (MS Office 16). This constituted step four (charting the data) of the scoping review framework process. Characteristics such as author, title, country of origin, research design, year, journal of publication, and outcome measured were recorded.

4. Results

This section reflects the concluding steps of the framework: collating, summarizing, reporting results and consultation. Next, the discussion section was utilized to expand on some areas.

4.1. Study Selection and Description

The technology-based search rendered a total of 2983 (2616 from the first search and 367 from the second search) relevant studies. Selection of studies was manually conducted, on an independent peer-reviewed basis, by the authors (AFV and JMM). Duplicates (282 total, 263 in first search and 19 in second search) were initially identified and excluded from the list. The selection of studies was completed in three steps and carried out simultaneously by both authors. First, titles were screened, and most (2394) papers were excluded for having to do with pathological/clinical scenarios. Second, the abstracts of the 307 articles deemed relevant were screened for eligibility, also on a peer-reviewed basis. Two hundred and thirty six papers were discarded based on the information on their abstract. Lastly, those papers that could not be excluded upon abstract check (58 from first search and 13 from second search) were deemed eligible for full text reading. In total, 71 papers were fully read and 58 of them were excluded during the full-text screening phase (Figure 1). All-stage decisions by the authors as to whether papers should be included or excluded for review were placed in common at the end of each stage. Disagreements were discussed one by one until consensus was reached. A total of 13 studies (6 studies from the first search and 7 studies from the second search) studies were finally deemed eligible. Most full texts (n = 23) were excluded due to their interventions being delivered in person and not by means of eHealth technologies. Only papers which included the use of technology for either the implementation of a PA/exercise intervention or its follow-up were considered eligible. A list of all reasons for exclusion is presented in Figure 1 for review.

The selected studies included 5 randomized controlled trials (RCTs), 2 pilot or feasibility studies, 2 RCT protocols, 2 observational studies, 1 formative research, and 1 congress abstract. Table 1 summarizes the key characteristics in the selected studies. Issuing countries included Australia [30,31], Greece [32], Spain [33,34], The Netherlands [35], Germany [36], United States of America [37,38], United Kingdom [28,39], China [40] and Taiwan [41]. A noticeable increase in the number of publications could be seen for 2021 and 2022.

Table 1. Scoping review matrix used for the collection of publication data from the reviewed articles.

Author [Ref]	Abridged Title	Year	Country	Research Design	Technology Type	Outcome	Operationalization
Albergoni [35]	Factors influencing walking and exercise ADH in healthy older adults ...	2020	The Netherlands	Exploratory (pilot) study with no control group	The app did not deliver exercises. Served as registry and motivation	Adherence to walking and exercise (difference based on heart rate count) program based on guidelines and adherence to exercise volume	Exercise and walking program ADH *: days per week the target was reached divided by the target training frequency. Exercise volume ADH: minutes per week divided by weekly target volume
Alley [31]	Web-based video-coaching to assist an automated computer-tailored physical activity ...	2016	Australia	RCT *	Web-based	ADH to PA intervention and engagement to website	ADH to PA intervention: % of actual vs. planned participation. Website engagement: Number of visits and minutes spent on website
Calvo Sánchez [33]	Experience in the use of videos for the promotion of physical exercise at home in online mode ...	2022	Spain	Observational, descriptive, nonexperimental, cross-sectional study	Videos on Vimeo and Youtube platforms	ADH to exercises in videos	Frequency (number per week) of video use; total use time (days)
Dawson [38]	Quantification of adherence in a mobile health exercise intervention for cardiometabolic health	2021	USA	Congress abstract on a pilot trial	Synchronous and asynchronous video sessions online	Adherence to exercise	Exercise ADH: ratio of completed to planned sessions performed/wk. ADH to exercise training dose: through heart rate-based training zones
Feng [37]	Feasibility of an at-home, web-based, interactive exercise program for older adults.	2019	USA	RCT, two-site, single-blind	Secure website	Adherence to exercise intervention	Number of completed sessions divided by total possible sessions (only for finishers).
Jansons [30]	Delivery of home-based exercise interventions in older adults facilitated by Amazon Alexa ...	2022	Australia	Feasibility study: prospective single-arm	Amazon Alexa skill application called Teletrainer and Buddy link web-based exercise prescription portal	Adherence to exercise program	Percentage of the total prescribed exercises completed

Table 1. *Cont.*

Author [Ref]	Abridged Title	Year	Country	Research Design	Technology Type	Outcome	Operationalization
Jossa-Bastidas [34]	Predicting physical exercise adherence in fitness apps using a deep learning approach	2021	Spain	Observational, retrospective, pilot study	Mobile app	Prediction model	Original app did not define ADH. This retrospective study considered participants as nonadherent if training was interrupted for 4+ continuous weeks
Konstantinidis [32]	Design, implementation, and wide pilot deployment of FitForAll ...	2016	Greece	RCT	Computer based with Nintendo Wii devices	Adherence to exercise protocol	Number of participation sessions over the number of planned sessions (%)
Liang [39]	Feasibility and acceptability of home-based exercise snacking and tai chi snacking ...	2022	United Kingdom	RCT	Written and video instructions delivered via email	Adherence to exercise program	Percentage of completed vs. prescribed intervention exercises
Morris [28]	Rise and recharge: exploring employee perceptions of and contextual factors ...	2021	United Kingdom	Feasibility study: 3-arm quasi-randomized intervention	Mobile app	Adherence to app-delivered prompts	Operationalization of ADH not specified. Study mentioned operationalization for participant compliance to both prompt and review questions, as calculated as the total number of participant responses (reported).
NCT02844296 [40]	Short-bout handgrip exercise for smoking cessation	2016	China	RCT protocol: single-blinded, two-arm	Mobile app with a single instructional video, used to send reminders and as an electronic daily diary	Adherence to suggested single exercise (PA is additionally assessed but not part of the intervention)	Frequency and duration of a single exercise (handgrip).

Table 1. *Cont.*

Author [Ref]	Abridged Title	Year	Country	Research Design	Technology Type	Outcome	Operationalization
Pischke [36]	Implementation and effects of information technology-based and print-based interventions …	2020	Germany	RCT protocol with crossover design	Study compared program internet vs. printed-out delivery modes, both modes being complemented with in-person sessions	Changes in PA levels	Adherence measures or operationalization not mentioned. Study used WHO guidelines as a reference
Sun [41]	Motivating adherence to exercise plans through a personalized mobile health app …	2021	Taiwan	Formative research	Mobile app	Adherence to exercise plan	Percentage of the exercise plan completed

* RCT: Randomized controlled trial. * ADH: Adherence.

4.2. Range of Conceptualizations for Adherence in the Reviewed Papers

In general, this review comprised a range of technologies and measures applied to the evaluation of adherence (Table 1). The technologies used included computers [32], internet or websites [31,36,37], Amazon Alexa and internet [30], video platforms [33,38,39], and mobile applications [28,34,35,40,41]. See Figure 2.

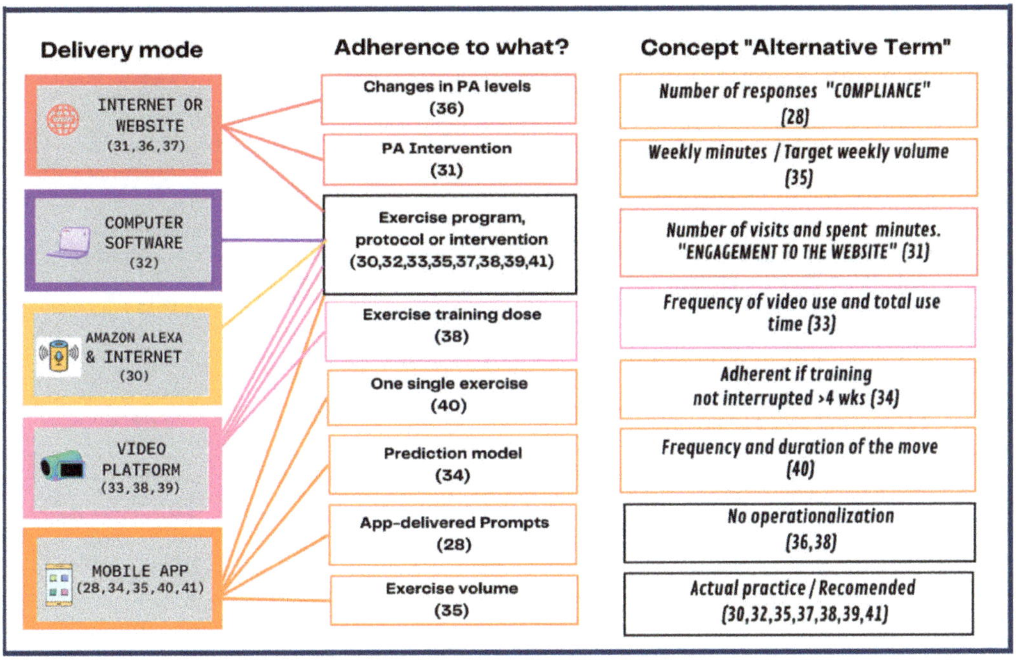

Figure 2. How has technology-delivered physical activity/exercise been defined in the literature [28,30–41].

As is customary in scoping reviews, the nature of the studies reviewed was heterogeneous, not only due to the different technologies used but also in regard to the choice of intervention, delivery, and registry mode, among other things. Most (8 out of 13) of the reviewed articles assessed adherence to exercise programs, protocols or interventions [30,32,33,35,37–39,41]; one focused on adherence to changes in PA levels [36], one focused on adherence to app-delivered prompts [28], one assessed adherence to a single exercise [40], one measured adherence to a PA intervention [31], and one focused on establishing a prediction of adherence based on a previously published pilot study [34]. In addition to measuring adherence to the exercise program, one of the studies also aimed to assess adherence to exercise volume [35] and yet another aimed to assess adherence to the exercise training dose [38]. Other than that, still related to the concept of adherence, one of the reviewed papers additionally measured engagement on a website, as the number of visits and minutes spent on it [31].

The majority of the reviewed papers that focused on assessing adherence to exercise programs did so by operationalizing the term as a percentage of actual practice over the recommended or planned amount of practice [30,32,35,37–39,41]. Of those, one of the studies specified that calculations had only been done for those participants who had completed the intervention [37]. A similar operationalization (i.e., percentage of actual versus planned participation) was used to assess adherence to PA by Alley et al. [31]. Only one of the papers which focused on adherence to an exercise program conceptualized the term adherence based on the mere frequency of video use and total use time [33].

One of the studies included in this scoping review did not effectively specify their operationalization of adherence [36], although they did mention that they focused on assessing changes in PA levels, while holding the WHO guidelines as the standard recommendation. One study focused on exercise volume adherence, by operationalizing it as the number of weekly minutes the person exercised, divided by the target weekly volume [35]. Another study reported adherence to exercise training dose and specified it would be monitored through heart rate-based training zones [38]. However, the precise operationalization of adherence in this case remained unclear.

One study operationalized adherence to a suggested single exercise by the frequency and duration of the move (handgrip) [40]. The study by Morris et al. focused on adherence to app-delivered prompts, as opposed to app-delivered exercises. They interchangeably use the term "participant compliance" and operationalized adherence to the prompts as the total number of participant responses [28]. Lastly, the study by Jossa-Bastidas et al. consisted of a deep-learning-developed prediction model for adherence to a given exercise app. The authors, in this case, operationalized adherence as a binary variable, according to whether the participant interrupted their training for a period of 4 weeks or more (nonadherent) or not (adherent) [34].

4.3. Adherence Operationally Defined as Related to Technology Design

Table 2 provides details as to how each of the reviewed articles categorized adherence to the technology, based on recommendations by Yang et al. [8] and Sieverink et al. [7]. Detailed information on these categories has also been included in the Adherence to eHealth for General PA and Exercise section, above.

Table 2. Operationalization of reviewed papers as per Yang et al. and Sieverink et al.'s classifications of adherence to eHealth technologies.

Author	Dimension as per Yang et al. [8]	Categorization as per Sieverink et al. [7]
Albergoni [35]	N/a *: App did not deliver exercises. App registered minutes of exercise as recorded by wearable device. Adherence measured in minutes.	N/a. App did not deliver intervention.
Alley [31]	N/a: Internet, not app.	Category A (for web use): Expected use not specified/the more use the better.
Calvo Sánchez [33]	N/a: Video platform, not app.	Category A (for video platform): expected use not specified.
Dawson [38]	N/a: Video platform, not app.	Category A (for videos): expected use not specified/the more use the better.
Feng [37]	N/a: Internet, not app.	Category B (for web use): Expected use specified, not justified.
Jansons [30]	N/a: Amazon Alexa, not app.	Category C (for Alexa plus video program): expected number of exercises specified, as justified by exercise recommendations.
Jossa-Bastidas [34]	N/a. Retrospective study.	N/a. Retrospective study.
Konstantinidis [32]	N/a: Computer, not app.	Category A (for computer use): Expected use of technology not specified.
Liang [39]	N/a: video platform, not app.	Category A (for exercises and prompting): expected use not specified/the more use the better.
NCT02844296 [40]	N/a: Study app was used for participant feedback, not intervention.	N/a. App does not deliver intervention. For participant motivation and feedback purposes: Cat. B—Expected use of "registry" app specified but not justified.
Morris [28]	N/a. Adherence to app not assessed.	Category A (for app use): expected use not specified.
Pischke [36]	N/a: Internet, not app.	Category A (for web use): Expected use of technology not specified.
Sun [41]	N/a. Adherence to app not assessed.	Category A (for app use): expected technology use not specified.

* N/a: not applicable.

The authors were unable to categorize any of the reviewed articles into any of the four categories described by Yang et al. in 2020 [8], as reflected by the n/a (not applicable) indications in Table 2. In most (8 out of the 13 reviewed studies) cases, the reason for this was that the reviewed articles evaluated interventions delivered by technology types other than mobile applications (i.e., computers, internet, Amazon Alexa, or videos), which, in essence, were not within the aim or scope of Yang's [8] publication. Other reasons included, in two instances, the app not delivering the intervention, in two instances, adherence to the app not being assessed or reported, and in one instance, the study not actually being of an interventional nature.

In regard to the classification of findings according to the eHealth categories established by Sieverink et al. in their 2017 systematic review [7]: most (8 out of 13) studies fell within Category A, meaning that an expected use of the technology was not specified in the reviewed papers so that a 'the more use, the better' approach was assumed. Of those articles which fell into Category A, one of the interventions was computer-delivered [32], two were internet-based [31,36], two were app-based [28,41] and three consisted of videos [33,38,39]. One paper, which involved an internet-delivered intervention [37], was identified as falling within Category B. One paper [30] offered explanation of intended use and justification for that choice, therefore falling into Category C. Three papers [34,35,40] could not be classified into any of Sieverink et al.'s pre-established categories.

5. Discussion

The purpose of this scoping review was to gain insight into how the concept of adherence has been used in previous eHealth interventions involving healthy adults. Our initial hypothesis, based on sound previous research, was that the term adherence was used in a variety of forms, conceptualizations and or definitions, therefore hindering direct comparison of measurements between studies. We began this research with the question of whether the trend toward eHealth interventions required an update of the traditional definition of the term adherence. Based on our observations and also on those of other researchers [6–8], both assumptions (i.e., variety of uses of the term adherence and a need for reconceptualization in light of increased technology use in healthcare) seem to have been confirmed.

5.1. Principal Findings

We included 13 studies in this review, all published between 1 January 2016 and 13 March 2022. Most interventions were delivered via smartphone application, followed by video platforms. A drift toward apps seemed apparent as we compared our results with those of Sieverink et al., who found that up until 2017, most digital interventions were web-based or mobile apps. Eight out of the thirteen studies reviewed focused on adherence to exercise programs. The fact that they most commonly included some kind of suggested program pinpointed a gap in the literature as far as voluntary, nonprescribed exercise was concerned. Our results also highlighted the fact that operationalizations of the term adherence were often based on the assumption that more use was better and did not include a threshold for intended use. This seemed to be in line with Sieverink et al.'s findings from 2017. We were surprised to find that few of the studies we reviewed were specific on the expected use of the technology, in contrast to the results previously found by Sieverink et al., in their review.

Most of the studies included in this scoping review measured adherence as the percentage of actual practice over the recommended or planned amount. Indeed, the most extended conceptualization of adherence in the published literature was that of the WHO, which established it as "the extent to which a person's behavior—taking medication, following a diet, and/or executing lifestyle changes—corresponds with agreed recommendations from a health care provider" [42]. This definition could be somewhat confusing, since adherence to prescribed therapies or recommendations is also known as compliance, as per the original conceptualization by Sacket et al. [43,44], which then led to the WHO implementing a new iteration of their definition. The WHO's preference for the term adherence aimed to better reflect the autonomy of the patient and the influences of their environment, experiences, knowledge, or resources [5]. Within our own results, the term compliance was found to be used interchangeably with adherence on one occasion.

Previous evidence has pointed at many other confusing terms being commonly used in research. In the past, exercise adherence has been used interchangeably with the terms intervention adherence, study adherence [45], commitment [46], retention [30,47,48], compliance [44], consistency [49], engagement [17,50,51], and feasibility [52]. When studying adherence to therapeutic exercise for musculoskeletal pain, Bailey et al. additionally found other terms to have been used interchangeably, such as concordance, agreement, cooperation, partnership, and therapeutic alliance [6]. The scientific community also lacks a clear operationalization of the term adherence to physical activities, even in clinical settings. Most studies which have defined adherence in their work have used frequency of exercise completion as the measuring parameter of adherence [5]. However, even frequency was not always measured the same way; it consisted variably of exercise repetitions, blocks of exercise time, or a variety of time frames (e.g., exercises per day, week or month) [5]. Other studies in the field of musculoskeletal pain have measured adherence based on behavioral parameters, session attendance, session completion, exercise exertion, or intensity or quality of execution [5]. Moreover, there is a third term that should be brought to mind; if adherence is the amount of exposure that people receive when using an intervention, then it could also be referred to as dose [46]. To this regard, Cugelman et al. considered that, for interventions that were voluntary, users received a dose that was proportional to their chosen level of adherence [46]. This is just another example of the terminological jigsaw puzzle researchers face, which will hopefully be solved with more standardized scientific reporting. Moreover, none of the included studies dealt directly with all four parameters (i.e., frequency, duration, intensity and accuracy) that the WHO believed characterized rehabilitation prescriptions [5].

This paper showed that the reviewed interventions frequently lacked a justification of the exercise prescription. This was also the case in Sieverink's review [7], which spanned from 2006 to 2017. In some cases, the reviewed papers did provide some type of intervention rationale. Albergoni [35], as well as Konstantinidis [32], specified that they were adhering to published PA guidelines. Sun [41] explained that they devised their own exercise plans. Even then, when talking about eHealth, researchers encountered yet another challenge: being able to differentiate between adherence to the intervention and adherence to the technology being used. In fact, 8 out of the 13 studies reviewed did not specify any intended dose of use of the technology.

5.2. Implications and Recommendations

This scoping review identified ongoing challenges regarding the conceptualization of the term adherence in health, and eHealth in particular. Exercise implies a personalized objective setting, which adds to the difficulty of reaching some homogenization of the concept. We seem to be facing a need to develop specific definitions for specific scenarios (according to purpose, population group, voluntary vs. prescribed, etc.).

Technology plays an important role and could be valuable in obtaining objective usage data. However, for eHealth interventions to be successful, future researchers and developers should focus on user perception of technology use—for instance, by using the System Usability Scale or a similar tool.

While some consensus for the use of the term adherence was reached, the authors of this review recommend that future studies clearly specify characteristics of their chosen technology, operationalization, expected user behavior toward both the intervention and the technology, and the existence or absence of a rationale to their selections.

6. Strengths and Limitations

In the conduction of the scoping review, the authors faced a number of limitations worth taking into consideration. Regarding the search query used, we started with the realization that MeSH did not have an adherence term that focused specifically on life behavior change, which required more creativity and therefore a risk of bias. Additionally, the MeSH terms "exercise therapy" and "telemedicine" were avoided, given that their definition was circumscribed to pathological conditions. Excluding those papers focusing on health issues, pain, or other rehabilitation environments may have caused some selection bias. Similarly, the MeSH terms "sports" and "physical fitness" were also avoided. We made every effort to include as many papers and study designs as possible in our scoping review and decided, when in doubt, to include studies. However, we were compelled to slightly change the search equations for different databases, which, in itself, constituted some limitation to the procedure. Another limitation arose from the fact that we specifically searched for the term adherence, while other authors may have published work using different terms to refer to the same user behaviors. Additionally, the search terms were limited to title, abstract, and keywords for a number of databases. Restricting the search in this way enabled us to select those studies that specifically focused on adherence to PA/exercise in eHealth, but could have left some undetected.

This scoping review encompassed a timespan of 6 years and 3 months. The authors considered this adequate, as it constituted a follow-up to Sieverink et al. and their 2016 work. Moreover, the COVID-19 pandemic caused an increased use of eHealth technologies; thus, in 2021 and 2022, there was an increase in related publications. This work aimed to reflect advances in the matter.

For the conduction of this scoping review, efforts were made to incorporate databases of a complementary nature, which focused, not only on healthcare, but also on exercise and sports. We believe this to have been a relevant decision as efforts were made to provide a general overview of all the existing literature. Having chosen not to restrict the search to any specific language may have helped to strengthen the results, as well.

This scoping review was carried out with a focus on detecting all potential conceptualizations of the term adherence to PA/exercise interventions delivered via eHealth. It contributes, therefore, to narrowing the focus of the concept of adherence to eHealth, and to finding valid, reliable, and acceptable measures of adherence to different physical activity or exercise interventions.

7. Conclusions

This review highlightes the fact that a well-defined and unanimous use of the term adherence to exercise is lacking. Traditional approaches which consider adherence as a fraction of prescribed dosage could possibly be suitable for prescription exercise, when performed onsite. Yet, if scientists aim to adhere to the specifications put forth by the WHO, special attention will need to be placed on adequate monitorization of frequency, duration, intensity, and accuracy of the exercises or exercise sessions.

One of the challenges we observed lay in establishing what exactly constituted adherence to voluntary exercise and how it could be measured. Our findings, as well as those by researchers before us, suggest a wide heterogeneity of conceptualizations in the literature. The second challenge we identified had to do with the addition of technologies to interventions, and their remote, asynchronous delivery. Sieverink et al. suggested that "adherence to eHealth technology is an underdeveloped and often improperly used concept". Our findings, six years later, did not contradict this.

This review calls for an improved definition of adherence to prescribed exercise, adherence to voluntary exercise and adherence to eHealth technologies. This is likely to be a necessary step towards reaching full comparability and applicability.

Author Contributions: Conceptualization, A.F.-V.; methodology, A.F.-V. and J.M.; validation, A.F.-V., M.G.-B., O.R.-N., J.J.-R. and J.M.; formal analysis, A.F.-V.; investigation, A.F.-V.; resources, A.F.-V.; data curation, A.F.-V.; writing—original draft preparation, A.F.-V.; writing—review and editing, A.F.-V., M.G.-B., O.R.-N., J.J.-R. and J.M.; supervision, J.J.-R. and J.M.; project administration, J.M.; funding acquisition, J.M. and O.R.-N. All authors have read and agreed to the published version of the manuscript.

Funding: This scoping review was conducted independently by a research team at Ramon Llull University. It was completed with research funds provided by Aristos Campus Mundus projects (ACM2021_02 and ACM2022_25) and Fundació Naccari-Ravà 2022. The authors would also like to acknowledge the support of the university Blanquerna-URL in providing funds for the employment of the principal author.

Institutional Review Board Statement: Not applicable.

Informed Consent Statement: Not applicable.

Data Availability Statement: Raw data of this article are available upon request to corresponding author.

Conflicts of Interest: The authors declare no conflict of interest.

Abbreviations

ADH	adherence
eHealth	electronic health
DHI	Digital health intervention
MeSH	medical subject heading
PA	physical activity
RCT	randomized controlled trial
WHO	World Health Organization

Appendix A

Keyword terms used within scientific database searches to determine the definitions of adherence to physical activity or physical exercise interventions delivered via eHealth.

Technology	Intervention	Adherence
"Mobile Health"	Exercis*	*Adheren*
mHealth	Train*	"treatment adherence and compliance"
"Mobile tech*"	Program*	
TeleHealth	Coach*	
eHealth	"Physical activity"	
Web*	"Physical fitness"	
Online*	"Resistance training"	
"information tech*"	"High-intensity interval training"	
Wearable*		
smartwatch		
Platform*		
"internet*based"		
App*		

Following are the exact search queries that were used for the retrieval of information in the different databases:

Cochrane Library:

(Exercis* OR "Physical activity" OR "Physical fitness" OR "Resistance training" OR "High-Intensity Interval Training") AND (*Adheren*) AND (teleHealth OR eHealth OR wearable* OR smartwatch OR APP* OR mHealth OR web)

Applied filters: Title Abstract Keywords; 1 January 2016 to 13 March 2022

Science Direct:

Adherence AND (Exercise OR "Physical activity") AND (APP OR eHealth OR mHealth OR Web OR online)

Applied filter: Title Abstract Keywords

Scielo:

(Exercis* OR "Physical activity" OR "Physical fitness" OR "Resistance training" OR "High-Intensity Interval Training") AND (*Adheren*) AND (teleHealth OR eHealth OR wearable* OR smartwatch OR APP* OR mHealth OR web)

Applied filters: none

Sport Discus:

(Exercis* OR "Physical activity" OR "Physical fitness" OR "Resistance training" OR "High-Intensity Interval Training") AND (*Adheren*) AND (teleHealth OR eHealth OR wearable* OR smartwatch OR APP* OR mHealth OR web)

Filter applied: 2016 to 2022

PubMed:

(Exercis* OR "Physical activity" OR "Physical fitness" OR "Resistance training" OR "High-Intensity Interval Training") AND (*Adheren*) AND (teleHealth OR eHealth OR wearable* OR smartwatch OR APP* OR mHealth OR web)

Filters applied: Humans; 1 January 2016 to 13 March 2022; 13 to 80+ years of age; all paper types including reviews.

Opengrey/Greynet International:

All attempted search queries retrieved zero relevant literature.

References

1. Guthold, R.; Stevens, G.A.; Riley, L.M.; Bull, F.C. Worldwide trends in insufficient physical activity from 2001 to 2016: A pooled analysis of 358 population-based surveys with 1·9 million participants. *Lancet Glob. Health* **2018**, *6*, e1077–e1086. [CrossRef]
2. World Health Organization. *Global Action Plan on Physical Activity 2018–2030: More Active People for a Healthier World*; World Health Organization: Geneva, Switzerland, 2018.
3. European Comission. Cluster 1: Health, Policy, Strategy, How to Apply and Work Programmes. Available online: https://ec.europa.eu/info/research-and-innovation/funding/funding-opportunities/funding-programmes-and-open-calls/horizon-europe/cluster-1-health_en (accessed on 5 February 2021).
4. Perski, O.; Blandford, A.; West, R.; Michie, S. Conceptualising engagement with digital behaviour change interventions: A systematic review using principles from critical interpretive synthesis. *Transl. Behav. Med.* **2017**, *7*, 254–267. [CrossRef] [PubMed]
5. Bailey, D.L.; Holden, M.A.; Foster, N.E.; Quicke, J.G.; Haywood, K.L.; Bishop, A. Defining adherence to therapeutic exercise for musculoskeletal pain: A systematic review. *Br. J. Sports Med.* **2020**, *54*, 326–331. [CrossRef]
6. Payne, J.E.; Turk, M.T.; Kalarchian, M.A.; Pellegrini, C.A. Defining Adherence to Dietary Self-Monitoring Using a Mobile App: A Narrative Review. *J. Acad. Nutr. Diet.* **2018**, *118*, 2094–2119. [CrossRef] [PubMed]
7. Sieverink, F.; Kelders, S.M.; Gemert-Pijnen, V. Clarifying the concept of adherence to ehealth technology: Systematic review on when usage becomes adherence. *J. Med. Internet Res.* **2017**, *19*, e402. [CrossRef]
8. Yang, X.; Ma, L.; Zhao, X.; Kankanhalli, A. Factors influencing user's adherence to physical activity applications: A scoping literature review and future directions. *Int. J. Med. Inform.* **2020**, *134*, 10439. [CrossRef]
9. Martinez, G.J.; Mattingly, S.M.; Robles-Granda, P.; Saha, K.; Sirigiri, A.; Young, J.; Chawla, N.; De Choudhury, M.; D'Mello, S.; Mark, G.; et al. Predicting Participant Compliance With Fitness Tracker Wearing and Ecological Momentary Assessment Protocols in Information Workers: Observational Study. *JMIR Mhealth Uhealth* **2021**, *9*, e22218. [CrossRef]
10. Bull, F.C.; Al-Ansari, S.S.; Biddle, S.; Borodulin, K.; Buman, M.P.; Cardon, G.; Carty, C.; Chaput, J.P.; Chastin, S.; Chou, R.; et al. World Health Organization 2020 guidelines on physical activity and sedentary behaviour. *Br. J. Sports Med.* **2020**, *54*, 1451–1462. [CrossRef]
11. Bullard, T.; Ji, M.; An, R.; Trinh, L.; MacKenzie, M.; Mullen, S.P. A systematic review and meta-analysis of adherence to physical activity interventions among three chronic conditions: Cancer, cardiovascular disease, and diabetes. *BMC Public Health* **2019**, *19*, 636. [CrossRef]
12. Sperandei, S.; Vieira, M.C.; Reis, A.C. Adherence to physical activity in an unsupervised setting: Explanatory variables for high attrition rates among fitness center members. *J. Sci. Med. Sport* **2016**, *19*, 916–920. [CrossRef]

13. Dasso, N.A. How is exercise different from physical activity? A concept analysis. *Nurs. Forum* **2019**, *54*, 45–52. [CrossRef] [PubMed]
14. Jordan, J.L.; Holden, M.A.; Mason, E.E.; Foster, N.E. Interventions to improve adherence to exercise for chronic musculoskeletal pain in adults. *Cochrane Database Syst. Rev.* **2010**, *2010*, CD005956. [CrossRef] [PubMed]
15. Garcia-Ortiz, L.; Recio-Rodriguez, J.I.; Agudo-Conde, C.; Patino-Alonso, M.C.; Maderuelo-Fernandez, J.A.; Gento, I.R.; Puig, E.P.; Gonzalez-Viejo, N.; Arietaleanizbeaskoa, M.S.; Schmolling-Guinovart, Y.; et al. Long-term effectiveness of a smartphone app for improving healthy lifestyles in general population in primary care: Randomized controlled trial (Evident II ki study). *JMIR Mhealth Uhealth* **2018**, *6*, e107. [CrossRef] [PubMed]
16. Martin, L.R.; Williams, S.L.; Haskard, K.B.; Dimatteo, M.R. The challenge of patient adherence. *Ther. Clin. Risk Manag.* **2005**, *1*, 189–199.
17. Mclaughlin, M.; Delaney, T.; Hall, A.; Byaruhanga, J.; Mackie, P.; Grady, A.; Reilly, K.; Campbell, E.; Sutherland, R.; Wiggers, J.; et al. Associations Between Digital Health Intervention Engagement, Physical Activity, and Sedentary Behavior: Systematic Review and Meta-analysis. *J. Med. Internet Res.* **2021**, *23*, e23180. [CrossRef] [PubMed]
18. Müller, A.M.; Maher, C.A.; Vandelanotte, C.; Hingle, M.; Middelweerd, A.; Lopez, M.L.; DeSmet, A.; Short, C.E.; Nathan, N.; Hutchesson, M.J.; et al. Physical Activity, Sedentary Behavior, and Diet-Related eHealth and mHealth Research: Bibliometric Analysis. *J. Med. Internet Res.* **2018**, *20*, e122. [CrossRef]
19. Schoeppe, S.; Alley, S.; Van Lippevelde, W.; Bray, N.A.; Williams, S.L.; Duncan, M.J.; Vandelanotte, C. Efficacy of interventions that use apps to improve diet, physical activity and sedentary behaviour: A systematic review. *Int. J. Behav. Nutr. Phys. Act.* **2016**, *13*, 127. [CrossRef]
20. Middelweerd, A.; Mollee, J.S.; van der Wal, C.N.; Brug, J.; Te Velde, S.J. Apps to promote physical activity among adults: A review and content analysis. *Int. J. Behav. Nutr. Phys. Act.* **2014**, *11*, 97. [CrossRef]
21. Fuente-Vidal, A.; Zahia, S.; Sánchez, N.; Roda, O.; Guerra, M.; Garcia-Zapirain, B.; Montane, J. Exercise Apps. A pilot study on how the use of big data for multivariable analysis can be applied in order to predict user behaviour and promote engagement. In Proceedings of the Abstract book for the ISBNPA 2021 Annual Meeting, International Society of Behavioral Nutrition and Physical Activity, online, 1 July 2021; p. 152.
22. Iribarren, S.J.; Cato, K.; Falzon, L.; Stone, P.W. What is the economic evidence for mHealth? A systematic review of economic evaluations of mHealth solutions. *PLoS ONE* **2017**, *12*, e0170581. [CrossRef]
23. Zhang, M.; Wang, W.; Li, M.; Sheng, H.; Zhai, Y.; Zhang, M.; Wang, W.; Li, M.; Sheng, H.; Zhai, Y. Citation: Efficacy of Mobile Health Applications to Improve Physical Activity and Sedentary Behavior: A Systematic Review and Meta-Analysis for Physically Inactive Individuals. *Int. J. Environ. Res. Public Health* **2022**, *19*, 4905. [CrossRef]
24. World Health Organization. *Monitoring and Evaluating Digital Health Interventions: A Practical Guide to Conducting Research and Assessment*; World Health Organization: Geneva, Switzerland, 2016.
25. Chan, A.; Chan, D.; Lee, H.; Ng, C.C.; Yeo, A.H.L. Reporting adherence, validity and physical activity measures of wearable activity trackers in medical research: A systematic review. *Int. J. Med. Inform.* **2022**, *160*, 104696. [CrossRef] [PubMed]
26. Stonerock, G.L.; Blumenthal, J.A. Role Of Counseling To Promote Adherence In Healthy Lifestyle Medicine: Strategies to Improve Exercise Adherence and Enhance Physical Activity. *Prog. Cardiovasc. Dis.* **2017**, *59*, 455. [CrossRef] [PubMed]
27. Risling, T.; Martinez, J.; Young, J.; Thorp-Froslie, N. Evaluating Patient Empowerment in Association With eHealth Technology: Scoping Review. *J. Med. Internet Res.* **2017**, *19*, e329. [CrossRef] [PubMed]
28. Morris, A.S.; Mackintosh, K.A.; Owen, N.; Dempsey, P.C.; Dunstan, D.W.; McNarry, M.A. Rise and recharge: Exploring employee perceptions of and contextual factors influencing an individual-level e-health smartphone intervention to reduce office workers' sedentary time at work. *Int. J. Environ. Res. Public Health* **2021**, *18*, 9627. [CrossRef] [PubMed]
29. Levac, D.; Colquhoun, H.; O'Brien, K.K. Scoping studies: Advancing the methodology. *Implement. Sci.* **2010**, *5*, 69. [CrossRef]
30. Jansons, P.; Dalla Via, J.; Daly, R.M.; Fyfe, J.J.; Gvozdenko, E.; Scott, D. Delivery of Home-Based Exercise Interventions in Older Adults Facilitated by Amazon Alexa: A 12-week Feasibility Trial. *J. Nutr. Health Aging* **2022**, *26*, 96–102. [CrossRef]
31. Alley, S.; Jennings, C.; Plotnikoff, R.C.; Vandelanotte, C. Web-based video-coaching to assist an automated computer-tailored physical activity intervention for inactive adults: A randomized controlled trial. *J. Med. Internet Res.* **2016**, *18*. [CrossRef]
32. Konstantinidis, E.I.; Billis, A.S.; Mouzakidis, C.A.; Zilidou, V.I.; Antoniou, P.E.; Bamidis, P.D. Design, implementation, and wide pilot deployment of FitForAll: An Easy to use exergaming platform improving physical fitness and life quality of senior citizens. *IEEE J. Biomed. Heal. Inform.* **2016**, *20*, 189–200. [CrossRef]
33. Sánchez, M.F.C.; Ureta, C.R.; BasualtoAlfaro, P.; García-Huidobro, G.B.; Giné, M.C. Experiencia en el uso de videos para la promoción de ejercicio físico en el hogar en modalidad online en personas mayores en Chile durante la pandemia COVID-19. *Rev. Esp. Geriatr. Gerontol.* **2022**, *57*, 79–84. [CrossRef]
34. Bastidas, O.J.; Zahia, S.; Fuente-Vidal, A.; Férez, N.S.; Noguera, O.R.; Montane, J.; Garcia-Zapirain, B. Predicting physical exercise adherence in fitness apps using a deep learning approach. *Int. J. Environ. Res. Public Health* **2021**, *18*, 10769. [CrossRef]
35. Albergoni, A.; Hettinga, F.J.; Stut, W.; Sartor, F. Factors Influencing Walking and Exercise Adherence in Healthy Older Adults Using Monitoring and Interfacing Technology: Preliminary Evidence. *Int. J. Environ. Res. Public Health* **2020**, *17*, 6142. [CrossRef] [PubMed]

36. Pischke, C.R.; Voelcker-Rehage, C.; Peters, M.; Ratz, T.; Pohlabeln, H.; Meyer, J.; Von Holdt, K.; Lippke, S. Implementation and Effects of Information Technology-Based and Print-Based Interventions to Promote Physical Activity Among Community-Dwelling Older Adults: Protocol for a Randomized Crossover Trial. *JMIR Res. Protoc.* **2020**, *9*, e15168. [CrossRef] [PubMed]
37. Feng, N.C.; Ryan, E.; Kidane, M.; Tusch, E.S.; McFeeley, B.M.; Carlsson, R.; Mohammed, A.H.; Håkansson, K.; Daffner, K.R. Feasibility of an at-home, web-based, interactive exercise program for older adults. *Alzheimer's Dement. Transl. Res. Clin. Interv.* **2019**, *5*, 825–833. [CrossRef]
38. Dawson, J.; Ede, A.; Nguyen, V.; Sequeira, A.; Donlin, A. Quantification Of Adherence In A Mobile Health Exercise Intervention For Cardiometabolic Health. *Med. Sci. Sport. Exerc.* **2021**, *53*, 234. [CrossRef]
39. Liang, I.J.; Perkin, O.J.; McGuigan, P.M.; Thompson, D.; Western, M.J. Feasibility and Acceptability of Home-Based Exercise Snacking and Tai Chi Snacking Delivered Remotely to Self-Isolating Older Adults During COVID-19. *J. Aging Phys. Act.* **2021**, *30*, 33–43. [CrossRef] [PubMed]
40. Lam, T. Clinical Trial Protocol: Efficacy of a Short-Bout Handgrip Exercise Intervention for Smoking Cessation: A Pilot Randomized Controlled Trial. Available online: https://clinicaltrials.gov/ct2/show/NCT02844296 (accessed on 5 February 2021).
41. Sun, R.-T.; Han, W.; Chang, H.-L.; Shaw, M.J. Motivating Adherence to Exercise Plans Through a Personalized Mobile Health App: Enhanced Action Design Research Approach. *JMIR Mhealth Uhealth* **2021**, *9*, e19941. [CrossRef] [PubMed]
42. Burkhart, P.V.; Sabaté, E. Adherence to Long-Term Therapies: Evidence for Action. *J. Nurs. Scholarsh.* **2003**, *35*, 207. [CrossRef]
43. Du, H.; Venkatakrishnan, A.; Youngblood, G.M.; Ram, A.; Pirolli, P. A Group-based mobile application to increase adherence in exercise and nutrition programs: A factorial design feasibility study. *JMIR Mhealth Uhealth* **2016**, *4*, e4. [CrossRef]
44. Sackett, D.L.; Haynes, R.B.; Gibson, E.S.; Taylor, D.W.; Roberts, R.S.; Johnson, A.L. Patient compliance with antihypertensive regimens. *Patient Couns. Health Educ.* **1978**, *1*, 18–21. [CrossRef]
45. Cugelman, B.; Thelwall, M.; Dawes, P. Online interventions for social marketing health behavior change campaigns: A meta-analysis of psychological architectures and adherence factors. *J. Med. Internet Res.* **2011**, *13*, e17. [CrossRef]
46. Sanatkar, S.; Baldwin, P.A.; Huckvale, K.; Clarke, J.; Christensen, H.; Harvey, S.; Proudfoot, J. Using cluster analysis to explore engagement and e-attainment as emergent behavior in electronic mental health. *J. Med. Internet Res.* **2019**, *21*, e14728. [CrossRef] [PubMed]
47. Pratap, A.; Neto, E.C.; Snyder, P.; Stepnowsky, C.; Elhadad, N.; Grant, D.; Mohebbi, M.H.; Mooney, S.; Suver, C.; Wilbanks, J.; et al. Indicators of retention in remote digital health studies: A cross-study evaluation of 100,000 participants. *NPJ Digit. Med.* **2020**, *3*, 21. [CrossRef] [PubMed]
48. Pekmezi, D.; Ainsworth, C.; Holly, T.; Williams, V.; Joseph, R.; Wang, K.; Rogers, L.Q.; Marcus, B.; Desmond, R.; Demark-Wahnefried, W. Physical Activity and Related Psychosocial Outcomes From a Pilot Randomized Trial of an Interactive Voice Response System–Supported Intervention in the Deep South. *Heal. Educ. Behav.* **2018**, *45*, 957–966. [CrossRef]
49. Hutchesson, M.J.; Tan, C.Y.; Morgan, P.; Callister, R.; Collins, C. Enhancement of Self-Monitoring in a Web-Based Weight Loss Program by Extra Individualized Feedback and Reminders: Randomized Trial. *J. Med. Internet Res.* **2016**, *18*, e82. [CrossRef] [PubMed]
50. Guertler, D.; Vandelanotte, C.; Kirwan, M.; Duncan, M.J. Engagement and Nonusage Attrition With a Free Physical Activity Promotion Program: The Case of 10,000 Steps Australia. *J. Med. Internet Res.* **2015**, *17*, e176. [CrossRef]
51. Liew, S.J.; Gorny, A.W.; Tan, C.S.; Müller-Riemenschneider, F. A mobile health team challenge to promote stepping and stair climbing activities: Exploratory feasibility study. *JMIR Mhealth Uhealth* **2020**, *8*, e12665. [CrossRef]
52. de Souto Barreto, P.; Pothier, K.; Soriano, G.; Lussier, M.; Bherer, L.; Guyonnet, S.; Piau, A.; Ousset, P.-J.; Vellas, B. A Web-Based Multidomain Lifestyle Intervention for Older Adults: The eMIND Randomized Controlled Trial. *J. Prev. Alzheimer's Dis.* **2021**, *8*, 142–150. [CrossRef]

International Journal of
Environmental Research and Public Health

MDPI

Review

Biomechanical Risks Associated with Foot and Ankle Injuries in Ballet Dancers: A Systematic Review

Fengfeng Li [1], Ntwali Adrien [1,2] and Yuhuan He [1,3,4,*]

1 Faculty of Sports Science, Ningbo University, Ningbo 315211, China; lifengfeng1999@hotmail.com (F.L.); ntwaliadrien@yahoo.com (N.A.)
2 Savaria Institute of Technology, Eötvös Loránd University, 9700 Szombathely, Hungary
3 Department of Physical and Health Education, Udon Thani Rajabhat University, Udon Thani 41000, Thailand
4 CEEC Economic and Trade Cooperation Institute, Ningbo University, Ningbo 315211, China
* Correspondence: heyuhuan@nbu.edu.cn; Tel.: +86-574-87600456

Abstract: Professional ballet dancers can be classified as dance artists and sports performers. This systematic review aims to consider the biomechanical risk factors for foot and ankle injuries in ballet dancers, as this could potentially reduce the impact that 'cost of injury' may have on ballet companies. An additional outcome was to examine the effects of injury on the career of ballet dancers. This study searched articles in four electronic databases for information in peer-reviewed journals. The included articles examined the relationships between biomechanical factors and the relationship between ballet shoes and foot performance. There were 9 articles included in this review. Among these articles, two focused on the peak force of the foot using two types of pointe shoes, three focused on overuse injuries of the ballet dancer's foot, one article focused on the loading of the foot of a dancer, and three articles focused on the function and biomechanics of the foot in dancers. This review also found that the pointe shoe condition was the most important factor contributing to a foot injury; overuse injury related to high-intensity training and affected both the ankle and the foot; and metatarsophalangeal joint injury related to the function and structure of the foot. Finally, strengthening the lower extremity muscle is also a recommendation to improve muscle coordination and reduce injuries.

Keywords: ballet dance; foot and ankle injuries; lower limb biomechanics

1. Introduction

The lower extremities continue to be a research issue in sports sciences [1]. Dancing may be termed a special competitive sport and dancers perform an activity in both open and closed kinetic chains [2]. The open-chain suggests that when performing a movement, the foot is not involved in any weight-bearing activity but moves freely in the air [2]. The closed chain indicates that in a dance movement the foot is subjected to weight-bearing and that all the joints are involved [3]. All dance movements comply with biomechanical rules and laws otherwise there are consequences in terms of injuries, including both chronic and acute injury. Kinetics analysis can also identify injury status using musculoskeletal modeling [4–6]. Additionally, in a dance movement, the dancers are required to maintain full ankle plantarflexion and extend through the mid-foot to the toes. This occurs when the foot and ankle are in an abnormal position and increases the flexibility of the ankle [7]. When we consider that foot joints and ligaments are not designed to accept excessive loading, the changes in a dance movement could result in the compression of the soft tissue structure and therefore joint injury [8].

Professional ballet dancers are dance artists, and due to the high-intensity training required and the technical discipline and difficulty needed for dance performance, "dance injury" is common in ballet dancers [9–11]. All forms of dance contain highly demanding movements, with an injury incidence of up to 95% over a dancer's lifetime [12–15]. Studies have focused on the injury of the knee joint and upper limbs; however, studies are lacking on the intense physical demands of dancing that exposes dancers' feet to a high risk of injuries such as hallux valgus, metatarsal injury, and subsequent ankle pain [16–19]. Although clinical examination often points to the underlying cause, injury prevention is often necessary to decrease dance company costs and ensure longevity in the dancers' careers [20]. As a theatrical performance, ballet is considered a global art [21] requiring dance companies to improve the technique of dancers to provide performances at high technical levels. As a result, injury rehabilitation costs are a significant part of the total expenses for a ballet dance company [22]. The human musculoskeletal system refers to the system having its muscles attached to an internal skeletal system. This structure is crucial for humans to perform complex activities, and because of the complex movements in ballet, injuries are common in ballet dancers. Previous studies have revealed that the injury incidence rate reaches 67–95% in ballet dancers [12–15,23]. Ballet dancers have a higher incidence of dance injury among all dancers.

Among all the reported injuries, foot and ankle injuries account for a large percentage of all musculoskeletal injuries and are particularly vulnerable to secondary damage suffered by dancers. This is primarily caused by the maximum dorsiflexion or a maximum effort in a turned-out position. For example, the excess force of rotation or turnout of the en pointe (shown in Figure 1) can lead to ankle and foot injuries and cause strain of structures around the ankle [24–26]. However, the full extent of the risk factors for foot and ankle injuries in dancers has not yet been summarized. In addition to the upper body and knee injuries, foot- and ankle-related injuries in ballet dancers are high. Foot and ankle function is complicated and needs detailed discussion to determine the mechanisms of injury. It is essential to reach a consensus regarding the benefits of injury prevention among ballet dancers, as this could potentially reduce the impact 'cost of injury' may have on ballet companies. Therefore, the purpose of this systematic review was to provide an up to date biomechanical assessment of studies on injury prevention among ballet dancers.

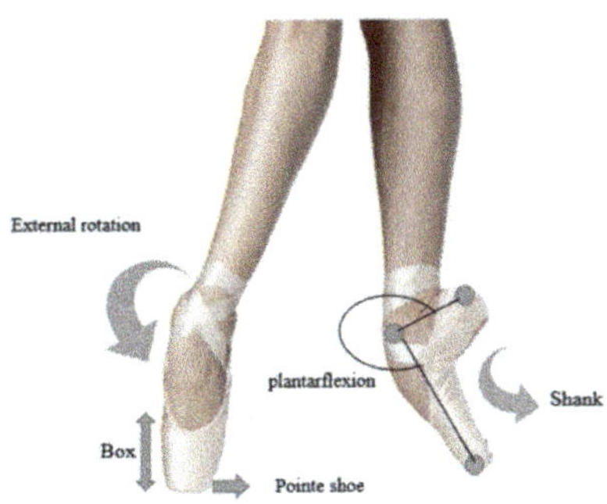

Figure 1. Dancing in the en pointe phase (pointe shoes: the shoes worn by ballet dancers during performance or training; Box: a shoe box that wraps and supports the toes at the front of the shoe; Shank: a piece of rigid shoe bone that reinforces the sole for more support).

2. Materials and Methods

2.1. Search Strategy

The authors reviewed the literature published from 1900 through December 2021, on foot and ankle injuries in ballet dance. To identify relevant articles, the research was conducted using five databases: Medline, Web of Science, Web of Science, Research Gate, Embase, and Scopus. The detailed electronic search used the following keywords: "ballet dance", "dancers", injury", "ankle injuries", "biomechanics injury", "biomechanics", "lower limb", "foot", "problems", "foot injury", "pointe shoes", and "injury risk". Among these, "ballet dance", "foot", and "injury" were connected with [and]; "biomechanics", "pointe shoes", "problems", and "ankle injury" were connected with [or]. All keywords were searched on each database individually and in combination. Figure 2 shows the detailed search strategy, and Table 1 shows the basic information of the included articles.

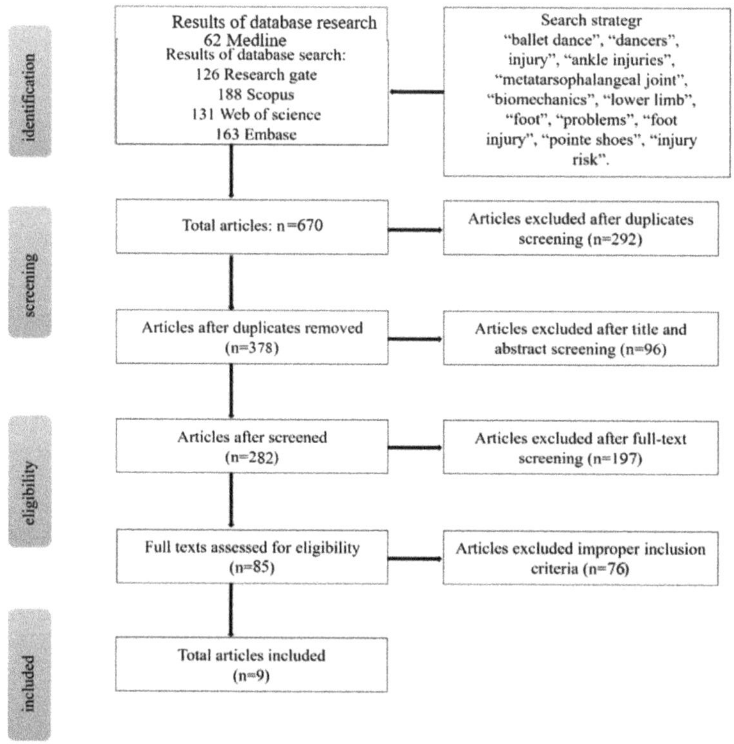

Figure 2. The detailed search strategy of the review.

Table 1. Basic information of the included articles.

Number	Author/Date	Title	Journal	Concentration
1	Bickle et al., 2018	The effect of pointe shoe deterioration on foot and ankle kinematics and kinetics in professional ballet dancers	Human movement science	Pointe shoes
2	Aquino et al., 2019	Biomechanical Comparison of "Dead" and "New" Pointe Shoes in Female Professional Ballet Dancers	The sport journal	Pointe shoes
3	Prochazkova et al., 2014	Analysis of foot load during ballet dancer's gait	Acta of Bioengineering and Biomechanics	Foot loading
4	Alyssa et al., 2019	Ground Reaction Forces in Ballet Differences Resulting from Footwear and Jump Conditions	Journal of Dance Medicine & Science	Foot loading
5	Liederbach et al., 2014	Comparison of landing biomechanics between male and female dancers and athletes, part: influence of fatigue and implications for anterior cruciate ligament injury	The American Journal of Sports Medicine	Overuse
6	Lin et al., 2016	Fatigue-Induced Changes in Movement Pattern and Muscle Activity During Ballet Releve on Demi-Pointe	Journal of Applied Biomechanics	Overuse
7	Rippetoe et al., 2020	Multi-Segment Assessment of Ankle and Foot Kinematics during Relevé Barefoot and En Pointe	Pereforming arts foot & ankle	Overuse
8	Jarvis et al., 2016	Kinematic and kinetic analyses of the toes in dance movements	Journal of sports sciences	Foot
9	Astone et al., 2019	Comparison of gait kinematics and kinetics between qualified dancers and non-dancers	Journal of Physical Education and Sport	Foot

2.2. Study Selection

Duplicate studies were identified from the different databases and removed. Then, the potential for bias was minimized. Following this, the first two authors independently performed article screening, which included the title, abstract, full-text, and data extraction examination. If disagreement occurred, a third reviewer was identified to review the opinion to reconcile differences.

2.3. Data Extraction and Eligibility Criteria

The data were retrieved from the selected articles: the author, publication years, participants' characteristics, ballet footwear condition, measured variables, purpose, and result. In data extraction, in case of disagreement, another reviewer was included in the discussion to reach a consensus.

2.4. Data Eligibility Criteria

The eligibility of selecting papers was estimated according to the following inclusion criteria: (1) the article had to focus primarily on healthy dancer participants wearing pointe shoes; (2) the literature was published in English; (3) the articles focused on the risk factors for the biomechanics of foot injuries in ballet dancers; (4) full articles were based on foot biomechanics injury risk of ballet dancers; and (5) the articles had to be retrievable. When the abstract did not sufficiently present the details for any of the eligibility criteria, the author would browse the full text. The article would be disregarded if it failed to meet the eligibility criteria. The included articles' characteristics and results are presented in Table 2.

Table 2. The characteristics and results of included articles.

First Author, Publication Year	Participants (Age: Year; Height: m; Weight: kg)	Experimental Measurements and Purposes	Results
Bickle, 2018	n = 15 age: 26 ± 4 height: 1.63 ± 0.61 weight: 51.7 ± 3.8	A 2D video camera, A force platform (Kistler 9287BA Force Platform, Kistler Instruments Ltd., Hampshire, UK), A pedobarograph (RSScan 0.5 m USB2 Plate, RS Scan Ipswich, UK) Purpose: investigating the differences in the kinetic and kinematic of the foot and ankle between a new and a worn pointe shoe.	There is a significantly greater mid-foot flexion and plantarflexion existing in the worn shoes as compared to new shoes,
Aquino, 2019	n = 13 age: 20.9 ± 1.9 height: 1.64 ± 0.35 weight: 52.1 ± 5.6	All data using an AMTI force plate collected (sampling rate of 960 Hz) Purpose: Examine the ground reaction forces and center of pressure differences between a "new" and "dead" shoe.	The way area of oscillation was significantly higher in "dead" shoes and the training time of the pointe shoe was related to an overuse injury in female ballet dancers.
Astone, 2019	n = 6 age: medial 22.83 height: medial 1.64 weight: 56	An optoelectronic system with six infrared cameras, two force platforms (BTS P6000) Purpose: comparing the gait kinematics and kinetics between professional dancers and non-dancers.	The dance movement they performed caused some differences in their motor skills. Dancers apply for compensation during their gait cycle that makes their gait as effective as possible.
Prochazkova, 2014	n = 13 (professional dancers) age: 24.1 ± 3.8 height: 1.70 ± 0.85 weight: 58.3 ± 11.2 n = 13 (non-dancers) age: 26.1 ± 5.3 height: 1.73 ± 0.73 weight: 74.1 ± 12.5	the Footscan gait software (version 7.97) purpose: comparing the peak pressure, total loading, and duration of the loading in the selected areas of the foot between the experimental group and control group.	There are greater peak pressure values in the big toe and higher values in the areas of the medial heel in professional dancers. The heel areas have a significantly longer duration of contact with the floor in both two groups.
Liederbach et al., 2014	n = 40 (female 20; male 20)	purpose: analyzing dancers and team atheletes' resistance and its effect on the biomechanics of single-legged landings.	Dancers took longer to reach fatigue, and female athletes are more prone to ACL injury after fatigue.

Table 2. *Cont.*

First Author, Publication Year	Participants (Age: Year; Height: m; Weight: kg)	Experimental Measurements and Purposes	Results
Lin et al., 2016	*n* = 20 (female) age: 17.98 ± 1.51 height: 1.60 ± 0.57 weight: 49.8 ± 5.4	A motion analysis system (Motion Analysis Corporation, Santa Rosa, CA, USA) Purpose: This article aims to evaluate the impact of fatigue on the performance of ballet dancers	Over-training has been seen as the most common risk factor for fatigue, which would result in impaired movement control and may therefore increase the risk of dance injury.
Rippetoe, 2020	*n* = 11 age: 21 height: 1.68 weight: 55.11	12-camera Qualisys™ Motion Analysis System and AMTI Force plates Purpose: describe the biomechanical differences between the barefoot and en pointe conditions while balancing in relevé and the differences between the barefoot and en pointe shoes.	There is a greater sagittal movement, and a greater midfoot, forefoot, arch height, and rotation movement when a dancer balances barefoot.
Jarvis, 2016	*n* = 10 age: 27.6 ± 3.2 height: 1.60 ± 0.1 weight: 56.3 ± 6.9	An 11-camera three-dimensional motion analysis system, AMTI force plate Purpose: comparing the motion and moments of the metatarsophalangeal joints during three common dance movements.	The peak joint moments related to the dance movement, and the largest values were found during saut de chat leaps, and the smallest value was found during relevés. Many dance movements place high demands on the foot and ankle joints.
Alyssa, 2019	*n* = 21 age: 19.28 ± 1.00 height:1.67 ± 0.44 weight: 52.74 ± 3.42	A recessed force plate (AMTI Accugait System Model ACG, Watertown, MA, USA) with a 2.5 m runway, a video camera (Sony Electronics Inc., San Diego, CA, USA) Purpose: (1) Investigating the maximal ground reaction force when dancer lands from two jump conditions in pointe shoes, barefoot and flat shoes; (2) exploring the specific pointe shoes characteristics effect on ground reaction force.	There is no significant difference in maximum ground reaction force between the three shoe conditions. A significant difference was found between the two types of jump conditions. The jumping distance was greater in the grand jeté but the jumping height was greater in assemble.

3. Results

The bibliographical database search identified 670 citations: 62 in Medline, 126 in Research Gate, 131 in Web of Science, 163 in Embase, and 188 in Scopus. This left a total of 378 articles for evaluation after duplications were removed. Two hundred and eighty-two studies were eliminated following the scanning of the titles and abstracts of the papers. The content of these papers did not reach the required standards for this review. The remaining 85 full-text studies were extracted for detailed review. Seventy-six studies were excluded, as these papers failed to meet the inclusion criteria. A total of nine cross-sectional studies were eventually used and all fully met the inclusion criteria.

Recommendations for decreasing the negative impact of the injury on ballet dancers include three important parameters: (1) shoe condition, (2) overuse injury, and (3) foot biomechanics and function. The investigation on foot and ankle injuries involved biomechanical changes in the lower extremities. Kinematics, such as plantar pressure and peak force in different regions of the foot were investigated. One included study involved the testing of the gait of ballet dancers to compare the difference in foot loading between professional dancers and non-dancers to further analyze risk factors for ballet dancers.

Two studies included several experiments to determine a foot injury for ballet dancers. Based on three different ballet movements (relevé, sous-sus, and pirouette), Aquino et al. assessed the effect of 'dead' and 'new' pointe shoes on peak forces generated by the foot in professional ballet dancers [27]. The results indicated that the sway area of the swing was significantly higher in the 'dead' shoes compared to the 'new' shoes. The peak force was significantly higher in the forefoot and hindfoot in the "new" shoe condition when compared to the "dead" shoe condition. Having a higher sway area suggests that a lack of support may contribute to less stability in the foot and ankle joint for ballet dancers when performing routines on their toes. However, there was no difference in peak force between the "new" and "dead" shoes in Bickle et al.'s study. Bickle et al. assessed the differences in the foot and ankle of ballet dancers' kinetics and kinematics between new and worn pointe shoes [28]. The mid-foot flexion in the "new" and "worn" shoe conditions were significantly different (New: 89.7 ± 5.5°; Old: 96.1 ± 3.9°, $p = 0.002$, $\eta^2 = 0.516$). The mean results indicated that a significantly greater mid-foot flexion and plantarflexion existed in the worn shoes compared to the new shoes. The mean results indicated that a significantly greater mid-foot flexion and plantarflexion existed in the worn shoes when compared to new shoes. The study also observed that having a greater mid-foot flexion and plantarflexion may be a factor contributing to a higher incidence of ankle and foot injury in ballet dancers [29].

Three studies demonstrated that a fatigue-induced overuse injury is common in ballet dancers. A dancer who requires a long training period has a greater risk of a dance-related injury. In their study, Liederbach et al. concluded that a longer training duration may lead to fatigue, moreover, female athletes were more prone to ACL injury after fatigue [30]. Additionally, Rippetoe et al. determined that a repeated balance technique in the performance of relevé could place atypical stresses and pressure on the joints as well as the tissues of the foot and ankle [31]. The force affected the foot and ankle while performing a dance movement, possibly contributing to injuries among dancers. Previous studies have suggested that around 30% of dancers suffering from acute ankle sprain would develop chronic ankle instability with recurring sprain [32]. Classical ballet requires the dancer to move the ankle between maximum weight-bearing dorsiflexion and maximum weight-bearing plantarflexion. The movements are repeatedly executed during the performance, in daily training, and during rehearsals. Lin et al. mentioned in their research that over-training has been seen as the most common risk factor for fatigue, which would result in impaired movement control and may therefore increase the risk of dance injury [33]. The results suggested that the length of training time in ballet was associated with an increase in the angular values of the left and the right foot, and had a tendency for worsening with increased training time.

Two articles mentioned that understanding the loading distribution strategies of a ballet dancer's foot is crucial in determining the incidence of foot injury or deformity in the dancer. Prochazkova et al. used a 2 m pressure plate (RSscan International, Olen, Belgium) to collect the gait data of participants (professional dancers and non-dancers) [34]. The results indicated that, compared with non-dancers, the values of the pressure impulse of the big toe and the first metatarsus areas in professional ballet dancers were observed to be significantly higher. The study also revealed that the loading duration of the foot was mainly concentrated on the big toe in ballet dancers. McPherson et al. compared two types of jumping styles (assemble, grand jeté) and three different foot and shoe conditions (flat shoes, pointe shoes, and barefoot) to investigate the maximum ground reaction forces in ballet dancers [35]. The results found that the grand jeté condition had a significantly higher GRFmax than the assemble condition. However, the three shoe and foot conditions showed no significant differences.

Rigidus of the hallux is an arthritic condition of the metatarsophalangeal joint, and excessive pronation of the foot is an important risk factor in the development of hallux valgus. Ballet dancers need 80 to 100 dorsiflexion while performing the act of relevés onto demi-pointe; this is a significantly disabling condition for a ballet dancer. In addition, the stiffness of the foot joint encourages a dancer to roll onto the lateral metatarsals which supports the most bodyweight. Jarvis et al. observed participants performing three different dance movements (relevés, sautés, and saut de chat leaps), and collected data; the article suggested that the focus of relevés is controlling the maximum ankle plantar flexion and metatarsophalangeal joint extension [36]. The greatest range of motion of the metatarsophalangeal joint is required in a ballet dance movement such as relevés. While the peak moment of the metatarsophalangeal joint, observed in the previous study, is small compared to other lower extremity joints, it is essential to consider the metatarsophalangeal joint in a dance injury [37]. Additionally, for the metatarsophalangeal joints, there is a higher demand for ballet dancers than in many other types of movements, which could potentially lead to pain in the foot or damaged toe conditions. Astone et al. examined the differences in the foot while ballet dancers walked compared with non-dancers, and observed that when the feet move, they move with an extra rotation during all walking cycles, reducing the energy expended [38].

4. Discussion

To reach a full understanding of the biomechanical risk factors associated with foot and ankle injuries in ballet dancers, knowledge of foot plantar pressure, footwear, and peak force are crucial. This systematic review identified nine articles which appraised either the effect of pointe shoes or overuse on lower limb injuries in ballet dancers. To determine the incidence of foot injury in ballet dancers, it is important to understand ballet position compensatory strategies. This review found that: (1) the pointe shoe condition is an important factor contributing to a foot injury; (2) overuse injury is related to high-intensity training and affected the ankle and foot; (3) metatarsophalangeal joint injury is related to the function and structure of the foot and results in swelling as the demands on the foot increase; and (4) footwear is also related to overuse injuries in professional ballet dancers.

Two studies met the inclusion criteria, the two articles identified the differences between "new" and "dead" pointe shoes. They used different methods, and a consensus emerged that a worn pointe shoe in a dance movement resulted in a significantly increased swing area, especially in the forefoot and mid-foot. Previous studies have found that injuries in ballet dancers can result from inadequate stabilization of the foot and ankle [39]. Pointe shoes are supportive of the foot, which provide stiffness with the compromise of the midfoot ligaments. Having a significant swing in the midfoot area may decrease stiffness and increase the lack of support in the dancer's foot, increasing the risk of lower limb injury. Previous studies suggested that during some specific dance movements, a repeated impact placed on the foot and ankle may possibly lead to a unique type of injury in a group of dance performers [25,31,40]. Although the peak ankle plantarflexion range of motion was not significantly different between dancers and non-dancers, it should be considered that the plantarflexion function and range of motion of ballet dancers needs measurably exceeded normative values than non-dancers (0 to 50 degrees) [7,41]. Thus, injury prevention is of great significance.

The human foot is an essential element of the locomotor system. It transports the power and the mass of the whole body while in contact with the ground. Ballet dancers use the foot to reach extreme external rotations and the foot and ankle need to twist in the air. As a result, the intense physical demands of dancing put dancers' feet at high risk of injuries such as hallux valgus, metatarsal injury, and ankle pain [16–19]. These injuries in a ballet dancer can result in two categories of injury: acute injury, and chronic injury. The structural differences among dancers may change lower limb kinetics and kinematics. The foot has been considered as a triple-arch structure, and the part of the lateral foot performs a rigid arch that supports our weight in a loaded position. Once the weight of the dancer is directed to the mid-foot, there will be consequences for the other parts of the foot. Additionally, to reach an extreme position in ballet, external rotation, especially at the ankle joint, is of great importance for dancers. The limitation of range of motion in the ankle may cause foot pronation (rolling in), and subsequently cause the foot to lose medial arch support. If the stability provided by the mid-foot begins to fail or decrease, dance performance will compensate to maintain the center of mass. Once the performer cannot compensate to keep the body in a correct position the dancer may fall out of the position, which can be the result of an acute injury. Therefore, the evaluation of dancers' foot injuries and pain should be included in clinical studies, and superimposed X-rays for assessing ankle and foot contributions to the extreme positions required of female ballet dancers offer insight into how these positions are attained [7].

Both the first metatarsophalangeal joint and the ankle are attached to the flexor hallucis longus [25,40,41], and flexor hallucis longus tendinopathy is common in ballet dancers. The metatarsophalangeal joints endure a repeated large range of motion and high peak joint moments may be a risk factor that contributes to the injury of the foot and ankle joints in dancing. Mattiussi et al. suggested that a greater percentage of injuries were classified as overuse injuries [42]. In addition, Shaw et al. noted in their study that older dancers in advanced groups were more likely to be injured [43]. Additionally, the lateral ligament complex of the ankle is the most frequently injured structure of a dancer's body. In many sports, ankle sprains do not develop into long-term disabilities, however, many patients do not resolve the problem well, which results in residual symptoms persisting for many years. In the continuous training and performance of dancers, repeatedly jumping and landing as well as the extreme plantarflexion or rotation is required. During these dance movements, the repeated shocks and pressure will impact the injured area, and the commonly reported symptoms in dancers include ankle re-injury and instability [44]. All of the articles reviewed mentioned that wearing a pointe shoe and overuse on their foot may accelerate rates of muscle fatigue and ankle sprains [25,45]. Once the forefoot strength decreases, the leg will externally rotate, and the support of the hip joint's muscle will be not stable when the heel is raised. As a result, all the joint chains will be affected, and ankle and foot re-injury is known to occur in many dancers.

In a ballet dance movement, executing the correct motion such as a simple heel raise of relevé when suffering frequent injuries to the lower limb is painful. Biomechanical analysis evaluating the function of muscles, bones, and tendons is essential in developing diagnostic tools to help identify the causes of injuries for any type of dancer, particularly ballet dancers. The footwear that is needed for each type of dance must also be determined, especially in ballet. It has been suggested that ballet dance footwear manufacturers should consider biomechanical design features in shoe manufacturing, as opposed to just focusing on the aesthetics of the shoes themselves [39]. In support of this, ground reaction force analysis has been seen as a variable of interest because of its potential correlation with increased injury rates. A reasonable design of dance footwear can reduce impact force and improve the stability of a dancer. An emergency stop is a basic technique for a professional dancer, therefor, the muscular lower extremity seems important in daily classes and needs preventive strategies to reduce the risk of injury. Biernack et al. suggested that lower limb strength is also an important factor leading to injuries in the lower extremities [46]. The long-term and intense extreme demands of the musculoskeletal system are relative to plantar pressure distribution in ballet dancers. Therefore, the dancers and dance trainers should reach a consensus that enhancing the controllability of the ankle and foot can reduce ankle restrains to a certain extent. In particular, the flexor hallucis longus and muscle strength enhancement can decrease tenosynovitis probability [47,48]. Dancers also create abnormal dynamic biomechanical forces when using various dance forms [49]. A thorough determination of these forces may inform the physician about the cause of the injures, especially specific overuse injuries. The knowledge provided here is important in the prevention of foot and ankle injuries in ballet dancers. Dance companies need to provide methodologies that reduce the incidence of injury, while improving the teaching quality of dance instruction. We suggest researching the corresponding dynamic effects for pointe shoes in further research. However, there are also some limitations in the current study. First, we focused on the lower limb biomechanics of ballet dancers. Secondly, this review presented some literature that has no specific data, and quantitative assessments cannot be carried out.

5. Conclusions

There is substantial evidence for ballet dance injury. Dance medical science, physical medicine, and sports science provide details about the importance of dance injury prevention in dance training. As an art form, ballet dancing requires tremendous physicality, and injury prevention is very important in this discipline. Foot and ankle problems are the predominant pathologies in dance medicine. Therefore, our study systematically reviewed research focused on the risk factors of ankle and foot injuries in ballet dancers. The elements of pointe shoes, overuse of the lower extremity, and the biomechanics and function of the foot are associated with lower limb injury. Improving the design of the shoes to provide stiffness with the compromise of the mid-foot ligaments to reduce injuries seems to be important. However, there are still some limitations in this review; due to the different methodologies used between all the included articles, the data presented in this review are limited. Further analysis is required, focusing on finite element model analysis and electromyography, combined with kinetic and kinematics analysis of the lower limb in ballet dancers. Moreover, we suggest studying the corresponding dynamic effects for pointe shoes in further research. This will provide a better understanding of ballet, and promote ballet dancing to the public while preventing the injury of ballet dancers.

Author Contributions: Conceptualization, F.L. and Y.H.; methodology, F.L.; software, N.A.; investigation, Y.H.; resources, F.L.; data curation, F.L. and N.A.; writing—original draft preparation, Y.H.; writing—review and editing, F.L.; supervision, Y.H. All authors have read and agreed to the published version of the manuscript.

Funding: This study was sponsored by the Key Project of the National Social Science Foundation of China (19ZDA352), and K. C. Wong Magna Fund in Ningbo University.

Conflicts of Interest: The authors declare that they have no conflict interest.

References

1. Xu, D.; Quan, W.; Zhou, H.; Sun, D.; Baker, J.S.; Gu, Y. Explaining the differences of gait patterns between high and low-mileage runners with machine learning. *Sci. Rep.* **2022**, *12*, 2981. [CrossRef]
2. Ahonen, J. Biomechanics of the foot in dance: A literature review. *J. Dance Med. Sci.* **2008**, *12*, 99–108. [PubMed]
3. Barnett, C.H.; Napier, J.R. The axis of rotation at the ankle joint in man. Its influence upon the form of the talus and the mobility of the fibula. *J. Anat.* **1952**, *86*, 1–9.
4. Xu, D.; Jiang, X.; Cen, X.; Baker, J.S.; Gu, Y. Single-leg landings following a volleyball spike may increase the risk of anterior cruciate ligament injury more than landing on both-legs. *Appl. Sci.* **2020**, *11*, 130. [CrossRef]
5. Xu, D.; Zhou, H.; Baker, J.S.; István, B.; Gu, Y. An investigation of differences in lower extremity biomechanics during single-leg landing from height using bionic shoes and normal shoes. *Front. Bioeng. Biotechnol.* **2021**, *9*, 679123. [CrossRef]
6. Zhou, H.; Chen, C.; Xu, D.; Ugbolue, U.C.; Baker, J.S.; Gu, Y. Biomechanical Characteristics between Bionic Shoes and Normal Shoes during the Drop-Landing Phase: A Pilot Study. *Int. J. Environ. Res. Public Health* **2021**, *18*, 3223. [CrossRef] [PubMed]
7. Russell, J.A.; Shave, R.M.; Kruse, D.W.; Koutedakis, Y.; Wyon, M.A. Ankle and foot contributions to extreme plantar-and dorsiflexion in female ballet dancers. *Foot Ankle Int.* **2011**, *32*, 183–188. [CrossRef]
8. Hedrick, M.R.; McBryde, A.M. Posterior ankle impingement. *Foot Ankle Int.* **1994**, *15*, 2–8. [CrossRef] [PubMed]
9. Shah, S.; Weiss, D.S.; Burchette, R.J. Injuries in professional modern dancers: Incidence, risk factors, and management. *J. Dance Med. Sci.* **2012**, *16*, 17–25. [PubMed]
10. Liederbach, M.; Dilgen, F.E.; Rose, D.J. Incidence of anterior cruciate ligament injuries among elite ballet and modern dancers: A 5-year prospective study. *Am. J. Sports Med.* **2008**, *36*, 1779–1788. [CrossRef] [PubMed]
11. Allen, N.; Nevill, A.; Brooks, J.; Koutedakis, Y.; Wyon, M. Ballet injuries: Injury incidence and severity over 1 year. *J. Orthop. Sports Phys. Ther.* **2012**, *42*, 748–821. [CrossRef] [PubMed]
12. Byhring, S.; Bø, K. Musculoskeletal injuries in the Norwegian National Ballet: A prospective cohort study. *Scand. J. Med. Sci. Sports* **2002**, *12*, 365–370. [CrossRef] [PubMed]
13. Nilsson, C.; Leanderson, J.; Wykman, A.; Strender, L.-E. The injury panorama in a Swedish professional ballet company. *Knee Surg. Sports Traumatol. Arthrosc.* **2001**, *9*, 242–246. [CrossRef] [PubMed]
14. Bronner, S.; Ojofeitimi, S.; Rose, D. Injuries in a modern dance company: Effect of comprehensive management on injury incidence and time loss. *Am. J. Sports Med.* **2003**, *31*, 365–373. [CrossRef]
15. Garrick, J.G. Early identification of musculoskeletal complaints and injuries among female ballet students. *J. Dance Med. Sci.* **1999**, *3*, 80–83.
16. Furia, J.P.; Juliano, P.J.; Wade, A.M.; Schaden, W.; Mittermayr, R. Shock wave therapy compared with intramedullary screw fixation for nonunion of proximal fifth metatarsal metaphyseal-diaphyseal fractures. *JBJS* **2010**, *92*, 846–854. [CrossRef] [PubMed]
17. Teitz, C.C. Hip and Knee injuries in dancers. *J. Dance Med. Sci.* **2000**, *4*, 23–29.
18. Bowling, A. Injuries to dancers: Prevalence, treatment, and perceptions of causes. *Br. Med. J.* **1989**, *298*, 731–734. [CrossRef] [PubMed]
19. Werber, B. Dance medicine of the foot and ankle: A review. *Clin. Podiatr. Med. Surg.* **2011**, *28*, 137–154. [CrossRef]

20. Jacobs, C.L.; Hincapié, C.A.; Cassidy, J.D. Musculoskeletal injuries and pain in dancers: A systematic review update. *J. Dance Med. Sci.* **2012**, *16*, 74–84.
21. Saleh, H.A.I.A. Lower limb Kinematic analysis to Le Petit Echappe´ by using two different Pointe Training Pointe and Professional Pointe in ballet. *Int. J. Sports Sci. Arts* **2021**, *17*, 51–70. [CrossRef]
22. Ramkumar, P.N.; Farber, J.; Arnouk, J.; Varner, K.E.; McCulloch, P.C. Injuries in a professional ballet dance company: A 10-year retrospective study. *J. Dance Med. Sci.* **2016**, *20*, 30–37. [CrossRef]
23. Wiesler, E.R.; Hunter, D.M.; Martin, D.F.; Curl, W.W.; Hoen, H. Ankle flexibility and injury patterns in dancers. *Am. J. Sports Med.* **1996**, *24*, 754–757. [CrossRef] [PubMed]
24. Khan, K.; Brown, J.; Way, S.; Vass, N.; Crichton, K.; Alexander, R.; Baxter, A.; Butler, M.; Wark, J. Overuse injuries in classical ballet. *Sports Med.* **1995**, *19*, 341–357. [CrossRef]
25. Kadel, N.J. Foot and ankle injuries in dance. *Phys. Med. Rehabil. Clin.* **2006**, *17*, 813–826. [CrossRef]
26. Quirk, R. Common foot and ankle injuries in dance. *Orthop. Clin. N. Am.* **1994**, *25*, 123–133. [CrossRef]
27. Aquino, J.; Amasay, T. Biomechanical comparison of "dead" and "new" pointe shoes in female professional ballet dancers. *Sport J.* **2019**, *21*, 305–316.
28. Bickle, C.; Deighan, M.; Theis, N. The effect of pointe shoe deterioration on foot and ankle kinematics and kinetics in professional ballet dancers. *Hum. Mov. Sci.* **2018**, *60*, 72–77. [CrossRef] [PubMed]
29. Hincapié, C.A.; Morton, E.J.; Cassidy, J.D. Musculoskeletal injuries and pain in dancers: A systematic review. *Arch. Phys. Med. Rehabil.* **2008**, *89*, 1819–1829. [CrossRef] [PubMed]
30. Liederbach, M.; Kremenic, I.J.; Orishimo, K.F.; Pappas, E.; Hagins, M. Comparison of landing biomechanics between male and female dancers and athletes, part 2: Influence of fatigue and implications for anterior cruciate ligament injury. *Am. J. Sports Med.* **2014**, *42*, 1089–1095. [CrossRef] [PubMed]
31. Rippetoe, J.; Ocsm, M.S. Multi-Segment Assessment of Ankle and Foot Kinematics during Relevé Barefoot and En Pointe. *Orthop. Phys. Ther. Pract.* **2020**, *32*, 167–175.
32. Zhang, B.; Lu, Q. A Current Review of Foot Disorder and Plantar Pressure Alternation in the Elderly. *Phys. Act. Health* **2020**, *4*, 95–106. [CrossRef]
33. Lin, C.-F.; Lee, W.-C.; Chen, Y.-A.; Hsue, B.-J. Fatigue-induced changes in movement pattern and muscle activity during ballet releve on demi-pointe. *J. Appl. Biomech.* **2016**, *32*, 350–358. [CrossRef]
34. Prochazkova, M.; Tepla, L.; Svoboda, Z.; Janura, M.; Cieslarova, M. Analysis of foot load during ballet dancers' gait. *Acta Bioeng. Biomech.* **2014**, *16*, 41–45. [PubMed]
35. McPherson, A.M.; Schrader, J.W.; Docherty, C.L. Ground reaction forces in ballet differences resulting from footwear and jump conditions. *J. Dance Med. Sci.* **2019**, *23*, 34–39. [CrossRef] [PubMed]
36. Jarvis, D.N.; Kulig, K. Kinematic and kinetic analyses of the toes in dance movements. *J. Sports Sci.* **2016**, *34*, 1612–1618. [CrossRef] [PubMed]
37. Petersen, J.; Nielsen, R.O.; Rasmussen, S.; Sørensen, H. Comparisons of increases in knee and ankle joint moments following an increase in running speed from 8 to 12 to 16 km·h(−1). *Clin. Biomech.* **2014**, *29*, 959–964. [CrossRef] [PubMed]
38. Astone, S.; Mignone, A.; Albano, D. Comparison of gait kinematics and kinetics between qualified dancers and non-dancers. *J. Phys. Educ. Sport* **2019**, *19*, 2289–2291.
39. Fong Yan, A.; Hiller, C.; Smith, R.; Vanwanseele, B. Effect of footwear on dancers: A systematic review. *J. Dance Med. Sci.* **2011**, *15*, 86–92.
40. Hamilton, W.G. Posterior ankle pain in dancers. *Clin. Sports Med.* **2008**, *27*, 263–277. [CrossRef]
41. Tao, D.; Gao, Y.; Li, F.; Liang, W.; Jiao, J.; Huang, W.; Supriya, R.; Baker, J. Physical education provision in schools, a role for dance. *Phys. Act. Health* **2022**, *6*, 38–41. [CrossRef]
42. Mattiussi, A.M.; Shaw, J.W.; Williams, S.; Price, P.D.B.; Brown, D.D.; Cohen, D.D.; Clark, R.; Kelly, S.; Retter, G.; Pedlar, C. Injury epidemiology in professional ballet: A five-season prospective study of 1596 medical attention injuries and 543 time-loss injuries. *Br. J. Sports Med.* **2021**, *55*, 843–850. [CrossRef] [PubMed]
43. Shaw, J.W.; Mattiussi, A.M.; Brown, D.D.; Williams, S.; Kelly, S.; Springham, M.; Pedlar, C.R.; Tallent, J. Dance exposure, individual characteristics, and injury risk over five seasons in a professional ballet company. *Med. Sci. Sports Exerc.* **2021**, *53*, 2290–2297. [CrossRef] [PubMed]
44. Ritter, S.; Moore, M. The relationship between lateral ankle sprain and ankle tendinitis in ballet dancers. *J. Dance Med. Sci.* **2008**, *12*, 23–31. [PubMed]
45. Beynnon, B.D.; Murphy, D.F.; Alosa, D.M. Predictive factors for lateral ankle sprains: A literature review. *J. Athl. Train.* **2002**, *37*, 376–380.
46. Biernacki, J.L.; Stracciolini, A.; Fraser, J.; Micheli, L.J.; Sugimoto, D. Risk factors for lower-extremity injuries in female ballet dancers: A systematic review. *Clin. J. Sport Med.* **2021**, *31*, 64–79. [CrossRef]
47. Gu, Y.D.; Li, J.S.; Lake, M.J.; Zeng, Y.J.; Ren, X.J.; Li, Z.Y. Image-based midsole insert design and the material effects on heel plantar pressure distribution during simulated walking loads. *Comput. Methods Biomech. Biomed. Eng.* **2011**, *14*, 747–753. [CrossRef]

48. Xiang, L.; Mei, Q.; Wang, A.; Shim, V.; Fernandez, J.; Gu, Y. Evaluating function in the hallux valgus foot following a 12-week minimalist footwear intervention: A pilot computational analysis. *J. Biomech.* **2022**, *132*, 110941. [CrossRef]
49. Tao, D.; Supriya, R.; Gao, Y.; Li, F.; Liang, W.; Jiao, J.; Baker, J. Dementia and dance: Medication or movement? *Phys. Act. Health* **2021**, *5*, 250–254. [CrossRef]

International Journal of
Environmental Research and Public Health

MDPI

Review

Computation of Fetal Kicking in Various Fetal Health Examinations: A Systematic Review

Yuwei Liu [1], Rongrong Xuan [2,*], Yuhuan He [1,3], Feng Ren [1,*] and Yaodong Gu [1,4]

1 Faculty of Sports Science, Ningbo University, Ningbo 315211, China; zoeliuyuwei@163.com (Y.L.); heyuhuan@nbu.edu.cn (Y.H.); guyaodong@nbu.edu.cn (Y.G.)
2 Affiliated Hospital of Medical School, Ningbo University, Ningbo 315020, China
3 Department of Physical and Health Education, Udon Thani Rajabhat University, Udon Thani 41000, Thailand
4 Faculty of Informatics, Eötvös Loránd University, H-9700 Szombathely, Hungary
* Correspondence: fyxuanrongrong@nbu.edu.cn (R.X.); renfengnb@yeah.net (F.R.)

Abstract: Fetal movement has always been considered an essential indicator to evaluate the health of the unborn fetus. Many factors affect fetal movement. The frequency of fetal kicking is an important measurement of whether fetal development is progressing and healthy. Various instruments and methods of detecting fetal movement have been used and each method has its advantages and disadvantages. Although limited by the fetal environment in utero, the finite element method and musculoskeletal model can be used to calculate fetal lower limb movement. This review aims to summarize the current detection techniques for fetal movement, especially in the lower limbs. These will be outlined by describing the different measurements of fetal movement, and the related biomechanical analyses of fetal lower limb skeletogenesis and the associated muscular development to better evaluate and calculate the movements of the fetus in the womb.

Keywords: fetal movement; kicking; ultrasound; cine-MRI; biomechanical

1. Introduction

Obstetricians discovered the relationship between fetal movement reduction and stillbirth in the 1970s [1]. Sudden alterations in fetal activity include a sudden increase or decrease, or the disappearance of any fetal movement; these changes are often related to adverse fetal outcomes, especially when the fetus is about to be born. Fetal dysplasia or excessive fetal growth during the third trimester is most likely to result in reduced fetal movement. The outcomes include extremely low fetal weight, fetal growth restriction sometimes resulting in premature labor, and fetal death [2–4]. Although examination and measurement of the movement of the fetus prior to birth does not cause any additional physical burden on the pregnant mother or the fetus itself, there is still no specific protocol, such as surgery or drug therapy, to solve the anomalous variations in quickening [5,6]. Extremely vigorous motion in the late gestational phase may indicate that the risk of stillbirth increases threefold; nevertheless, this type of strenuous activity is usually determined in retrospective investigations [5,7]. It has been observed that there is a relationship between unusually vigorous movements and stillbirth [4].

Alterations in fetal motion may be pathological or physiological. Physiologically, there are many causes of fetal movement restriction. As the fetus grows, fetal growth tends to be limited by the uterine environment in the third trimester, which leads to decreased fetal movement. Pathologically, if oxygen and nutrients in the placenta are inadequate, this can lead to the condition of fetal hypokinesis [8,9]. Hypoxia and nutrient consumption cause the brain and central nervous system to save energy physiologically, and as a result, the frequency and intensity of fetal movement decreases. Maternal diseases and chromosomal abnormalities also cause reduced or absent fetal movement [10]. In addition to this, some pathological causes, such as placental dysfunction syndrome, may also result in fetal movement restriction, which ultimately leads to decompensation, and even stillbirth of the fetus [5,6,8,11]. Occasionally, fetal epileptic seizures associated with increased fetal movement can be accompanied by a lack of oxygen, leading to heart failure and possible death [12]. The motor behaviors of neonates, such as posture and reflexes, positively correlate with neurologic impairment. Therefore, the detection of neuropathological conditions related to fetal movements and reactions in the early stage is very crucial [13–15].

The first involuntary fetal movement begins around 7 gestational weeks; independent voluntary movement, such as kicking, commences at 12 weeks as the neuromuscular unit continues to grow [16]. Distinct movement patterns, such as startle, hiccup, stretch, and head or eye movements usually occur at about 15 gestational weeks [17]. Maternal sensation of fetal motion normally occurs after 16 weeks [18]. From the 24th week until the 32nd week of pregnancy, the frequency of fetal movement tends to be steady until labor is about to begin. The evaluation of fetal lower extremities is crucial for the evaluation of neurological disorders and muscular and skeletal development. Therefore, the detection of movement during the period from the gestational age of 24 weeks to postpartum 16 weeks of prematurity plays an essential role in detecting fetal neurodevelopmental abnormalities [19]. The type of fetus movement may change as the pregnancy progresses; nonetheless, during this same period, the frequency does not decrease except for pathological reasons [20]. The regular movement of the fetus has been regarded as one of the indicators of fetal health and represents the normal function of the fetal central nervous system [21,22].

Research has demonstrated via the observation of the movement of a large number of fetuses that in the third trimester, the fetal general range of movement decreases with the progress of the pregnancy. As the fetus grows in size, its range of motion in the womb becomes more limited. The quality and quantity of fetal motion are affected by space constraints in the uterus and the uterine environment. This is particularly prominent as the amplitude of fetal motion decreases near the end of labor. By about 30 weeks of gestation, lower limb motion decreases significantly, which may be related to high flexion of the hip and knee joints. In addition, full-term infants have lower knee and ankle joint angles than term-equivalent age preemies, and are more prone to bending the lower limbs [23]. Although the mechanical stimulation mechanism is unknown, there is a causal link between fetal motion and joint morphology [24]. When neurological dysfunction appears in the early trimester of pregnancy, fetuses often have lower limb disarray and uncontrollable movements throughout the whole body [25]. Therefore, the evaluation of fetal movement is also a notable predictor of neuropathology disorders, not just cerebral palsy or hemiplegia [14,26]. The qualitative and quantitative assessment of general fetal movement is a compatible method for evaluating neurological disorders, diseases, and congenital malformations with growth constraints in the fetus.

Unnatural fetal movement has always been a concern and it is an influential index for evaluating the health of fetal development. A pathological reduction in fetal movement may lead to several diseases, such as dysplasia of the hip, fetal akinesia deformation sequence, and arthrogryposis. With the advent of objective measurement tools, maternal perception is no longer the primary method of assessing fetal movement. Assessment methods such as cardiotocography (CTG), the actograph, ultrasound, and cine-MRI have been used more recently.

These methods have proved to be effective methods to detect fetal movement in clinics. However, it difficult to quantitatively analyze fetal movements accurately using these measurements, especially during late gestation. Therefore, the accuracy and effectiveness of fetal motion assessment are especially important. The most common lower limb movement of the fetus, especially the kicking movement, is significant in the study of fetal maturation and movement. The biomechanical detection and measurement of fetal lower limb movement can provide more accurate data to support fetal whole-body movement and health evaluation. In this study, our aim was to conduct a systematic review to (i) summarize the existing measurement methods for assessing fetal kicking movement and (ii) determine to what extent each method can measure fetal lower limb movement.

2. Materials and Methods

This systematic review followed PRISMA (Preferred Reporting Item for Systematic Reviews and Meta-analysis) protocols [27]. The articles chosen for this review were acquired using searches on PubMed and the Web of Science up until March 2022. Outcomes of interest were conclusions about fetal movements or lower limbs. In the search strategy, the keywords consisted of fetal movement biomechanics and the terms using the Boolean operation keywords in this search were: (fetal OR foetus* OR embryo OR fetus OR foetal) AND (move* OR motion OR motility OR kick*) AND ("lower limb" OR "lower extremity" OR biomechanics* OR musculoskeletal). In total, 992 articles were found in the chosen databases and 11 were selected for this systematic review. Animal experiments and cadaver experiments did not meet the selection criteria of this paper and were excluded. Only English papers and journal papers are selected, and the paper screening process is shown in Figure 1. According to PICO principles (participants, interventions, comparisons, and outcomes), this study seeks the computation of fetal kicking in various fetal health examinations. Information was extracted from 11 selected studies based on the subjects' characteristics and biomechanical gait parameters. Data were collected, including the gestational age, numbers of fetus, reference method, ultrasonic scanning plane/MRI section thickness, and inspection area.

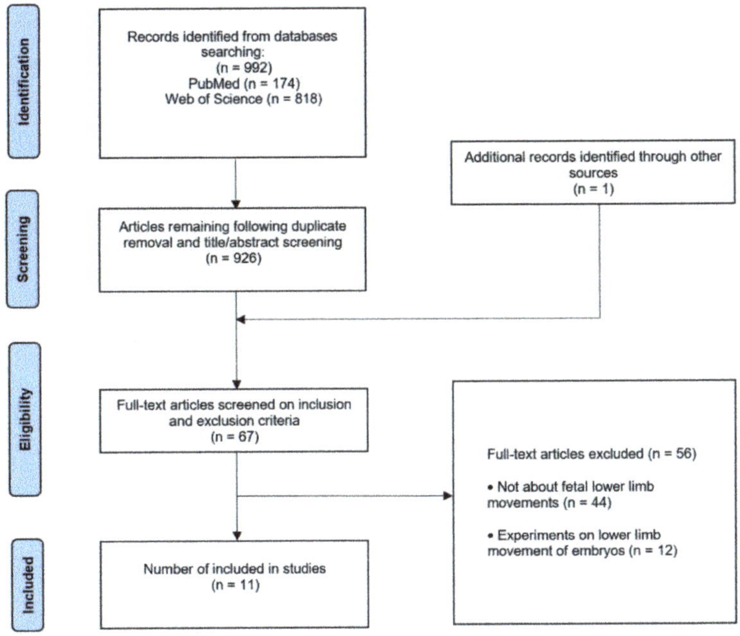

Figure 1. PRISMA flowchart of the process including the literature search and screening.

3. Results

An electronic database search of 992 articles on fetal movement was conducted and an additional study was found from a bibliography. Of these, 926 articles were discarded based on titles, abstracts, and duplication. The remaining 67 articles were read in total, and 56 were discarded according to the screening criteria. Finally, a total of 11 articles were included. The details are shown in Table 1.

Table 1. The detailed measurement of the fetal lower limb movement.

Studies	Gestational Age	Numbers	Reference Method	Ultrasonic Scanning Plane/MRI Section Thickness	Inspection Area
Rayburn et al., 1980 [28]	from 28 to 43 gestational weeks	24 pregnancies	ultrasound	along the longitudinal axis of the fetus	fetal abdomen and lower extremities
Budorick et al., 1998 [29]	from 16 to 32 gestational weeks	33 fetuses	ultrasound	corresponding to the coronal, sagittal, and axial planes	the lower leg bones and digits containing ossification centers; a vertical appearance to hindfoot; visualization of the forefoot, hindfoot, ossification centers in the hindfoot; a perpendicular orientation of the sole of the foot; a complete foot in the axial plane;
Nemec et al., 2011 [30]	from 18 + 4 to 31 + 1 gestational weeks	6 fetuses	MRI	coronal and sagittal T2-w sequences: 3–4 mm; dynamic steady-state free precession sequence: 30 mm; a three-dimensional thick-slab T2-w sequence: 30–50 mm	the whole fetus including the fetal extremities/musculoskeletal system
Giorgi et al., 2015 [31]	three in the early-middle (gestational weeks: 21, 22) stages; two in the late-middle (gestational weeks: 29, 34) stages.	5 fetuses	cine-MRI and Abaqus	30–40 mm	the whole fetus especially the prenatal hip joint
Carreras et al., 2016 [32]	from 18 and 26 gestational weeks	18 fetuses	B-mode ultrasound	sagittal plane	fetal lower limbs movements
Verbruggen et al., 2016 [33]	after 20 gestational weeks	3 fetuses	cine-MRI	30–40 mm	kicking sequences
Maroto et al., 2017 [34]	from 20.6–24.5 gestational weeks	28 fetuses	grey-scale (mode B) ultrasound	a sagittal plane	lower-limb movements
Verbruggen et al., 2018 [35]	20 weeks gestational age	341 fetuses	cine-MRI	30–40 mm	clear in-plane extension-flexion fetal kicks
Oliver et al., 2020 [36]	from 18 to 25 gestational weeks	404 fetuses	ultrasound and MRI	/	fetal lower-extremity
Chen et al., 2021 [37]	24, 27, 30 gestational weeks, respectively	3 fetuses	ultrasound	/	lower-limb movements

4. Discussion

A series of methods have been used previously to quantify fetal movements, such as cardiotocography, ultrasound, or MRI, but each method requires localization, and it is difficult to determine a gold standard. Each test has its advantages and disadvantages; previously popular methods, such as CTG, for detecting fetal movement have proven ineffective and not reliable. As technology advances, it is becoming easier to capture fetal movement patterns more accurately and distinguish fetal movement from maternal sensation. Through the modeling of skeletal muscle, there is the potential to develop specific simulations of the force of fetal kicking.

4.1. Maternal Sensation

Maternal sensation was the most common method used to assess fetal movement. Mothers are able to judge the health of their baby by perceiving its movements. Pregnant females sense the movement of the fetus through the uterine and associated abdominal wall muscles, and the mother easily recognizes a reduction in the fetus' movement. Factors such as fetal weight, fetus placental position, and maternal psychology all affect the maternal perception of fetal movement [38]. On account of the different approaches to counting the frequency of fetal movements, it is difficult to assign appropriate standard for evaluating normal fetal movement in late gestation [39,40]. Reduced fetal movement frequency perceived by the mother is associated with an increased risk of fetal stillbirth [41]. The fetal movement perceived by the mother is particularly evident in the fetal trunk and fetal lower limbs [18]. The actual fetal movement frequency is generally influenced by factors such as the mother's body position, maternal activity, anxiety neurosis and food intake [42–44]. The increased strength and frequency of fetal motion presumably reflects a general trend across the previous two weeks instead of a simple uncharacteristic warning signal [45]. Excessive fear from the expectant mother may be why the pregnant woman feels the fetal movement is extremely intense [7,46].

Several observational studies have demonstrated that any additional changes in fetal activity prior to delivery may affect neonatal outcomes. When seizure-like fetal hyperactivity occurs, a number of potential causes of injury need to be considered. Harmful stimuli, abnormal spasms, and infection also need to be considered and distinguished from fetal movement increases [7,46,47]. The hypokinetic movement repertoire of most fetuses is often accompanied by low velocity and a reduction in the frequency of activity. Conversely, if the fetus appears to produce a sudden rapid action, this often prompts the occurrence of epilepsy. In follow-up visits of women with stillborn infants, sudden changes in the exaggerated activity in infants are sometimes described as crazy motions, as distinguished from some of the general movements of early infants [7,40]. About a quarter of women had negative outcomes such as stillbirth or preterm childbirth when fetal movements decreased. Reduced perception of fetal movement can usually be seen as a warning of intrauterine death [2,5,48].

4.2. Maternal Wearable Devices

Maternal wearable devices can be independent of expensive laboratory equipment such as ultrasound, and can detect fetal movement over a more extended period instead of a short clinical measurement period [49]. Most accelerometer-based systems such as capacitive accelerometers and tri-axial accelerometers are not able to distinguish between fetal and maternal voluntary movements. Some study results show that startle movements and other forms of activity can be differentiated by acoustic sensor systems in association with accelerometers, effectively eliminating inconsistent noisy data resulting from maternal movements [50]. The acoustic measurement of fetal movement outcomes is not as accurate as ultraphonic scans or MRI.

4.3. Cardiotocography (CTG)

Cardiotocography (CTG) is a well-developed test for detecting fetal movement. This technique is potentially essential in that compensatory ultrasound is used to identify heart rate to predict fetal hypoxia [51]. It can be used externally and internally to observe and preserve the fetal heart rate and contraction or deviation of the mother's uterus placement. The results of the CTG test can be used to describe four features of fetal movement: fetal heart rate variability (FHRV), baseline fetal heart rate, acceleration, and deceleration. Although the CTG can measure fetal movement, the noise affecting the recordings make it less accurate; when the CTG is inclusive of accelerations, the results are practically in accordance with real-time ultrasonic imaging [52]. Intrauterine epilepsy is difficult to distinguish from the normal movement of the fetus and can only be confirmed when using ultrasound and CTG to check out the epilepsy phenomena at delivery [53]. Although the clinical effect of fetal movement reduction is not accurate and is strongly associated with stillbirth, CTG as a routine clinical method is mostly (about 80–90%) used with ultrasound to detect fetal motion reduction [54]. Recent research suggests that using CTG as a routine procedure for detecting fetal movement does not provide great advantage for diagnosis [55].

4.4. Actograph

The actograph is an objective method to quantify the data from CTG, and is positively associated with antenatal ultrasound assessment [56]. It can be used to distinguish high-frequency signals such as fetal heart activity and regards low-frequency signals as fetus movement [57]. Although the subtle movements of the fetus, such as breathing are not enough to produce any signals, the vast majority of fetal movement signals can be detected by the actograph [58]. The size of the fetus has a positive correlation with fetal movement using quantified actograph output. Actograph exhibits a high false-positive rate when it is included in most CTG devices, so it is not widely used [56].

4.5. Ultrasound

Two-dimensional sonography images were first used in the 1970s to observe the intrauterine environment of the fetus for real-time imaging [59]. Most maternal perceptions of fetal movement are usually so subjective that it is easily confused; only a few motions can be captured by the doppler device [60]. Modern brightness B-mode ultrasonography uses a curvilinear array of transducers to capture the three-dimensional image and video of the fetus in continuous motion. During an ultrasound examination, the obstetrician is required to apply the conductive gel to the appropriate examination area and record the relevant features of the fetal conditions. In order to minimize the exposure, the operator needs to monitor fetal movements for a brief period. Nevertheless, measurement of the fetal movement is generally not part of a routine prenatal ultrasonic examination. The variable speed, amplitude, direction of fetuses' general movement disorders can be detected and analyzed by using sonographic imaging; this is an important tool for obstetricians to judge whether the fetus is healthy or not [61].

The volume of fetal growth fluid in the uterus detected by ultrasound to recognize placental insufficiency is closely related to fetal movement restriction and stillbirth [62]. Sonography is an optimum method to measure fetal movement. The only limitation to this approach isa segmentary view of the fetus' gross movement around first 20 weeks [63]. In late gestation, Doppler ultrasound is not able to capture the whole fetus for clinicopathological examination due to the increase in fetal volume; natimortality of the fetus is still an intractable problem [57]. Therefore, the accuracy of fetuses' motor evaluation in the later stages of pregnancy is hard to guarantee [64]. Ultrasound is still regarded as the best standard in fetal movement detection and is frequently used to produce quite clear two-dimensional images. The fetus' general movement is usually suitable for ultrasound measurement, and is comprised of spontaneous motor behavior that is stable and sustainable from the first trimester of pregnancy and is maintained three to five months after delivery [61]. It was found that with the increase in gestational age, the frequency of all movement patterns decreased, which may be related to the uterine volume [65]. Although the measurement of fetal movements is momentous in fetal neurological measurements, with the restriction of using ultrasound during the second and third trimesters, it is not able to cover the whole movement using the standard method to measure the whole fetal movement [66]. Using ultrasound to observe fetal movement and intervention has reduced the fetal mortality rate; thus, it can also be inferred that using ultrasound and intervention therapy can effectively reduce fetal mortality [67].

4.6. Cine-MRI

The development of dynamic cine-MRI sequences in the field of MRI has led to improved techniques for detecting fetal movement during recent years. Cine-MRI scans are a novel and valuable technique that can directly observe the entire fetal movement using MRI technology [68]. The rendered image of cine-MRI can precisely capture the fetus' gross body movement patterns and monitor the fetus in detail, especially in the equivalent period of delivery of the fetus [64]. Cine-MRI can provide more comprehensive imageology information of the intrauterine environment. Through the use of cine-MRI, it was found that changes in fetal motor behavior were positively related to the uterine cavity volume during pregnancy [33,69]. Cine-MRI can be used to identify premature and neonatal outcomes by distinguishing regular and unusual images of fetal movement [64]. Cinematography is considered the most suitable imageology method for fetal motion since its balanced steady-state free alignment makes the image more detailed and precise [70]. The cine-MRI has a lower absorption rate, and a higher signal-to-noise ratio compared to other alternative imaging methods under the same conditions. Moreover, it can also clearly display fluid and tissue boundaries, rendering images with strong contrast characteristics [68,70]. At around 28 gestational weeks, the fetus begins to have limited movement in the womb; cine-MRI can more easily distinguish changes in fetal position, as well as some bending and stretching, than other measuring methods. The fetus may occupy approximately 90% uterine content at near term, which decreases the movement of the fetus because the volume of the fetus in the uterine cavity increases [66].

Inborn brain impairments increase the risk of neurodevelopmental abnormalities after birth [71]. Evaluation of the pattern and frequency of movement during pregnancy is an efficacious method for neurological screening of fetuses with congenital brain injury [71]. Biomechanical testing combined with the cine-MRI and musculoskeletal modeling methods attempt to characterize fetal movement quantitatively. Finite element analysis and musculoskeletal measurement can quantify the kick forces and associated muscle forces, as well as fetal bone stress and strains [35,72,73]. The lower limb muscle forces generated by kicking at a certain gestational age can be quantified using the finite element analysis and adult musculoskeletal modeling method. Quantifying the strike alteration in the kicking force and muscle force produced by a simple stretching during pregnancy reveals that the stresses and strain stimuli of the fetus show an increasing trend in the second half of pregnancy [33]. At about 35 weeks, the uterine wall is much less deformed than in the first trimester; the fetal bone stresses and strains basically remain unchanged [35]. When the stress and strain stimulation of fetal lower limbs were significantly higher, the intramuscular force, particularly the kicking force, increased. In the third trimester, due to the uterine environment and constrained fetal position, the fetal kicking range decreases while kicking force increases [35]. The growth and development of skeleton is basically driven by cells; through the biomechanical stimulation of fetal tissue, such as stress and strain, the bone gradually mineralizes and forms [74]. With the development of tissue engineering, the existing research is able to simulate the production of engineered skeleton and gristle tissue by studying the natural developmental processes of chondrogenesis and endochondral ossification [75]. The calculation of stress and strain in lower limb bones has also made a great contribution to biomaterials.

4.7. Biomechanics of Fetal Lower Limb Movement

Fetal movement can be effectively inferred through monitoring fetal lower limb movement to assess the fetus' health. Numerous studies have investigated the relationship between fetal lower limb movements and healthy fetus development, as summarized in Table 1. The lower limb movement of the fetus and the whole-body movement of the fetus were firstly distinguished sonographically. The measures included strong movements like fetal trunk movements with kicking and weak movements such as isolated limb motion [28]. The data from 2D ultrasound and 3D ultrasound were used to observe the number of bones and fingers in the lower limb of the fetus through the coronal plane, sagittal plane, and transverse plane, respectively [29]. Abnormal lower limb movements such as limb reduction defects are generally associated with a number of diseases such as skeletal dysplasia or neuromuscular disorders, or neural tube defects. Ultrasound examination of neural tube defects shows the abnormal fetal lower limb starts at 10 weeks onwards, and as a result, isolated lower limb motion occurs [32]. Ultrasound proved to be an effective way to detect deformities and abnormalities in the lower extremities. Compared with MRI detection, real-time ultrasound examination has a certain timeliness because ultrasound can hardly obtain the full body image of the fetus in the third trimester. By comparing different ultrasound views of fetal leg movement in the late trimester, the fetal lower limb movement profile was adequately evaluated with the front of the legs facing the anterior ultrasound probe [32,34]. Combining MRI and ultrasound to confirm the condition of talipes or lower-extremity impairment is highly associated with myelomeningocele or open spinal dysraphism [36]. The Simi Motion System is a software commonly used in sports to measure the motion angles of lower limb joints. Using this software to process ultrasound imaging data, we were able to clearly calculate the change in fetal lower limb movement angle in a pilot experiment [37].

The use of MRI as an adjunct measurement to ultrasound in multiple fetal anomalies has shown beneficial effects, particularly in central nervous disorders. MRI may be valuable for differentiating the etiological heterogeneity that leads to arthrogryposis and fetal akinesia-hypokinesia deformation sequences and identifying related central nervous system abnormalities. Prolonged restriction of fetal movement in the third trimester has a favorable prognosis with the appropriate orthopedic intervention. Conversely, most fetal motor disorders due to congenital neuropathy result in an adverse pregnancy outcome due to hypoplastic lung [30]. Some neurological diseases, such as fetal akinesia deformation sequences, do not respond well to prenatal DNA diagnosis; therefore, prenatal imaging diagnosis plays a vital role in discovering and detecting these diseases [76]. With the improvement in the level of detection accuracy, cine-MRI began to be used to detect the whole fetal movement [69]. On this basis, the examination of fetal lower limbs is becoming increasingly accurate. Developmental hip dysplasia can be analyzed and calculated by cine-MR image sequences to capture the motion at the hip joint [31]. Dysplasia of the hip is the most common abnormal joint shape disease, especially when fetal breech presentation happens with fetal abnormal movement, which then affects prenatal musculoskeletal development and joint shape development [35]. Studies have used adult models and the 2D FE method to calculate fetal lower limb kicking force, and lower limb muscle exertions, stresses and strains [33,35,77]. The average uterus displacements for kicking in utero were calculated using a custom tracking software and the finite element method, then using the musculoskeletal model to predict fetal kicking of the hip joint and knee surrounding maximum muscle forces [33]. By observing the uterine wall deformation and fetal skeleton development, it was found that stress and strain stimulation increases over the second half of pregnancy [77,78]. Altered biomechanical stimulus by stress and strain in the hip joint and kick forces may reveal the link between the risk of developmental dysplasia of the hip and the specific endouterine environment [35]. A series of measurement methods can effectively improve the measurement of fetal lower limb movement.

5. Conclusions

After comparing the advantages and disadvantages of different measuring instruments, it is not difficult to conclude that no method is the most ideal for the observation of fetal movement because each method has some limitations. Maternal sensation is the most basic and original method for recording fetal movement, but the data obtained is not reliable due to the intense subjectivity. At present, some maternal wearable devices can capture fetal movements much more accurately than maternal sensation and are not limited by experimental instruments and sites. However, these methods are difficult to distinguish the different fetal movements compared with the imaging information such as ultrasound and MRI. The CTG has been proven not to be a reliable test of fetal movement based on the fetus' heart rate mode. The actograph is a method that combines the data of CTG and ultrasound. Although ultrasound is the most commonly used fetal monitoring method, it is difficult to thoroughly investigate fetal movement patterns in the third trimester of pregnancy; this problem occurs for the actograph as well. Compared with ultrasound, the cine-MRI may be a better way to quantitatively evaluate fetal movement. However, cine-MRI has its limitations. Because of the limitations and equipment, most pregnant women choose this method only when they feel abnormality in the fetus, so it is difficult to use MRI to obtain more extensive maternal data. Combined with cine-MRI and an adult model to calculate fetal limb movement data, it provides a novel perspective to understand the closed mechanical environment of the uterus. However, adult lower limb biomechanics and in utero fetal movement data still have significant differences, while using the corresponding infant data to simulate the fetal movement may provide more reliable simulation results.

In summary, this review briefly explored the effects of fetus movement on fetal growth and development, the outcomes of fetal movement reduction, as well as methods for measuring fetal movement conditions. This review has a potential role in guiding the treatment and diagnosis of fetal movement reduction and presents a foundation model for the quantification and calculation of fetal movement in the future.

Author Contributions: All authors have made substantial contributions to the manuscript. Y.L. and R.X. were responsible for the conception and design of the study. Y.L. was responsible for data acquisition and data processing. R.X., Y.H., F.R. and Y.G. were responsible for data analysis and interpretation and drafting the article. R.X. and F.R. critically revised the manuscript. All authors have read and agreed to the published version of the manuscript.

Funding: This study is supported by Zhejiang Province Medical and Health Science and Technology Plan Project (2018KY710), Ningbo Public Welfare Science and Technology Plan Project (2019C50095), Health Youth Technical Talent Cultivation Special Fund Project (2020SWSQNGG-01), Ningbo Medical Science and Technology Plan (2020Y14), Young Cultivation Fund Project of the Affiliated School of Medicine of Ningbo University (FYQM-KY-202003), and Open Fund Project of Institute of Human Biomechanics of Ningbo University (CJ-HBIO202112).

Data Availability Statement: The data that support the findings of this study are available from the corresponding author upon reasonable request.

Conflicts of Interest: The authors declare no conflict of interest.

References

1. Sadovsky, E.; Yaffe, H. Daily fetal movement recording and fetal prognosis. *Obstet. Gynecol.* **1973**, *41*, 845–850. [PubMed]
2. Efkarpidis, S.; Alexopoulos, E.; Kean, L.; Liu, D.; Fay, T. Case-control study of factors associated with intrauterine fetal deaths. *Medscape Gen. Med.* **2004**, *6*, 53.
3. Leader, L.; Baillie, P.; Van Schalkwyk, D.J. Fetal movements and fetal outcome: A prospective study. *Obstet. Gynecol.* **1981**, *57*, 431–436. [PubMed]
4. Resnik, R. Intrauterine growth restriction. *Obstet. Gynecol.* **2002**, *99*, 490–496.
5. O'sullivan, O.; Stephen, G.; Martindale, E.; Heazell, A.J.J.O.O. Predicting poor perinatal outcome in women who present with decreased fetal movements. *J. Obstet. Gynaecol.* **2009**, *29*, 705–710. [CrossRef]

6. Sinha, D.; Sharma, A.; Nallaswamy, V.; Jayagopal, N.; Bhatti, N. Obstetric outcome in women complaining of reduced fetal movements. *J. Obstet. Gynaecol.* **2007**, *27*, 41–43. [CrossRef]
7. Stacey, T.; Thompson, J.M.; Mitchell, E.A.; Ekeroma, A.; Zuccollo, J.; McCowan, L.M. Maternal perception of fetal activity and late stillbirth risk: Findings from the Auckland Stillbirth Study. *Birth* **2011**, *38*, 311–316. [CrossRef]
8. Warrander, L.K.; Heazell, A.E. Identifying placental dysfunction in women with reduced fetal movements can be used to predict patients at increased risk of pregnancy complications. *Med. Hypotheses* **2011**, *76*, 17–20. [CrossRef]
9. Maulik, D.; Figueroa, R. Doppler velocimetry for fetal surveillance: Adverse perinatal outcome and fetal hypoxia. In *Doppler Ultrasound in Obstetrics and Gynecology*; Springer: Berlin/Heidelberg, Germany, 2005; pp. 363–374.
10. Velazquez, M.D.; Rayburn, W.F. Antenatal evaluation of the fetus using fetal movement monitoring. *Clin. Obstet. Gynecol.* **2002**, *45*, 993–1004. [CrossRef]
11. Rayburn, W.F. Clinical implications from monitoring fetal activity. *Am. J. Obstet. Gynecol.* **1982**, *144*, 967–980. [CrossRef]
12. Bennet, L.; Roelfsema, V.; Pathipati, P.; Quaedackers, J.; Gunn, A. Relationship between evolving epileptiform activity and delayed loss of mitochondrial activity after asphyxia measured by near-infrared spectroscopy in preterm fetal sheep. *J. Physiol.* **2006**, *572*, 141–154. [CrossRef] [PubMed]
13. Prechtl, H.F.; Einspieler, C.; Cioni, G.; Bos, A.F.; Ferrari, F.; Sontheimer, D. An early marker for neurological deficits after perinatal brain lesions. *Lancet* **1997**, *349*, 1361–1363. [CrossRef]
14. Guzzetta, A.; Mercuri, E.; Rapisardi, G.; Ferrari, F.; Roversi, M.; Cowan, F.; Rutherford, M.; Paolicelli, P.; Einspieler, C.; Boldrini, A. General movements detect early signs of hemiplegia in term infants with neonatal cerebral infarction. *Neuropediatrics* **2003**, *34*, 61–66. [PubMed]
15. Hadders-Algra, M.; Mavinkurve-Groothuis, A.M.; Groen, S.E.; Stremmelaar, E.F.; Martijn, A.; Butcher, P.R.J.C.R. Quality of general movements and the development of minor neurological dysfunction at toddler and school age. *Clin. Rehabil.* **2004**, *18*, 287–299. [CrossRef] [PubMed]
16. Piontelli, A. *Development of Normal Fetal Movements*; Springer: Berlin/Heidelberg, Germany, 2014.
17. Vries, J.I.P.D.; Fong, B.F. Normal fetal motility: An overview. *Ultrasound Obstet. Gynecol.* **2010**, *27*, 701–711. [CrossRef] [PubMed]
18. Sadovsky, E.; Mahler, Y.; Polishuk, W.; Malkin, A. Correlation between electromagnetic recording and maternal assessment of fetal movement. *Lancet* **1973**, *301*, 1141–1143. [CrossRef]
19. Cioni, G.; Ferrari, F.; Einspieler, C.; Paolicelli, P.B.; Barbani, T.; Prechtl, H.F. Comparison between observation of spontaneous movements and neurologic examination in preterm infants. *J. Pediatr.* **1997**, *130*, 704–711. [CrossRef]
20. Rådestad, I.; Lindgren, H. Women's perceptions of fetal movements in full-term pregnancy. *Sex. Reprod. Healthc.* **2012**, *3*, 113–116. [CrossRef]
21. Sival, D.; Visser, G.; Prechtl, H. The effect of intrauterine growth retardation on the quality of general movements in the human fetus. *Early Hum. Dev.* **1992**, *28*, 119–132. [CrossRef]
22. Visser, G.; Laurini, R.; De Vries, J.; Bekedam, D.; Prechtl, H. Abnormal motor behaviour in anencephalic fetuses. *Early Hum. Dev.* **1985**, *12*, 173–182. [CrossRef]
23. Heriza, C.B. Comparison of leg movements in preterm infants at term with healthy full-term infants. *Phys. Ther.* **1988**, *68*, 1687–1693. [CrossRef]
24. Sandell, L.J. Etiology of osteoarthritis: Genetics and synovial joint development. *Nat. Rev. Rheumatol.* **2012**, *8*, 77–89. [CrossRef] [PubMed]
25. Bellussi, F.; Livi, A.; Saccone, G.; De Vivo, V.; Oliver, E.A.; Berghella, V. Fetal movement counting and perinatal mortality: A systematic review and meta-analysis. *Obstet. Gynecol.* **2020**, *135*, 453–462. [CrossRef] [PubMed]
26. Ferrari, F.; Cioni, G.; Einspieler, C.; Roversi, M.F.; Bos, A.F.; Paolicelli, P.B.; Ranzi, A.; Prechtl, H.F. Cramped synchronized general movements in preterm infants as an early marker for cerebral palsy. *Arch. Pediatr. Adolesc. Med.* **2002**, *156*, 460–467. [CrossRef] [PubMed]
27. Moher, D.; Liberati, A.; Tetzlaff, J.; Altman, D.G.; Medicine, P.G.J.A.o.i. Preferred reporting items for systematic reviews and meta-analyses: The PRISMA statement. *Ann. Intern. Med.* **2009**, *151*, 264–269. [CrossRef] [PubMed]
28. Rayburn, W.F. Clinical significance of perceptible fetal motion. *Am. J. Obstet. Gynecol.* **1980**, *138*, 210–212. [CrossRef]
29. Budorick, N.E.; Pretorius, D.H.; Johnson, D.D.; Nelson, T.R.; Tartar, M.K.; Lou, K.V. Three-dimensional ultrasonography of the fetal distal lower extremity: Normal and abnormal. *J. Ultrasound Med.* **1998**, *17*, 649–660. [CrossRef]
30. Nemec, S.F.; Höftberger, R.; Nemec, U.; Bettelheim, D.; Brugger, P.C.; Kasprian, G.; Amann, G.; Rotmensch, S.; Graham, J.M., Jr.; Rimoin, D.L.; et al. Fetal akinesia and associated abnormalities on prenatal MRI. *Prenat. Diagn.* **2011**, *31*, 484–490. [CrossRef]
31. Giorgi, M.; Carriero, A.; Shefelbine, S.J.; Nowlan, N.C. Effects of normal and abnormal loading conditions on morphogenesis of the prenatal hip joint: Application to hip dysplasia. *J. Biomech.* **2015**, *48*, 3390–3397. [CrossRef]
32. Carreras, E.; Maroto, A.; Illescas, T.; Melendez, M.; Arevalo, S.; Peiro, J.L.; Garcia-Fontecha, C.G.; Belfort, M.; Cuxart, A. Prenatal ultrasound evaluation of segmental level of neurological lesion in fetuses with myelomeningocele: Development of a new technique. *Ultrasound Obstet. Gynecol.* **2016**, *47*, 162–167. [CrossRef]
33. Verbruggen, S.W.; Loo, J.H.; Hayat, T.T.; Hajnal, J.V.; Rutherford, M.A.; Phillips, A.T.; Nowlan, N.C. Modeling the biomechanics of fetal movements. *Biomech. Model. Mechanobiol.* **2016**, *15*, 995–1004. [CrossRef] [PubMed]

34. Maroto, A.; Illescas, T.; Melendez, M.; Arevalo, S.; Rodo, C.; Peiro, J.L.; Belfort, M.; Cuxart, A.; Carreras, E. Ultrasound functional evaluation of fetuses with myelomeningocele: Study of the interpretation of results. *J. Matern.-Fetal Neonatal Med.* **2017**, *30*, 2301–2305. [CrossRef] [PubMed]
35. Verbruggen, S.W.; Bernhard, K.; Shelmerdine, S.C.; Arthurs, O.J.; Hajnal, J.V.; Rutherford, M.A.; Phillips, A.T.M.; Nowlan, N.C. Altered biomechanical stimulation of the developing hip joint in presence of hip dysplasia risk factors. *J. Biomech.* **2018**, *78*, 30037582. [CrossRef] [PubMed]
36. Oliver, E.R.; Heuer, G.G.; Thom, E.A.; Burrows, P.K.; Didier, R.A.; DeBari, S.E.; Martin-Saavedra, J.S.; Moldenhauer, J.S.; Jatres, J.; Howell, L.J.; et al. Myelomeningocele sac associated with worse lower-extremity neurological sequelae: Evidence for prenatal neural stretch injury? *Ultrasound Obstet. Gynecol.* **2020**, *55*, 740–746. [CrossRef]
37. Chen, H.; Song, Y.; Xuan, R.; Hu, Q.; Baker, J.S.; Gu, Y. Kinematic Comparison on Lower Limb Kicking Action of Fetuses in Different Gestational Weeks: A Pilot Study. *Healthcare* **2021**, *9*, 1057. [CrossRef]
38. Bradford, B.; Maude, R. Maternal perception of fetal movements in the third trimester: A qualitative description. *Women Birth* **2018**, *31*, e287–e293. [CrossRef]
39. Frøen, J.F. A kick from within–fetal movement counting and the cancelled progress in antenatal care. *J. Perinat. Med.* **2004**, *32*, 13–24. [CrossRef]
40. Heazell, A.P.; Frøen, J. Methods of fetal movement counting and the detection of fetal compromise. *J. Obstet. Gynaecol.* **2008**, *28*, 147–154. [CrossRef]
41. Mangesi, L.; Hofmeyr, G.J.; Smith, V.; Smyth, R.M.D. Fetal movement counting for assessment of fetal wellbeing. *Cochrane Database Syst. Rev.* **2015**, *15*, CD004909. [CrossRef]
42. Eller, D.P.; Stramm, S.L.; Newman, R.B. The effect of maternal intravenous glucose administration on fetal activity. *Am. J. Obstet. Gynecol.* **1992**, *167*, 1071–1074. [CrossRef]
43. Dlugosz, L.; Belanger, K.; Hellenbrand, K.; Holford, T.R.; Leaderer, B.; Bracken, M.B. Maternal caffeine consumption and spontaneous abortion: A prospective cohort study. *Epidemiology* **1996**, *7*, 250–255. [CrossRef] [PubMed]
44. Sjöström, K.; Valentin, L.; Thelin, T.; Maršál, K. Maternal anxiety in late pregnancy: Effect on fetal movements and fetal heart rate. *Early Hum. Dev.* **2002**, *67*, 87–100. [CrossRef]
45. Heazell, A.E.; Warland, J.; Stacey, T.; Coomarasamy, C.; Budd, J.; Mitchell, E.A.; O'Brien, L.M. Stillbirth is associated with perceived alterations in fetal activity–findings from an international case control study. *BMC Pregnancy Childbirth* **2017**, *17*, 369. [CrossRef] [PubMed]
46. Warland, J.; O'Brien, L.M.; Heazell, A.E.; Mitchell, E.A. An international internet survey of the experiences of 1,714 mothers with a late stillbirth: The STARS cohort study. *BMC Pregnancy Childbirth* **2015**, *15*, 172. [CrossRef] [PubMed]
47. Heazell, A.E.; Stacey, T.; O'Brien, L.M.; Mitchell, E.A.; Warland, J. Excessive fetal movements are a sign of fetal compromise which merits further examination. *Med. Hypotheses* **2018**, *111*, 19–23. [CrossRef]
48. Dutton, P.J.; Warrander, L.K.; Roberts, S.A.; Bernatavicius, G.; Byrd, L.M.; Gaze, D.; Kroll, J.; Jones, R.L.; Sibley, C.P.; Frøen, J.F. Predictors of poor perinatal outcome following maternal perception of reduced fetal movements–a prospective cohort study. *PLoS ONE* **2012**, *7*, e39784. [CrossRef]
49. Delay, U.; Nawarathne, B.; Dissanayake, D.; Ekanayake, M.; Godaliyadda, G.; Wijayakulasooriya, J.; Rathnayake, R. Non Invasive Wearable Device for Fetal Movement Detection. In Proceedings of the 2020 IEEE 15th International Conference on Industrial and Information Systems (ICIIS), Rupnagar, India, 26–28 November 2020; pp. 285–290.
50. Jonathan, L.; Richard, W.; Yuriy, A.; Qurratul, A.M.; Lees, C.C.; Ravi, V.; Nowlan, N.C.; Marco, A. Performance of a wearable acoustic system for fetal movement discrimination. *PLoS ONE* **2018**, *13*, e0195728.
51. Grivell, R.M.; Alfirevic, Z.; Gyte, G.M.L.; Devane, D. Antenatal cardiotocography for fetal assessment. *Cochrane Database Syst. Rev.* **2015**, *12*, CD007863. [CrossRef]
52. Rabinowitz, R.; Persitz, E.; Sadovsky, E. The relation between fetal heart rate accelerations and fetal movements. *Obstet. Gynecol.* **1983**, *61*, 16–18.
53. Landy, H.J.; Khoury, A.N.; Heyl, P.S. Antenatal ultrasonographic diagnosis of fetal seizure activity. *Am. J. Obstet. Gynecol.* **1989**, *161*, 308.
54. Heazell, A.E.; Green, M.; Wright, C.; Flenady, V.; Frøen, F. Midwives' and obstetricians' knowledge and management of women presenting with decreased fetal movements. *Acta Obstet. Gynecol. Scand.* **2008**, *87*, 331–339. [CrossRef] [PubMed]
55. Alfirevic, Z.; Devane, D.; Gyte, G.M.L. Continuous cardiotocography (CTG) as a form of electronic fetal monitoring (EFM) for fetal assessment during labour. *Cochrane Database Syst. Rev.* **2013**, *31*, CD006066. [CrossRef]
56. Maeda, K. New ultrasonic Doppler fetal actograph and continuous recording of fetal movement. *Nihon Sanka Fujinka Gakkai Zasshi* **1984**, *36*, 280–288. [PubMed]
57. Lai, J.; Nowlan, N.C.; Vaidyanathan, R.; Visser, G.H.; Lees, C.C. The use of actograph in the assessment of fetal well-being. *J. Matern.-Fetal Neonatal Med.* **2020**, *33*, 2116–2121. [CrossRef] [PubMed]
58. Besinger, R.E.; Johnson, T.R.B. Doppler recording of fetal movement: Clinical correlation with real-time ultrasound. *Obstet. Gynecol.* **1989**, *74*, 277–280. [PubMed]
59. Fitzgerald, D.; Drumm, J. Non-invasive measurement of human fetal circulation using ultrasound: A new method. *Br. Med. J.* **1977**, *2*, 1450–1451. [CrossRef]

60. Johnson, T.; Jordan, E.T.; Paine, L.L. Doppler recordings of fetal movement: II. Comparison with maternal perception. *Obstet. Gynecol.* **1990**, *76*, 42–43.
61. De Vries, J.; Fong, B. Changes in fetal motility as a result of congenital disorders: An overview. *Ultrasound Obstet. Gynecol.* **2007**, *29*, 590–599. [CrossRef]
62. Frøen, J.F.; Tveit, J.V.H.; Saastad, E.; Børdahl, P.E.; Stray-Pedersen, B.; Heazell, A.E.P.; Flenady, V.; Fretts, R.C. Management of Decreased Fetal Movements. *Semin. Perinatol.* **2008**, *32*, 307–311. [CrossRef]
63. Whitworth, M.; Bricker, L.; Mullan, C. Ultrasound for fetal assessment in early pregnancy. *Cochrane Database Syst. Rev.* **2015**, *14*, CD007058. [CrossRef]
64. Hayat, T.T.; Martinez-Biarge, M.; Kyriakopoulou, V.; Hajnal, J.V.; Rutherford, M.A. Neurodevelopmental correlates of fetal motor behavior assessed using cine MR imaging. *Am. J. Neuroradiol.* **2018**, *39*, 1519–1522. [CrossRef] [PubMed]
65. Roodenburg, P.; Wladimiroff, J.; Van Es, A.; Prechtl, H. Classification and quantitative aspects of fetal movements during the second half of normal pregnancy. *Early Hum. Dev.* **1991**, *25*, 19–35. [CrossRef]
66. Kurjak, A.; Miskovic, B.; Stanojevic, M.; Amiel-Tison, C.; Ahmed, B.; Azumendi, G.; Vasilj, O.; Andonotopo, W.; Turudic, T.; Salihagic-Kadic, A. New scoring system for fetal neurobehavior assessed by three-and four-dimensional sonography. *J. Perinat. Med.* **2008**, *36*, 73–81. [CrossRef]
67. Tveit, J.V.H.; Saastad, E.; Stray-Pedersen, B.; Børdahl, P.E.; Flenady, V.; Fretts, R.; Frøen, J.F. Reduction of late stillbirth with the introduction of fetal movement information and guidelines—A clinical quality improvement. *BMC Pregnancy Childbirth* **2009**, *9*, 32. [CrossRef] [PubMed]
68. Guo, W.-Y.; Ono, S.; Oi, S.; Shen, S.-H.; Wong, T.-T.; Chung, H.-W.; Hung, J.-H. Dynamic motion analysis of fetuses with central nervous system disorders by cine magnetic resonance imaging using fast imaging employing steady-state acquisition and parallel imaging: A preliminary result. *J. Neurosurg. Pediatr.* **2006**, *105*, 94–100. [CrossRef]
69. Hayat, T.T.A.; Nihat, A.; Martinez-Biarge, M.; Mcguinness, A.; Allsop, J.M.; Hajnal, J.V.; Rutherford, M.A. Optimization and initial experience of a multisection balanced steady-state free precession cine sequence for the assessment of fetal behavior in utero. *AJNR Am. J. Neuroradiol* **2011**, *32*, 331–338. [CrossRef]
70. Carr, J.C.; Simonetti, O.; Bundy, J.; Li, D.; Pereles, S.; Finn, J.P. Cine MR angiography of the heart with segmented true fast imaging with steady-state precession. *Radiology* **2001**, *219*, 828–834. [CrossRef]
71. Einspieler, C.; Prechtl, H.F. Prechtl's assessment of general movements: A diagnostic tool for the functional assessment of the young nervous system. *Ment. Retard. Dev. Disabil. Res. Rev.* **2005**, *11*, 61–67. [CrossRef]
72. Gao, Y.; Ren, S.; Zhou, H.; Xuan, R. Impact of Physical Activity During Pregnancy on Gestational Hypertension. *Phys. Act. Health* **2020**, *4*, 32–39. [CrossRef]
73. Xuan, R.; Yang, M.; Gao, Y.; Ren, S.; Li, J.; Yang, Z.; Song, Y.; Huang, X.-H.; Teo, E.-C.; Zhu, J.; et al. A Simulation Analysis of Maternal Pelvic Floor Muscle. *Int. J. Environ. Res. Public Health* **2021**, *18*, 10821. [CrossRef]
74. Nowlan, N.C.; Sharpe, J.; Roddy, K.A.; Prendergast, P.J.; Murphy, P. Mechanobiology of embryonic skeletal development: Insights from animal models. *Birth Defects Res. Part C Embryo Today Rev.* **2010**, *90*, 203–213. [CrossRef] [PubMed]
75. Quintana, L.; zur Nieden, N.I.; Semino, C.E. Morphogenetic and regulatory mechanisms during developmental chondrogenesis: New paradigms for cartilage tissue engineering. *Tissue Eng. Part B Rev.* **2009**, *15*, 29–41. [CrossRef] [PubMed]
76. Witters, I.; Moerman, P.; Fryns, J.P. Fetal akinesia deformation sequence: A study of 30 consecutive in utero diagnoses. *Am. J. Med. Genet.* **2002**, *113*, 23–28. [CrossRef] [PubMed]
77. Verbruggen, S.W.; Kainz, B.; Shelmerdine, S.C.; Hajnal, J.V.; Rutherford, M.A.; Arthurs, O.J.; Phillips, A.T.M.; Nowlan, N.C. Stresses and strains on the human fetal skeleton during development. *J. R. Soc. Interface* **2018**, *15*, 20170593. [CrossRef]
78. Ren, S.; Gao, Y.; Yang, Z.; Li, J.; Xuan, R.; Liu, J.; Chen, X.; Thirupathi, A. The Effect of Pelvic Floor Muscle Training on Pelvic Floor Dysfunction in Pregnant and Postpartum Women. *Phys. Act. Health* **2020**, *4*, 130–141. [CrossRef]

International Journal of
Environmental Research and Public Health

MDPI

Systematic Review

Full-Day Physical Activity and Sedentary Behaviour Levels of Typically Developing Children and Adolescents in the Middle East: A Systematic Review

Esraa Burahmah, Sivaramkumar Shanmugam and Ben Stansfield *

School of Health and Life Sciences, Glasgow Caledonian University, Cowcaddens Road, Glasgow G4 0BA, UK; esraa.burahmah@gcu.ac.uk (E.B.); sivaram.shanmugam@gcu.ac.uk (S.S.)
* Correspondence: ben.stansfield@gcu.ac.uk

Abstract: Physical activity (PA) and sedentary behaviour (SB) are important components of physical behaviour associated with long-term health outcomes. Environmental and cultural factors may influence physical behaviour. To explore full day PA and SB in children and adolescents (2–18 years old) in the Middle East, a systematic literature review was performed including 183 journal articles. A wide range of PA and SB outcomes were reported, in some cases making synthesis of results difficult. As a consequence, results were generally reported narratively (MVPA time, total PA, SB time). Meta-regression of daily step count revealed females took 4600 fewer steps than males, with 3000 fewer steps on weekdays than weekends, and overweight individuals taking 2800 fewer steps/day. Steps decreased with age. Meta-regression for TV viewing time demonstrated an increase by 0.04 h per year of age. Even though environmental and cultural conditions may be different, PA and SB of children and adolescents in the Middle East were largely comparable to those of Europeans and North Americans. The wide range of data collection instruments used (both self-report questionnaire and body-worn devices) and heterogeneity of data made synthesis of reported data across studies very difficult, suggesting a need for greater standardisation of data collection methods.

Keywords: physical activity; sedentary behaviour; Middle East; children; adolescents; physical behaviour; self-report; body-worn sensor; environment; culture

1. Introduction

The World Health Organisation (WHO) recommends that, to maintain health, children and adolescents aged 5–17 years of age should engage in 60 min of moderate to vigorous physical activity (MVPA) per day, vigorous-intensity aerobic activities three times per week and limit sedentary time [1]. Both physical activity (PA) and sedentary behaviour (SB) are important components of physical behaviour as they have been independently associated with long-term health outcomes [2,3]. Establishing the volume of children and adolescents' physical behaviour requires some form of assessment using either self-reporting (e.g., International Physical Activity Questionnaire (IPAQ) [4]), reporting by an observer (e.g., parent or carer) or the use of body-worn monitors.

The globally recognised recommendations for PA and SB provide minimum values associated with the maintenance of good health and the prevention of the development of non-communicable diseases (e.g., diabetes type II). When establishing the physical behaviour levels of groups, it is possible to assess behaviour against the minimum recommendations (e.g., % performing > 60 min of MVPA per day [5]). However, this does not provide a description of the actual volume of the behaviour. To more clearly define actual behaviour, reporting of volume indicators (e.g., actual hours per day of PA) allows evidence of behaviour time distributions to be explored.

Physical behaviour is context-specific and may vary depending on a number of environmental as well as socio-cultural factors. For example, extreme ranges of temperature will influence the amount of time that can be spent outside [6]. and cultural norms may influence types of behaviour that are acceptable [7]. Different regions of the world have different climates and different cultural norms, so it might be expected that children and adolescents exhibit different physical behaviour patterns in different regions. Additionally, groups within populations may face differing challenges to engaging with PA. For example, contextual factors may impact on males and females differently [8], or those who live in rural and urban areas [9].

Although there is no universally accepted definition of the region of the world considered to be the 'Middle East', it is possible to identify a group of countries which might be considered to have similar socio-cultural characteristics (primary Muslim, Arab) [10] and environmental characteristics. The Middle East has an environment that is characterised by very high summer temperatures, making outdoor activity challenging in some regions in the summer months [11]. Extreme temperature events in this region appear to be on the increase [12], possibly leading to even greater restrictions on PA engagement. Gender and cultural norms are highlighted as barriers to PA participation throughout the region [11]. Therefore, it is possible, due to cultural and environmental reasons, that PA and SB characteristics of children and adolescents in this region are different from those living in Europe and North America, for example. Numerous reports of physical behaviour of children and adolescents in Middle Eastern countries are available through large studies such as the CASPIAN series and through use of the ATLS instrument [13,14]. However, to date, there has been no systematic review of this material and, specifically, no extraction of daily volumes of PA and SB measures.

The aim of this systematic review of the literature was therefore to provide a summary of the daily volumes of PA and SB of children and adolescents (2–18 years of age) in the Middle East region as recorded using both self/observer-reporting and body-worn monitors. The objective was not to explore the proportion meeting physical behaviour guidelines but to characterise the absolute volume of physical behaviours.

2. Materials and Methods

A systematic review was conducted of published literature on daily volume of physical activity and sedentary behaviour of children and adolescents (2–18 years old) in Middle Eastern countries. The Preferred Reporting Items for Systematic Reviews and Meta-Analyses (PRISMA 2020) guidelines were used to guide implementation of the review (Supplementary Table S1).

2.1. Geographical Area of Interest: The Middle East

For the purposes of this review the Middle East region was defined to include countries of the Arabian Peninsula (Yemen and the Gulf Cooperation Council (GCC) countries: Bahrain, Kuwait, Oman, Qatar, Saudi Arabia, UAE) and the modern Levant area (Iraq, Israel, Jordan, Lebanon, Palestine, Syria) [15]. Additionally, areas that have historically been associated with the Middle East (Egypt, Turkey, Cyprus) were included. Cyprus is viewed as a European country; however, geographically and historically, it is located in the Middle East [16]. Although the term Middle East and North Africa (MENA) is used to define a region, an extended list of North African countries was not included in the current review due to diverging cultural and socio-economic patterns from the core Middle Eastern countries.

2.2. Information Sources and Search Strategy

The Cumulative Index to Nursing and Allied Health Literature (CINAHL), Medical Literature Analysis and Retrieval System Online (MEDLINE), Web of Science and PsychINFO were used for this literature review. Both terms associated with physical activity (including 'steps') and sedentary behaviour (including 'sitting') were used alongside explicit reference to children or adolescents within the country context of interest (full search terms available in Supplementary Material S2). The search was conducted in April 2021.

2.3. Eligibility Criteria

Population: young people (children and adolescents) between the ages of 2 and 18 years old living in the Middle East and typically developing were the target population. Inclusion of participants above the age of 18 or below 2 years old did not exclude studies as long as the mean/mid group age for reported data was in this range. For data to be included, it was necessary for details of the age distribution to be included. As a minimum, the range of data was accepted. If data for a country (or region) of interest could not be isolated, it was not included. Only children and adolescents without any reported motor, developmental or cognitive disability were included.

Outcome measure: to be eligible for the review, publications had to provide a measure of physical activity or sedentary behaviour which could be interpreted as a whole-day measure.

Study design: any form of study design was accepted (e.g., cross-sectional, longitudinal, intervention, etc.) as long as original data were reported.

No restriction was placed on publication year. Primary data published in peer-reviewed English language journals were included.

2.4. Selection Process

Details of identified studies were imported to Mendeley reference manager (version 1.19.8), where duplicates were removed. Subsequently, references were uploaded to Rayyan [17], where titles and abstracts were reviewed against the inclusion and exclusion criteria by two reviewers independently (two from EB, BS, SS). Articles considered to be irrelevant by two reviewers were excluded at this stage; all others were taken forward.

Full texts of all papers were retrieved where possible and reviewed independently by two reviewers (two from EB, BS, SS). Where conflicts arose as to whether to include the paper, agreement was reached through discussion. Reasons for rejection were recorded and are reported via a PRISMA flow chart [18].

2.5. Data Extraction Process

Data were manually extracted from the papers and entered into an Excel spreadsheet. Data were checked by a second reviewer (EB, BS). Participant characteristics (sample size, M/F, age, BMI, medical conditions) were extracted. Based on possible influence on the level of physical activity and sedentary behaviour, a number of additional participant and study characteristics were extracted (country, region, urban/rural, public or private school, year of data collection, season/months of data collection). To characterise the PA or SB, additional descriptive variables were extracted (specific PA/SB definition, data collection instrument, number of weekday/weekend days of data recording).

For interventional studies, baseline data were extracted, as they represented a typical population before intervention. Where papers referred to other sources for the definition of outcomes, details were extracted where possible from the original source. All relevant PA and SB outcomes were extracted. If the children and adolescents' condition was not mentioned, they were assumed to be typically developing.

2.6. Quality Assessment

The quality of all selected papers was assessed against an adapted version of the quality appraisal tool proposed by Chaabane et al. [19]. This included characteristics related to population, outcome definition, methodology, setting, timing, sampling and response rate, to give a total score out of 18 (see Supplementation Material S3). Quality assessment was performed by two reviewers and any differences resolved through discussion (EB, BS). All available data have been reported with quality score used to identify weakly reported data. However, no data were excluded based on reporting quality.

2.7. Synthesis Methods

The intention of the analysis was to implement meta-regression analysis of each PA or SB outcomes against a number of possible covariates, using weighting of the study data standard error. Backward stepwise selection of covariates was used to identify significant contributors to the description of the outcome of interest. Beta coefficients with 95% confidence intervals describe confidence in model fit. I^2 was used to evaluate the heterogeneity of included study results. Where necessary, subgroup analysis was considered. SPSS version 28.0.1.1 (IBM Corporation, Armonk, NY, USA) was used for all statistical analysis. If statistical analysis was not possible, a narrative synthesis was planned.

As it has previously been demonstrated that physical behaviour may be related to various characteristics, the intention was to include the following characteristics in the meta-regression: age [20,21], gender [20,22], weight status [23,24], the nature of the educational establishment (state/public or private) [25,26], location of residence (urban or rural) [27,28] and the data collection time period (week or weekend [29], season [30,31] and year [32,33]).

Conversion of Reported Outcomes to Allow Standardised Presentation

In anticipation of a range of reporting methods, a uniform method of presenting a summary across data was required. To achieve this, outcomes reported in the literature were adapted as indicated in Tables 1 and 2.

Table 1. Conversions of reported age variables to allow standardised presentation.

Available Data	Mid Age	Age Min	Age Max	+Error Bar	−Error Bar
Range and mean	Mean	range min	Range max (if whole number round to next whole number)	(Age max) − (Mid age)	(Mid age) − (Age min)
Range only	(Age min) + (Age max − Age min)/2				
Mean and SD	Mean	(Mid age) − (2 × SD)	(Mid age) + (2 × SD)	2 × SD	2 × SD

SD = standard deviation, min = minimum, max = maximum.

Table 2. Conversions of outcomes to mean and SD values where necessary to allow standardised presentation. Non-parametric distribution characteristics were converted to the equivalent normal distribution characteristics to allow presentation of data within the same graphical display.

Original PA or SB Outcome	Converted Outcome
Median (using equivalent normal distribution)	Mean
IQR/1.35 (using equivalent normal distribution)	SD
95%CI/4 (assumed 95% CI ≈ 4 × SD)	SD
Range/6 (assumed 99% CI ≈ 6 × SD)	SD
SE × square root of sample size (Based on definition of SE)	SD

IQR = interquartile range, SD = standard deviation, CI = confidence interval, SE = standard error.

When reporting the age range, all maximum ages with fractions were used exactly as they were. However, if a range was given, the maximum ages were rounded to the next whole number, i.e., if the age range was 10–12 years, minimum age was reported as 10 years and maximum age was reported as 13.

Bubble plots were used to illustrate relative sample size associated with each data point. Where overall sample size for a study was reported and data presented split into subcategories of study participants, for illustrative purposes if no sample size of subgroups was provided, an equal split to each sub-group was assumed.

3. Results

3.1. Study Selection

After duplicates had been removed, 6665 studies were identified as relevant to the topic area (Figure 1). Following abstract and title screening, 2022 studies remained. Of these, it was possible to retrieve all but 28 full texts (there was no response from any authors for copies of full texts or additional data). Based on full text review, a substantial number of the studies (777) did not report daily measures of PA or SB, 533 did not have data specifically associated with a country of interest, 464 reported data on participants with groups of mid-age outside 2–18 years (typically young adult populations), 54 reported data not in the English language and 53 reported only data on non-typically developing children. A total of 183 individual journal article reports were included in the final data summary (a full list of all references is available in Supplementary Information Table S4) [34–215]. The eligible studies were all published after 2000 with 6, 25, 53 and 73 articles published between 2000–2004, 2005–2009, 2010–2014 and 2015–2019, respectively. Twenty six articles were published from 2020 onwards. The vast majority of study designs were cross-sectional in nature with a small number of experimental intervention studies (baseline data presented in this report) and longitudinal studies [98,169,201,205].

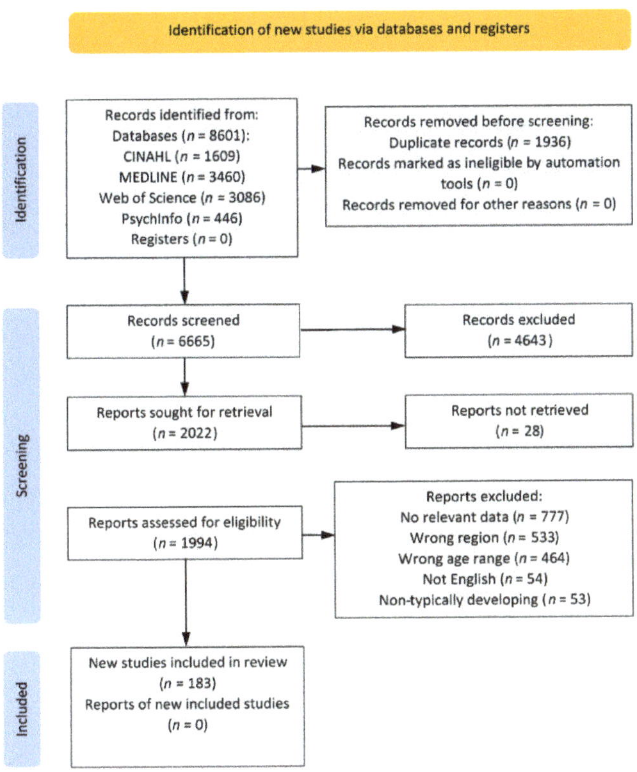

Figure 1. PRISMA flow chart of the number of journal articles included at each stage of the review process [18]. Within 'Screening', records were first screened by title and abstract, followed by retrieval of full texts and assessment of eligibility based on the full text.

Of particular note in terms of reasons for exclusion was the large number of studies where reports of PA were in relation to meeting specific daily targets. Reports typically presented % of samples reaching specific PA targets. For this review, the daily volume of PA or SB was required. Percentages of participants meeting specified targets did not meet this inclusion criteria, as the specific level of PA was usually not reported.

The number of studies and total sample size varied widely between countries (Table 3) with the largest number of studies (68) and total sample size (>100,000) being from Iran. Data by country are reported in Table 3 under various sub-categories of PA and SB.

Table 3. The number of studies, sample size, and PA and SB measurements reported by country.

Country *	Number of Studies	Total Sample Size (Duplicate Samples Combined)	PA Measure Category					SB Measure Category					
			Steps 1	Kcal/ Total EE 3	Counts 4	Time 5	METs 8	TV/DVD/Video 1	Computer/ Computer Games/Internet 2	Combination of Screen Time 3	Total Screen Time/ Electronic Use 4	Time 6	METs 8
Cyprus	13	4482	6	0	0	5	0	4	1	2	4	1	0
Egypt	2	363	0	2	1	0	0	0	0	0	0	0	0
Iran	68	101,611	1	5	1	28	19	15	14	7	11	8	1
Iraq	3	913	0	0	1	1	1	1	0	1	0	0	0
Israel	8	5223	0	0	0	3	0	1	1	0	3	2	0
Jordan	4	4358	0	0	0	0	2	3	1	0	1	0	0
Kuwait	4	1292	0	1	0	3	1	1	1	0	0	2	0
Lebanon	5	7923	0	0	0	2	0	1	1	1	1	1	0
Oman	6	2114	0	0	0	4	0	0	0	3	2	1	0
Palestine	1	378	0	0	0	1	0	0	0	0	0	0	0
Qatar	1	1161	0	0	0	0	1	0	0	0	1	0	0
Saudi Arabia	27	10,627	5	3	0	8	10	9	7	4	6	7	0
Turkey	37	18,208	7	7	0	13	8	4	1	1	2	11	0
UAE	3	666	0	1	0	1	0	1	0	0	0	3	0

* There were no sources including Bahrain, Syria or Yemen. One source was mixed Palestine, Jordan and Israel. EE = energy expenditure, METs = metabolic equivalents.

3.2. PA and SB Outcomes

The number of papers included in this review was 183. Of these, 63 reported both PA and SB, 80 reported only PA and 40 reported SB variables only. PA and SB were reported using various terminologies. The full range of reported outcomes is listed in Table 4. A total of over 1100 reportable PA or SB items were found in the 183 papers.

Table 4. Variables reported in the literature characterising daily volumes of PA or SB. Both objective (device-measured) and subjective (self/observer-reported) data types are listed.

	Objective or Subjective	Variable	Sub-Categories	Base Units *
PA	Objective	Steps		Steps
		Energy expenditure	TEE, DEE, AEE	Kcal or kJ
		Counts		Counts
		Time		Mins
	Subjective	METs	Light, Moderate, Vigorous, Moderate + Vigorous	MET mins
		Time	Light, Moderate, Vigorous, Moderate + Vigorous Exercise/sport	Mins
		Postures	Upright, transitions	Mins or number
SB	Objective	Time		Mins
	Subjective	Screen-based activity time	Either one or a combination of the following: TV/DVD/video/video games/computer/computer games/internet/smart phone/tablet	Mins
		Sedentary-based activity time	Sedentary time/physical inactivity/doing home-work/sitting/reading books/desk work	Mins
		METs		MET mins

* Base units used in description of variable (per day or per week). TEE = Total energy expenditure, DEE = Daily energy expenditure, AEE = Activity energy expenditure, and MET = Metabolic equivalent, mins = minutes.

All outcomes extracted from all papers are included in Supplementary Data (Table S5). The reader is referred to the Supplementary Data should they wish to extract data on the full range of variables listed in Table 4. Only those variables with sufficiently consistent definitions and for which there were suitable volumes of available data are reported here.

Of all variables reported in the literature, there was only sufficient, consistent information to warrant reporting for the following variables:

- PA: steps, MVPA (time), total PA (METs mins/day, IPAQ, and ATLS questionnaires).
- SB: TV screen time (overall and specifically for the ATLS and CASPIAN questionnaires), time (body-worn devices).

3.3. Study Quality

There was a wide range of study quality reported (median 11, IQR 4-13 out of a maximum score of 18) (Table 5). Generally, the quality scores suggested most studies used well-defined outcomes, although 9% were not well defined. Most studies (75%) used subjective data collection methods with only 21% using objective device-recorded outcomes. The setting was often not clearly reported with specific location only given in 34% of cases and only combined with information on urban/rural in 10% or cases. No information on time of data collection was present in 33% of cases, but year only (27%) and additionally season (39%) were reported across the majority of studies. Sampling typically included some element of random selection (68%), although response rate was often not reported (55%).

Table 5. Quality assessment of included studies (percentage per score).

	Quality Assessment Criteria					
Grade	Outcome Definition	Data Collection Instrument	Setting	Timing	Sampling	Response Rate
0	not defined	not defined	not defined	not stated	not stated	not defined
1	unclear non-standard	non-validated	region/city (+1)		self-selected or unclear	<50%

Table 5. *Cont.*

	Quality Assessment Criteria					
Grade	**Outcome Definition**	**Data Collection Instrument**	**Setting**	**Timing**	**Sampling**	**Response Rate**
2	clear non-standard	validated	specific location (+1)	Year	clear non-random	50–79%
3	standard	objective	urban/rural (+1)	year and season	random (by location or within location)	80%+
Grade			Percentage per criterion			
0	1	4	10	33	15	55
1	8	24	46	1	7	1
2	39	51	34	27	10	11
3	53	21	10	39	68	33

3.4. Sample Characteristics

Only a small number of papers (ten articles) reported data for children with mid-age less than 6 years. There were 56 articles with mid-age >6 and ≤12 years, and 117 with mid-age >12 and ≤18 years old.

Details of participant characteristics were often absent from reports. Data were present in the following proportions across the studies: BMI (60.8%), urban/rural (41.3%), sex (78.7% identified as either M or F, remainder mixed sex), day of the week (PA/SB 88.7/69.3% identify either as weekday, weekend day or both, remainder unknown), number of days over which measurements taken (PA/SB 87.3/65.2%), year (72.2%), time of year (56.1% as either precise month or season), public/private schools (50.2%) and socio-economic status (20.1%, but often mixed). The lack of consistency of reporting of key participant characteristics made summary using meta-regression inappropriate for most variables. Additionally, data were often reported for groups of participants as averages across large age ranges (e.g., 6–13 years of age [184]).

The variables with the largest volume of data were step count (measured either using pedometers or accelerometers) and TV viewing time (measured using a range of different questionnaires). A meta-regression of these variables was performed grouping reports which did not present specific characteristics into an additional analysis category. For example, data were often presented as combined male and female data. This was considered a separate category to male and female in the meta-regression analysis. The expected effect of this was to reduce the likelihood of detecting significant effects of group characteristics on differences between groups, as including the mixed group increased the number of groups and the mixed group would fall between the other groups. A backward step-wise approach was taken to isolate significant covariates. This should be considered an exploratory analysis.

All other data are presented in a graphical and narrative form.

3.5. Physical Activity Measurements

3.5.1. Step Count

Reported step-count data were collected using a range of body-worn devices including both accelerometers and pedometers. A range of accelerometer types (SenseWear [216], Actigraph [49,66,67,123,124,145,161,168,213] ActivPAL [79]) and pedometer types (e.g., Yamax Digiwalker SW 701 [52] Omron HJ-112 [62], Kenz Lifecorder [95,194], Healer MP-22 [187], Silva [92], Oregon Scientific PE320 [78]) were used in data collection. A wide range of step-count values were reported across the age range studied (4000–23,000 steps per day) (Figure 2).

Overall, there appeared to be a trend for females to record lower step counts than males across the full age range. However, there were numerous studies with combined results for males and females where step count was reported as being relatively high. Additionally, there appeared to be a reduction in step count with higher age. This reduction in step count with higher age was particularly evident in one large cross-sectional study where data were collected within year groups from 6–13 years [92].

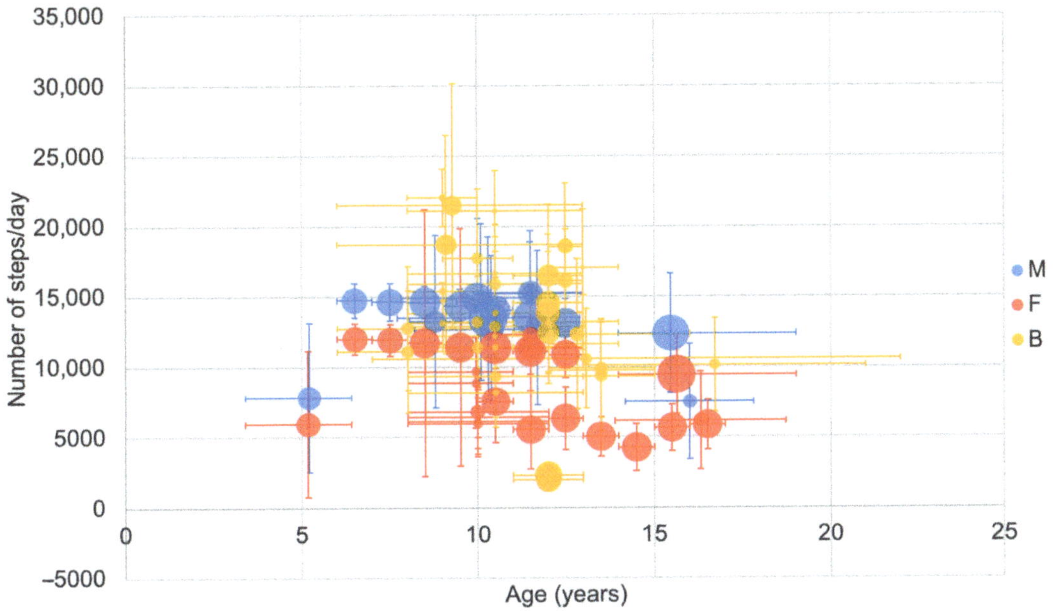

Figure 2. Number of reported daily steps by age. Mid age is used to present the data with range (see Table 1). Mean number of steps per day is presented ±SD (see Table 2). Bubbles indicate the relative sample size between studies. Data are presented as male (M), female (F) or both (B).

Meta-Regression Analysis of Step Count

For the journal papers reporting step count, there was a range of missing data in terms of the covariates of interest. The year of data collection was only reported in a small number of studies and could not be included in the analysis. Socio-demographic status was rarely reported and therefore not included. Nature of schooling, either public of private, was also poorly reported and therefore not included in analysis. Sex was always reported as either M/F or both. Mid age could always be calculated and was used in the analysis. Weight status was dichotomised as normal weight (assumed status if not specified) and overweight (where specified). Day of the week was categorised as either weekend, weekday or unspecified. Urban/rural was either specified as such or in an unspecified category. Similarly, season was either summer (April–September) or winter (October–March) with an additional unspecified category.

When all covariates (sex, weight status, day of week, age, urban/rural, season) were included in a meta-regression model of daily steps, urban/rural and season were not significant contributors. Therefore, the final model included sex, weight status, day of week and age (Table 6) (Figure 3). Age was centred at 12 years. A male of normal weight aged 12 years took on average 15,794 steps per day at the weekend. Females took 4602 fewer steps than males, being overweight was associated with 2799 fewer steps and 3098 fewer steps were taken on weekdays compared to weekends. The reports that combined both males and females appeared to show step count near to the values of males (only 212 higher on average). Where day of the week was unspecified, the step count appeared to be nearer to the weekday count than the weekend count.

Table 6. Meta-regression model of step count including sex, weight status, day of week and age as covariates. Note: age centred at 12 years.

Parameter		B Coefficient	95%CI	*p* Value
Intercept *		15,794	13,928, 17,663	$p < 0.001$
Sex	Female	−4602	−6131, −3074	$p < 0.001$
	Male + Female	212	−1263, 1686	0.776
Weight status	Overweight	−2799	−4832, −767	0.001
Day of week = week day	Week day	−3098	−4850, −1347	0.001
	Unspecified	−2282	−3985, −578	0.009
Age		−260	−513, −8	0.044

* Intercept value for male, normal weight, weekend, age of 12 years. CI = confidence interval.

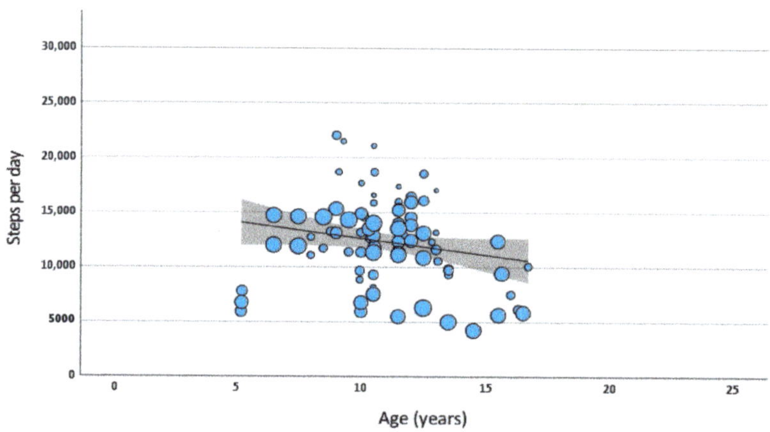

Figure 3. Meta-regression of steps per day by age (with adjustment for sex, weight status and day of week). Bubble size for each data point represents standard error. Prediction line and 95% confidence intervals are shown.

Exploration of the heterogeneity of results indicated that it was not possible to assume that all studies originated from the same underlying population ($I^2 = 99.9\%$). Examination of visual plots of data did not suggest any obvious subgroup analysis. These results suggest that there were differences in the underlying populations from which the samples were taken that were not captured by the variables included in the analysis.

3.5.2. MVPA Time (Body-Worn Device)

A number of reports were available on the time spent in moderate to vigorous physical activity derived using body-worn devices (Figure 4). The number of minutes per day that was reported varied widely. The methods of calculating the MVPA time depended on device-specific methods and the implementation of the method used by the authors. There was no clear trend across age groups or between the sexes in terms of minutes of MVPA per day, which ranged from virtually zero up to 170 min. Variation in device wear time, definition of MVPA within signal analysis algorithms and different data sources (e.g., use of acceleration—Actigraph [57], heart rate—Actical [217]) may have influenced outcomes differently between studies.

The large sample of children with mean age of 6 years was derived as part of the IDEFICS study with an undefined body-worn accelerometer device [179]. All papers reported that body-worn devices were kept on during waking hours, except one point

(130.83 min/day [113]), which reported 5 consecutive days' wear. It appeared that values measured using similar types of body-worn devices were clustered.

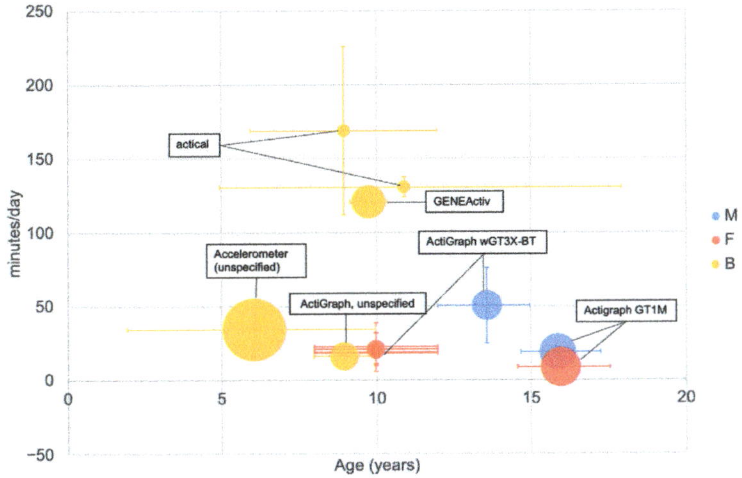

Figure 4. Minutes per day spent in MVPA by age measured using body-worn devices. The type of body-worn device used to measure the variable is illustrated. The largest bubble refers to a sample size of 484 [179]. See Figure 2 for explanation of plot.

3.5.3. Total PA (Mets min/day) (IPAQ Questionnaire)

The International Physical Activity Questionnaire [4] was used in a number of large studies to record overall daily physical activity in METs min/day (Figure 5).

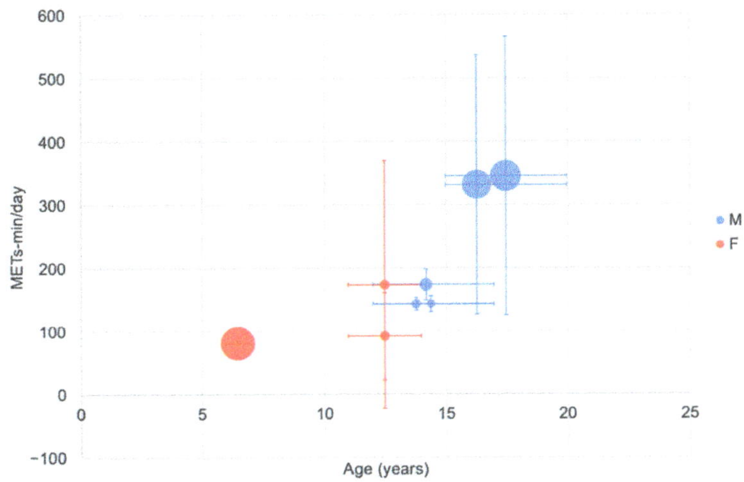

Figure 5. Total PA in METs min/day measured using the IPAQ by age. The largest bubble refers to a study with a sample size of 672 [34]. See Figure 2 for explanation of plot.

The data presented in Figure 5 represent the outcomes of large studies in Iran conducted between 2013 and 2019. Generally, males exhibited higher total PA in terms of METs min/day than females, although in the reported studies, males were generally older than females.

3.5.4. Total PA (METs Min/Day) (ATLS Questionnaire)

The ATLS (Arab Teens Lifestyle Study) [13] was used in a number of studies in Saudi Arabia, Kuwait, Qatar, and Jordan to report the total physical activity in METs min/day equivalents (Figure 6). Sample mean values appeared to indicate that males (400–700 METs min/day) were engaging in higher PA compared to females (100–350 METs min/day). The ATLS METs min/day values appeared to be generally higher than those reported for the IPAQ (Figure 5).

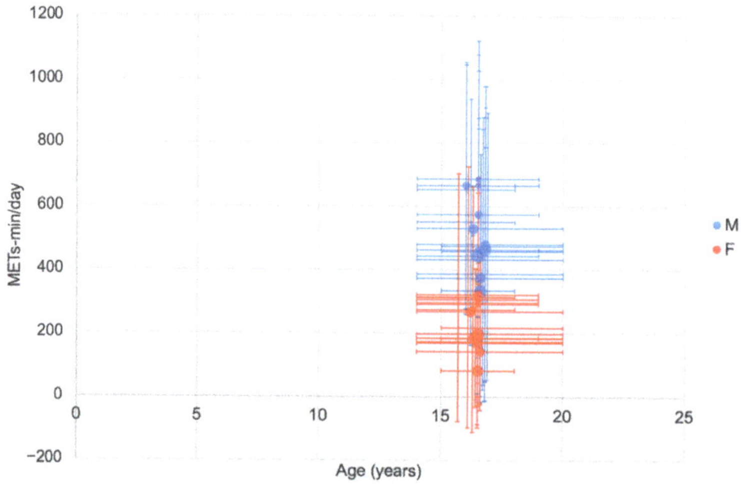

Figure 6. Physical activity as measured in METs min/day reported using the ATLS questionnaire by age. The largest bubble represents a sample size of 851 for girls and 797 for boys [57]. See Figure 2 for explanation of plot.

3.6. Sedentary Behaviour Measures

3.6.1. TV Viewing Time

There were numerous reports of TV viewing time with data collected using a range of different questionnaires. A meta-regression was implemented to predict TV viewing time with covariates urban/rural, year of data collection, season (summer/winter), age, sex (male, female or both), weight normal or overweight), and day of week (weekday, weekend or unidentified).

There were insufficient numbers of reports containing urban/rural (8/81) and day of week (6/81) to reasonably include these variables in the model. Again, socio-demographic status was not reported widely, or reported as mixed. Only age was a significant contributor in the prediction of volume of TV viewing time (Table 7) (Figure 7). For a 12-year-old, the average TV viewing time was 2.643 h per day. For every year older, 0.039 h more TV viewing time per day was predicted in the model.

There was extensive heterogeneity of results (I^2 = 99.3%), suggesting that across studies the data did not originate from the same underlying population. No clear subgroup analysis was warranted. It is possible that variables not captured in this review are important explanatory factors in TV viewing time.

Table 7. Meta-regression model of TV viewing time (hours/day) including age as a covariate. Note: age centred at 12 years.

Parameter	B Coefficient	95%CI	*p* Value
Intercept *	2.643	2.515, 2.771	<0.001
Age	0.039	0.008, 0.069	0.014

* Intercept value for age 12 years old. CI = confidence interval.

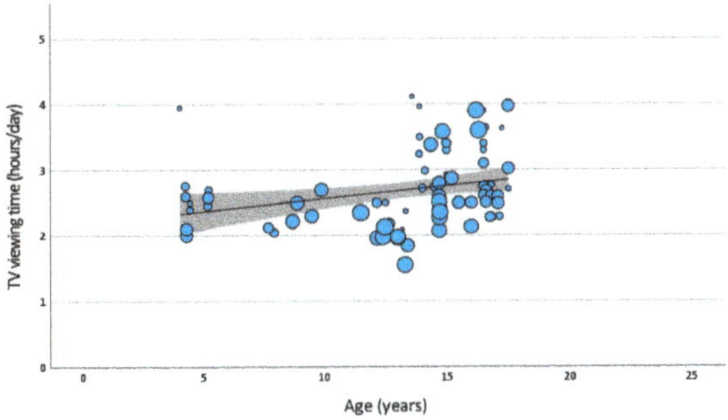

Figure 7. Meta-regression model of TV viewing time by age. Bubble size for each data point represents standard error. Prediction line and 95% confidence intervals are shown.

3.6.2. Screen/TV Time (ATLS, CASPIAN)

Two data collection tools used to collect information on screen/TV time were reported in several studies. These were the ATLS [13] and CASPIAN (Childhood and Adolescence Surveillance and Prevention of Adult Non-Communicable Disease in Iran [14]) study data collection tools.

TV Viewing/Screen Time (ATLS)

Questions asked in the ATLS questionnaire around TV viewing and screen time were "how long per day do you watch TV and/or DVD/Video during week days?", "how long per day do you watch TV and/or DVD/Video during weekends?", "how long per day do you spend on the computer and/or the internet (for leisure) during week days?" and "how long per day do you spend on the computer and/or the internet (for leisure) during weekends?".

For screen time and TV time reported using the ATLS questionnaire (Figure 8), two groupings of reported time (mins per day) are seen with screen time being higher than reported TV time. Reported data were predominantly derived from samples with wide age ranges. Screen time ranged from 171.6 to 450.6 min/day, and TV viewing time ranged from 136.8 to 234 min/day. There was no clear difference between males and females.

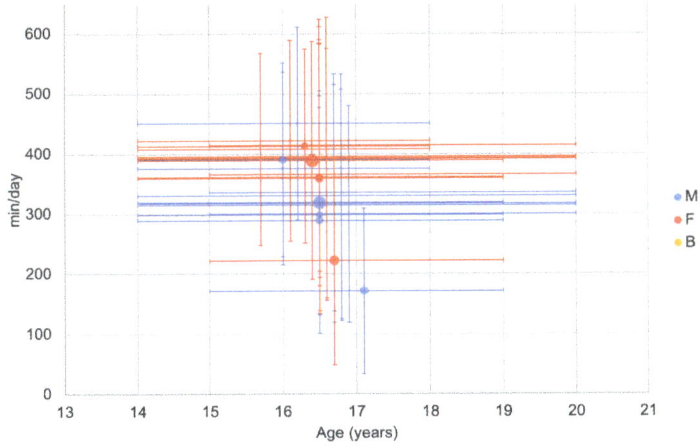

(a)

Figure 8. *Cont.*

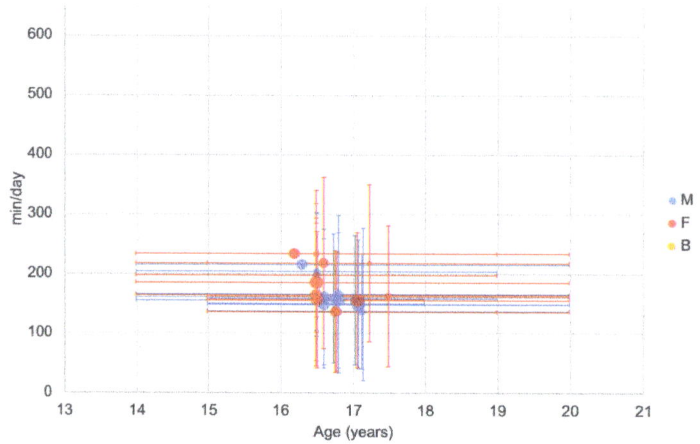

(b)

Figure 8. Minutes per day by age from the ATLS questionnaire of (**a**) screen time (largest bubble represents a sample size of 851 [62]); (**b**) TV viewing time (largest bubble represents a sample size of 663 [70]). See Figure 2 for explanation of plot.

3.6.3. Screen/TV Time (CASPIAN)

For the data reported using the CASPIAN data collection tool, screen time ranged from 74.22 to 186 min/day and TV watching time from 117.6 to 151.2 min/day (Figure 9). There were insufficient data to observe trends with age or gender.

3.6.4. Sedentary Time (Body-Worn Devices)

There were a number of reports on the daily volume of sedentary time (mins per day) as measured using body-worn devices (Figure 10). No clear trend was observed in sedentary time. Studies detailed a range of different protocols for defining sedentary time. This included variation in device wear time (i.e., full or waking day—see Figure 10).

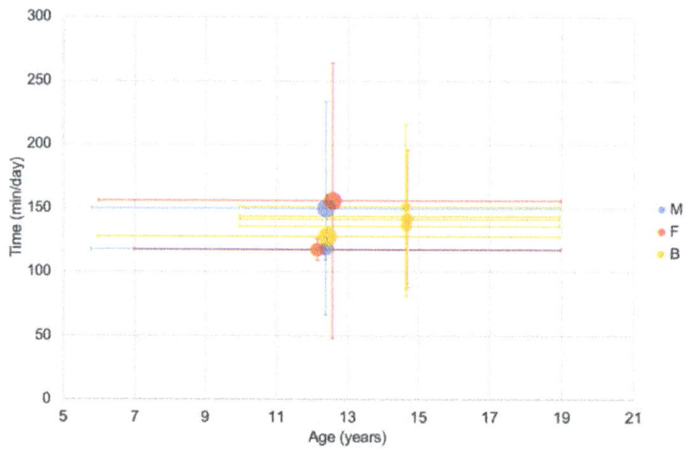

(a)

Figure 9. *Cont.*

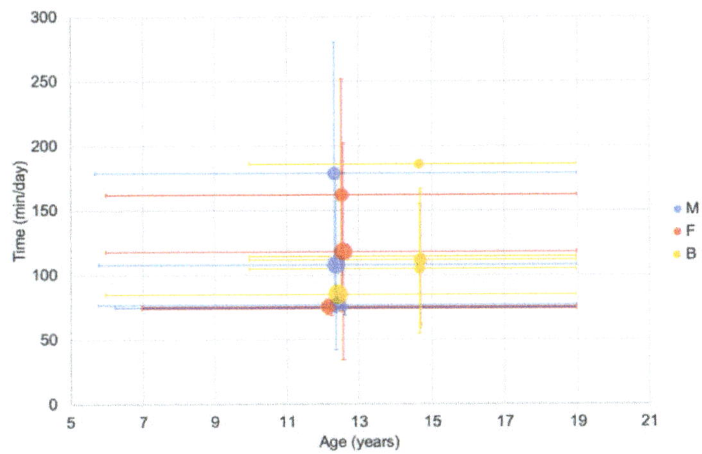

(b)

Figure 9. Minutes per day by age from the CASPIAN series of studies of (**a**) time spent watching a screen; (**b**) time spent watching TV. Largest bubbles represent a sample size of 13,486 [128]. See Figure 2 for explanation of plot.

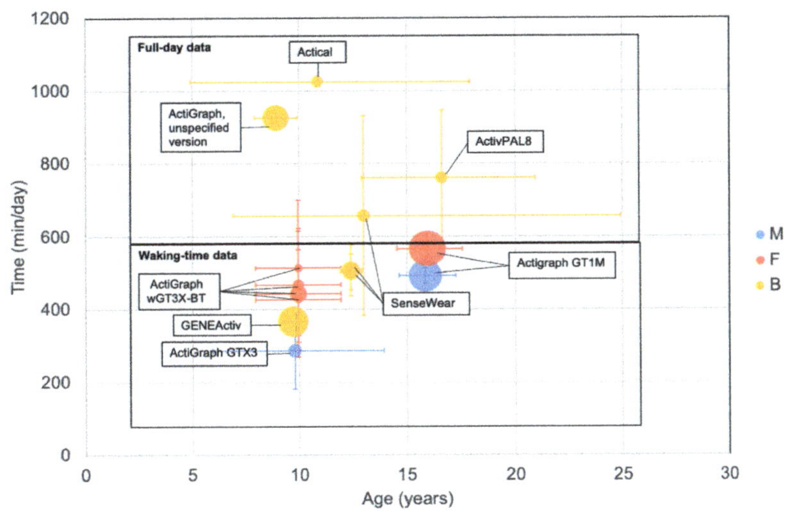

Figure 10. Minutes per day spent in sedentary behaviour derived using body-worn devices. The horizontal line delineates full-day data from waking-time data. Largest bubbles relate to a sample size of 189 for girls and 162 for boys [123]. See Figure 2 for explanation of plot.

All points below 600 min per day of sedentary time measured waking time only. All points above 600 measured full 24 h days. There was not a clear trend of sedentary behaviour measured using a body-worn device with age.

4. Discussion

This systematic literature review was performed to gather previously reported information on the daily volumes of PA and SB in children and adolescents 2–18 years old in Middle Eastern countries. This was done to provide a characterisation of physical behaviour in this area of the world that might be considered to have broadly similar environmental and cultural factors. Any measurements of PA and SB were considered acceptable for inclusion as long as they were representative of whole-day physical behaviour, derived using either objective body-worn devices or subjective self- or observer-reported questionnaires. A total of 183 journal articles reporting PA or SB were identified, reporting a range of outcome measures. Of all outcome measures reported, it was only possible to present a statistical analysis of daily step count and TV viewing time with other outcomes being described graphically and narratively due to small numbers of reports.

The search terms of the literature review were kept intentionally broad to ensure all reports of physical activity and sedentary behaviours were included.

The area of interest, the Middle East, was defined based on a range of countries where cultural influences and environmental influences might lead to similar constraints on and opportunities for PA and SB. While the authors acknowledge that the extent of the boundaries of the area considered to constitute the Middle East are not well defined, the choice of countries to include was justified based on historical, cultural and environmental considerations. To allow the reader to interpret results based on isolated countries, Supplementary Data is provided with a full list of all variables from all available literature (Supplementary Data S5).

The review identified a substantial body of literature reporting daily PA or SB measures (183 journal articles). However, reports were concentrated mainly in Iran (68 publications), Turkey (37) and Saudi Arabia (27) with none reporting data from Bahrain, Syria or Yemen. There were a number of large cohort studies associated with these concentrations of reporting (e.g., ATLS: Saudi Arabia (Al-Khobar, Jeddah, Riyadh, Al-Ahsa), Kuwait, Qatar, Iraq, Jordan, Oman; CASPIAN: Iran). The larger cohort studies provided evidence of random sampling across regions, and therefore, reported data should be representative of national trends in physical behaviour for the age groups studied. However, in other countries, the sample sizes were smaller and must be considered to be less representative of the broader national populations of children (e.g., Egypt, Iraq, Palestine, Qatar, UAE). An additional constraint on the reported data is that reports often grouped children and adolescents across broad age ranges [49,62,65], making identification of trends with age difficult.

The variables reported were of numerous types with many different quantities defined (Table 4). The intention to present meta-regression analysis could only be achieved for step count and TV viewing time due to the small number of studies on each PA or SB measure. It was possible to present a number of PA and SB measures graphically. Even within this limited selection of variables, there were several data collection methods used which made comparison between study outcomes difficult. For example, MVPA was measured using various different technologies (Figure 4) (e.g., incorporating data from accelerometry, body temperature [218], heart rate [219]). For identification of SB, the surrogate of TV viewing or screen viewing was reported in several studies. However, different definitions were used in different studies (e.g., ATLS, CASPIAN), making comparison between studies challenging.

A simple quality assessment was performed to identify key components of study reporting. Either unclear reporting or use of non-standardised outcome measures (without clear validity) was present in 47% of studies, highlighting difficulties in comparing outcomes between studies. This points to a need for the adoption of standardised and validated body-worn device outcomes or self-report measures across studies to allow data gathering and exploration of changes in PA and SB across ages and over time. Ambiguity in the exact questions asked in questionnaires concerning sedentary time (TV viewing, screen viewing, etc.) were particularly problematic for comparison of sedentary outcomes. Perhaps this difficulty has been compounded by a lack of foresight by researchers in anticipating changes in technology. Not all studies reported whether the setting was urban/rural or reported the time of year. Without reporting of such demographic and season data, it is difficult to understand differences between study results. While a majority of studies (68%) reported an element of randomisation in selection of their sample population, there was limited reporting of response rate, potentially introducing bias into the reported data.

An attempt was made to extract information on participant BMI, sex, socio-demographic status, day of week data was recorded for, and if study participants attended public or private schools. It is possible that all of these variables may influence physical behaviour, but they were not reported in all studies, again making inter-study comparison difficult.

4.1. Reports of Physical Activity

PA was reported using a wide range of quantities. This included time spent in postures (e.g., standing) and the number of steps taken per day. These are relatively unambiguous concepts that can be measured using body-worn devices. Additionally, PA was reported in relation to energy expenditure, either as daily energy expenditure or as time spent at set energy expenditure levels (e.g., moderate or vigorous intensity). The determination of these quantities was device- or questionnaire-dependent, causing difficulties with comparison between studies.

4.1.1. Stepping Activity

The most enduring measure of physical activity performance appears to be step count. Studies reported step count evaluation using body-worn devices including pedometer and other accelerometer-based devices (Figure 2). It was possible to perform a meta- regression analysis of step count, suggesting age, sex, weight status and day of the week were important in describing variance (Table 6). However, there was a high level of heterogeneity between study results, suggesting that there were differences in the underlying populations from which samples were taken. The step counts reported were broadly similar to those reported for other regions of the world: Male weekend daily step count for 12-year-olds (15,845) was higher compared to similarly aged children in America [220]. However, day of the week is often not specified, and there was an indication of ~3000 fewer steps being taken on weekdays. Females took fewer steps (−4602 per day), similar to observations in other parts of the world, for example in Australia [221] (10,463 for boys and 8940 for girls.), in Canada [222] (12,100 for boys and 10,300 for girls) and in Finland [8] (10,824 for boys and 9040 for girls). Additionally, those who were characterised as over-weight took fewer steps (−2799 per day), again similar to other regions, e.g., UK [223] and Ireland [224].

Based on the identified relationships between step count and gender, body weight, day of the week and age, there is evidence (although weak) to support similar patterns of activity in the Middle East to those in Europe and North America (as referenced previously). This would suggest that the effect of these factors on step count are similar even though the cultural and environmental contexts are different. It is possible therefore that the underlying reasons for differences between sub-groups of children and adolescents may be the same across the world, including the impact of differences in social interactions for boys and girls, the association of excessive body weight with activity levels, the importance of day of the week and the general decline in activity (stepping) with age. These similarities may suggest that components of interventions to increase stepping activity (e.g., enhanced social support [225]; enhanced psychological support [226]) could be similar across contexts, including the Middle East.

4.1.2. MVPA Time (Body-Worn Devices)

The reported values of MVPA time (Figure 4) highlight differences between different devices (e.g., actical, ActiGraph). It appeared that different wear time protocols and different algorithms for identifying MVPA time made values incomparable. Standardisation of measurements is required before data can be reasonably synthesised.

4.1.3. Total PA (METs min/day) IPAQ and ATLS

The IPAQ and ATLS have been used in large cross-sectional studies to determine daily PA time as METS min/day (Figures 5 and 6). Unfortunately, the data reported did not cover the age range of interest well and the IPAQ results appeared to be generally lower than the ATLS outcomes. Overall, however, it is possible to observe a higher total PA level for males than females. The total PA measured using IPAQ showed that males engage in more total PA compared to females, in agreement with Bauman et al. [227], which was conducted in 20 countries.

4.2. Reports of Sedentary Behaviour

4.2.1. Screen/TV Time

There were several different methods used to assess screen time. A common method was to ask questions about TV screen time ('TV watching', 'TV viewing', 'TV time'). Other combinations of screen time, including video, computer games and mobile phone, were reported (see Supplementary Material S5). However, it was difficult to compare between studies as technological changes reduced the relevance of chronological comparison. This evolution of terminology added a layer of complexity to comparing not only changing questions, but also changing meaning of the same question. For example, 'screen time', has developed from including only TV viewing to including progressively video, gaming devices, computers and mobile phone screens. To compound difficulties with exploration of these changing definitions, numerous studies did not report the year of data collection.

When TV viewing time was taken in isolation, a meta-regression analysis suggested that only age was an important predictor, indicating an increase of 0.039 (95% CI: 0.008, 0.069) hours per day per year of age. However, due to high levels of heterogeneity in study outcomes and no clear sub-group analysis pathway, these results must be treated with a high level of caution.

While TV viewing time is highlighted here as a possible daily SB quantity, a study conducted on teenagers in the UK suggests that TV viewing time does not reflect full-day sedentary time [228,229]. Also, McGrane Minton et al. [230] suggest not using full-day sitting time and TV viewing time interchangeably when measuring SB. TV viewing can therefore only be considered a partial surrogate for SB.

Unfortunately, due to the various definitions used in questionnaires, it was not possible to robustly examine total screen time across all studies. The changing self-report questions concerning screen-based device usage tend to reflect changing habits. For example, although Mullan [231] report a 30 min per day increased use of screen-based devices among 8–18-year-old children in the UK from 2000 to 2015, this was attributed to an increase in boys playing video games.

In a scoping review by Thomas et al. (2019), it was highlighted that total screen time (TV viewing, computer use, and playing video games) among 5–18-year-olds increased over time, but within this group, TV viewing declined a little. Thomas et al. [232] also showed an increase in overall screen time over a 4-year period (2010–2014) for Australian children aged 10–15 (TV viewing, computer use, and social networking and online communication). Differences in cultural norms and environmental factors may have made changes in the Middle East different to those seen in other continents [19,233,234]. Unfortunately, the inconsistent use of terminology between studies made exploration of changes with chronological time impossible.

4.2.2. SB Body-Worn Devices

The disparate results of sedentary behaviour time per day reported using body-worn devices point to a need for a standardisation of measurement in this area.

4.3. Limitations

There is no clearly identified region which constitutes the Middle East. However, for the current review, countries were included where it was anticipated cultural and environmental factors may be similar.

This review did not include an analysis of the grey literature. It is possible that, for example, governmental reports may add further insight into PA and SB levels in this region.

It was not possible to gain access to original data sets. No authors responded to requests for additional information. Gaining further details on study cohorts, timing of data collection and details of specific data collection instruments not included in reports would have been helpful in informing outcome analysis.

The use of a wide range of data collection instruments that were often poorly defined and lacked consistency of application between studies made synthesis of results difficult across most outcome measures.

It was common for studies to report outcomes for grouped results across wide age ranges; this may have masked age-related changes.

The meta-regression analyses reported identified heterogeneity of data and should be considered to be exploratory in nature.

5. Conclusions

There is extensive reporting of PA and SB in children and adolescents across the Middle East through small-scale studies, but also through relatively large-scale cross-sectional studies with randomised selection of participants. However, there is a lack of standardisation of outcome measures, making synthesis of findings across studies difficult. The absence of longitudinal studies prevents definitive conclusions on changes of behaviour with age, as shifting patterns of behaviour (e.g., screen viewing) may be the underlying cause of changes rather than age.

Where sufficient data were available, it was observed that those children and adolescents who were male, of normal weight and younger appeared to undertake more PA in terms of stepping activity. More stepping activity was undertaken at weekends. This was reinforced for questionnaire-based outcomes of PA energy expenditure in terms of METs min/day, where males tended to report more daily PA.

TV viewing time as a surrogate for sedentary behaviour suggested an increase with age. There was insufficient data of objectively measured sedentary time to allow synthesis and analysis of the influence of covariates.

Generally, trends in PA and SB between males and females were similar to those found in European/North American studies, although there may be greater differences in the Middle Eastern region. The observation of similar differences between sexes in different cultures and environments points to the possibility that there may be common behavioural, social and psychological factors affecting relative physical behaviour levels. This may imply that similar intervention strategies can be used across regions to enhance physical behaviour for improved long-term health.

Overall, while there were a large number of reports of PA and SB, the outcomes reported were disparate and confounded by changing behaviour in regard to engagement with technology (SB measured using TV/screen viewing). There is a need for further standardisation of measurement to ensure synthesis of report findings is possible in the future.

Supplementary Materials: The following supporting information can be downloaded at https://www.mdpi.com/article/10.3390/ijerph20206940/s1, Table S1: PRISMA Checklist; Table S2: Search terms used within the CINAHL, MEDLINE, Web of Science and PsychoINFO databases; Table S3: Quality assessment criteria with definitions used to facilitate scoring; Table S4: Reference list of all papers included in the review; Table S5: Extracted PA and SB data from all studies identified.

Author Contributions: Conceptualization, B.S. and S.S.; methodology, B.S. and E.B.; validation, B.S., E.B. and S.S.; formal analysis, B.S. and E.B.; investigation, B.S., E.B. and S.S.; data curation, E.B. and B.S.; writing—original draft preparation, E.B.; writing—review and editing, B.S. and E.B.; visualization, B.S. and E.B.; supervision, B.S. and S.S.; project administration, E.B. and B.S. All authors have read and agreed to the published version of the manuscript.

Funding: This research received no external funding.

Institutional Review Board Statement: As this was a review study of existing literature, it was not necessary to receive ethical approval to proceed.

Data Availability Statement: To enquire about access to the data used to develop outcomes in this paper, please contact the lead author or refer to Supplementary Material Table S5.

Conflicts of Interest: The authors declare no conflict of interest.

References

1. Bull, F.C.; Al-Ansari, S.S.; Biddle, S.; Borodulin, K.; Buman, M.P.; Cardon, G.; Carty, C.; Chaput, J.-P.; Chastin, S.; Chou, R.; et al. World Health Organization 2020 guidelines on physical activity and sedentary behaviour. *Br. J. Sports Med.* **2020**, *54*, 1451–1462. [CrossRef] [PubMed]
2. Posadzki, P.; Pieper, D.; Bajpai, R.; Makaruk, H.; Könsgen, N.; Neuhaus, A.L.; Semwal, M. Exercise/physical activity and health outcomes: An overview of Cochrane systematic reviews. *BMC Public Health* **2020**, *20*, 1724. [CrossRef] [PubMed]
3. Katzmarzyk, P.T.; Lee, I.-M. Sedentary behaviour and life expectancy in the USA: A cause-deleted life table analysis. *BMJ Open* **2012**, *2*, e000828. [CrossRef] [PubMed]
4. Hagströmer, M.; Oja, P.; Sjöström, M. The International Physical Activity Questionnaire (IPAQ): A study of concurrent and construct validity. *Public Health Nutr.* **2006**, *9*, 755–762. [CrossRef]
5. Baran, J.; Weres, A.; Wyszyńska, J.; Pitucha, G.; Czenczek-Lewandowska, E.; Rusek, W.; Leszczak, J.; Mazur, A. 60 Minutes Per Day in Moderate to Vigorous Physical Activity as a Natural Health Protector in Young Population. *Int. J. Environ. Res. Public Health* **2020**, *17*, 8918. [CrossRef]
6. Hussein, T.; Paasonen, P.; Kulmala, M. Activity pattern of a selected group of school occupants and their family members in Helsinki—Finland. *Sci. Total. Environ.* **2012**, *425*, 289–292. [CrossRef]
7. Al-Hazzaa, H.M. Physical Activity Research in the Gulf Cooperation Council Countries: Progress Made but Work Still to Do. *J. Phys. Act. Health* **2022**, *19*, 769–770. [CrossRef]
8. Jussila, A.-M.; Husu, P.; Vähä-Ypyä, H.; Tokola, K.; Kokko, S.; Sievänen, H.; Vasankari, T. Accelerometer-Measured Physical Activity Levels and Patterns Vary in an Age- and Sex-Dependent Fashion among Finnish Children and Adolescents. *Int. J. Environ. Res. Public Health* **2022**, *19*, 6950. [CrossRef]
9. Whitfield, G.P.; Carlson, S.A.; Ussery, E.N.; Fulton, J.E.; Galuska, D.A.; Petersen, R. Trends in Meeting Physical Activity Guidelines Among Urban and Rural Dwelling Adults—United States, 2008–2017. *MMWR Morb. Mortal. Wkly. Rep.* **2019**, *68*, 513–518. [CrossRef]
10. Schwedler, J. (Ed.) Frontmatter. In *Understanding the Contemporary Middle East*; Lynne Rienner Publishers: Boulder, CO, USA, 2013; pp. i–iv. [CrossRef]
11. Chaabane, S.; Chaabna, K.; Doraiswamy, S.; Mamtani, R.; Cheema, S. Barriers and Facilitators Associated with Physical Activity in the Middle East and North Africa Region: A Systematic Overview. *Int. J. Environ. Res. Public Health* **2021**, *18*, 1647. [CrossRef]
12. Ntoumos, A.; Hadjinicolaou, P.; Zittis, G.; Proestos, Y.; Lelieveld, J. Projected Air Temperature Extremes and Maximum Heat Conditions Over the Middle-East-North Africa (MENA) Region. *Earth Syst. Environ.* **2022**, *6*, 343–359. [CrossRef]
13. Al-Hazzaa, H.M.; Musaiger, A.O.; Arab Teens Lifestyle Study Research Group. Physical activity patterns and eating habits of adolescents living in major Arab cities. The Arab Teens Lifestyle Study. *Saudi Med. J.* **2010**, *31*, 210–211. [PubMed]
14. Kelishadi, R.; Gheiratmand, R.; Ardalan, G.; Adeli, K.; Gouya, M.M.; Razaghi, E.M.; Majdzadeh, R.; Delavari, A.; Shariatinejad, K.; Motaghian, M.; et al. Association of anthropometric indices with cardiovascular disease risk factors among children and adolescents: CASPIAN Study. *Int. J. Cardiol.* **2007**, *117*, 340–348. [CrossRef]
15. Marsh, D. *The Middle East Unveiled. Little*; Brown Book Group: Boston, MA, USA, 2011. Available online: https://books.google.co.uk/books?id=F4meBAAAQBAJ (accessed on 11 October 2023).
16. Ker-Lindsay, J. Europe's Eastern Outpost: The Republic of Cyprus and the Middle East. *Round Table* **2008**, *97*, 535–545. [CrossRef]
17. Ouzzani, M.; Hammady, H.; Fedorowicz, Z.; Elmagarmid, A. Rayyan—A web and mobile app for systematic reviews. *Syst. Rev.* **2016**, *5*, 210. [CrossRef] [PubMed]
18. Page, M.J.; McKenzie, J.E.; Bossuyt, P.M.; Boutron, I.; Hoffmann, T.C.; Mulrow, C.D.; Shamseer, L.; Tetzlaff, J.M.; Akl, E.A.; Brennan, S.E.; et al. The PRISMA 2020 statement: An updated guideline for reporting systematic reviews. *BMJ* **2021**, *372*, 71. [CrossRef]
19. Chaabane, S.; Chaabna, K.; Abraham, A.; Mamtani, R.; Cheema, S. Physical activity and sedentary behaviour in the Middle East and North Africa: An overview of systematic reviews and meta-analysis. *Sci. Rep.* **2020**, *10*, 9363. [CrossRef]
20. Bauman, A.E.; Reis, R.S.; Sallis, J.F.; Wells, J.C.; Loos, R.J.; Martin, B.W. Correlates of physical activity: Why are some people physically active and others not? *Lancet* **2012**, *380*, 258–271. [CrossRef]
21. O'Donoghue, G.; Perchoux, C.; Mensah, K.; Lakerveld, J.; van der Ploeg, H.; Bernaards, C.; Chastin, S.F.M.; Simon, C.; O'Gorman, D.; Nazare, J.-A.; et al. A systematic review of correlates of sedentary behaviour in adults aged 18–65 years: A socio-ecological approach. *BMC Public Health* **2016**, *16*, 163. [CrossRef] [PubMed]
22. Prince, S.A.; Roberts, K.C.; Melvin, A.; Butler, G.P.; Thompson, W. Gender and education differences in sedentary behaviour in Canada: An analysis of national cross-sectional surveys. *BMC Public Health* **2020**, *20*, 1170. [CrossRef]
23. Hills, A.P.; Andersen, L.B.; Byrne, N.M. Physical activity and obesity in children. *Br. J. Sports Med.* **2011**, *45*, 866–870. [CrossRef] [PubMed]
24. Biddle, S.H.J.; Bengoechea, E.G.; Wiesner, G. Sedentary behaviour and adiposity in youth: A systematic review of reviews and analysis of causality. *Int. J. Behav. Nutr. Phys. Act.* **2017**, *14*, 43. [CrossRef] [PubMed]
25. Pearman, S.N.; Valois, R.F.; Thatcher, W.G.; Drane, J.W. Physical Activity Behaviors of Adolescents in Public and Private High Schools. *Am. J. Health Behav.* **2001**, *25*, 42–49. [CrossRef] [PubMed]

26. Nascente, F.M.N.; Jardim, T.V.; Peixoto, M.D.R.G.; Carneiro, C.d.S.; Mendonça, K.L.; Póvoa, T.I.R.; Sousa, A.L.L.; Barroso, W.K.S.; Jardim, P.C.B.V. Sedentary lifestyle and its associated factors among adolescents from public and private schools of a Brazilian state capital. *BMC Public Health* **2016**, *16*, 1177. [CrossRef]
27. Prince, S.A.; Reed, J.L.; McFetridge, C.; Tremblay, M.S.; Reid, R.D. Correlates of sedentary behaviour in adults: A systematic review. *Obes. Rev.* **2017**, *18*, 915–935. [CrossRef]
28. Martin, S.L.; Kirkner, G.J.; Mayo, K.; Matthews, C.E.; Durstine, J.L.; Hebert, J.R. Urban, Rural, and Regional Variations in Physical Activity. *J. Rural. Health* **2005**, *21*, 239–244. [CrossRef]
29. Fairclough, S.J.; Boddy, L.M.; Mackintosh, K.A.; Valencia-Peris, A.; Ramirez-Rico, E. Weekday and weekend sedentary time and physical activity in differentially active children. *J. Sci. Med. Sport* **2014**, *18*, 444–449. [CrossRef]
30. Tucker, P.; Gilliland, J. The Effect of Season and Weather on Physical Activity: A Systematic Review. *Public Health* **2007**, *121*, 909–922. [CrossRef]
31. Turrisi, T.B.; Bittel, K.M.; West, A.B.; Hojjatinia, S.; Hojjatinia, S.; Mama, S.K.; Lagoa, C.M.; Conroy, D.E. Seasons, weather, and device-measured movement behaviors: A scoping review from 2006 to 2020. *Int. J. Behav. Nutr. Phys. Act.* **2021**, *18*, 24. [CrossRef]
32. Sasayama, K.; Adachi, M. Secular changes in total steps and moderate-to-vigorous physical activity among fourth-grade students in Japan in 2003/2004 and 2016/2017. *J. Sports Sci.* **2019**, *38*, 416–421. [CrossRef]
33. Dalene, K.E.; Kolle, E.; Steene-Johannessen, J.; Hansen, B.H.; Ekelund, U.; Grydeland, M.; Anderssen, S.A.; Tarp, J. Device-measured sedentary time in Norwegian children and adolescents in the era of ubiquitous internet access: Secular changes between 2005, 2011 and 2018. *Leuk. Res.* **2022**, *51*, 1556–1567. [CrossRef] [PubMed]
34. Eslami, A.A.; Abasi, M.H.; Rakhshani, F.; Shiri, M. A self-efficacy questionnaire regarding leisure time physical activity: Psychometric properties among Iranian male adolescents. *Iran. J. Nurs. Midwifery Res.* **2016**, *21*, 20–28. [CrossRef] [PubMed]
35. Eslami, A.A.; Abasi, M.H.; Rakhshani, F.; Shiri, M. Development and psychometric properties of a self-regulation scale about leisure time physical activity in Iranian male adolescents. *Iran. J. Nurs. Midwifery Res.* **2016**, *21*, 183–190. [CrossRef]
36. Abdulaziz, J.S.; Hassan, M.K. Nutritional status of children and adolescents with haemophilia in Basra, Iraq. *Haemophilia* **2019**, *25*, E353–E360. [CrossRef]
37. Abiri, B.; Sarbakhsh, P.; Vafa, M. Prevalence of overweight, obesity, and associated risk factors in healthy female adolescents in Tehran, Iran. *Cent. Asian J. Glob. Health* **2019**, *8*, 413. [CrossRef]
38. Khalid, M.E.; Ahmed, H.S.; Osman, O.M.; Ballal, M.; Al-Hashem, F.H. The association between physical activity and overweight and obesity in a population of children at high and low altitudes in Southwestern Saudi Arabia. *J. Fam. Community Med.* **2016**, *23*, 82–87. [CrossRef]
39. Akbulut, G.; Yildirim, M.; Sanlier, N.; van Stralen, M.M.; Acar-Tek, N.; Bilici, S.; Brug, J.; de Meij, J.S.; Gezmen-Karadag, M.; Koksal, E.; et al. Comparison of energy balance-related behaviours and measures of body composition between Turkish adolescents in Turkey and Turkish immigrant adolescents in the Netherlands. *Public Health Nutr.* **2013**, *17*, 2692–2699. [CrossRef]
40. Akman, M.; Akan, H.; İzbirak, G.; Tanrıöver, Ö.; Tilev, S.M.; Yıldız, A.; Tektaş, S.; Vitrinel, A.; Hayran, O. Eating patterns of Turkish adolescents: A cross-sectional survey. *Nutr. J.* **2010**, *9*, 67. [CrossRef] [PubMed]
41. Aktürk, S.; Büyükavcı, R.; Aktürk, Ü. Relationship between musculoskeletal disorders and physical inactivity in adolescents. *J. Public Health* **2018**, *27*, 49–56. [CrossRef]
42. Al Barwani, S.; Al Abri, M.; Al Hashmi, K.; Al Shukeiry, M.; Tahlilkar, K.; Al Zuheibi, T.; Al Rawas, O.; O Hassan, M. Assessment of aerobic fitness and its correlates in Omani adolescents using the 20-metre shuttle run test: A pilot study. *J. Sci. Res.* **2001**, *3*, 77–80.
43. Al Yazeedi, B. Childhood Obesity and Family Influence on Children's Nutrition Intake, Physical Activity Patterns, and BMI Z-Scores in Oman. Ph.D. Thesis, University of North Carolina at Chapel Hill Graduate School, Chapel Hill, NC, USA, 2018.
44. Alaca, N.; Yüksel, M. Comparison of physical functions and psychosocial conditions between adolescents with pectus excavatum, pectus carinatum and healthy controls. *Pediatr. Surg. Int.* **2021**, *37*, 765–775. [CrossRef] [PubMed]
45. Alamolhoda, M.; Heydari, S.T.; Ayatollahi, S.M.T.; Tabrizi, R.; Akbari, M.; Ardalan, A. A multivariate multilevel analysis of the risk factors associated with anthropometric indices in Iranian mid-adolescents. *BMC Pediatr.* **2020**, *20*, 191. [CrossRef]
46. Albarwani, S.; Al-Hashmi, K.; Al-Abri, M.; Jaju, D.; Hassan, M.O.; Andrade, S.; Ochoa-Avilés, A.; Lachat, C.; Escobar, P.; Verstraeten, R.; et al. Effects of Overweight and Leisure-Time Activities on Aerobic Fitness in Urban and Rural Adolescents. *Metab. Syndr. Relat. Disord.* **2009**, *7*, 369–374. [CrossRef] [PubMed]
47. Alghadir, A.H.; Gabr, S.A.; Al-Eisa, E. Effects of Physical Activity on Trace Elements and Depression Related Biomarkers in Children and Adolescents. *Biol. Trace Element Res.* **2015**, *172*, 299–306. [CrossRef] [PubMed]
48. Alghadir, A.H.; Gabr, S.A.; Iqbal, Z.A. Effects of sitting time associated with media consumption on physical activity patterns and daily energy expenditure of Saudi school students. *J. Phys. Ther. Sci.* **2015**, *27*, 2807–2812. [CrossRef]
49. Alghadir, A.H.; Gabr, S.A.; Rizk, A.A. Physical Fitness, Adiposity, and Diets as Surrogate Measures of Bone Health in Schoolchildren: A Biochemical and Cross-Sectional Survey Analysis. *J. Clin. Densitom.* **2018**, *21*, 406–419. [CrossRef]
50. Alghadir, A.H.; Iqbal, Z.A.; Gabr, S.A. Differences among Saudi and Expatriate Students: Body Composition Indices, Sitting Time Associated with Media Use and Physical Activity Pattern. *Int. J. Environ. Res. Public Health* **2020**, *17*, 832. [CrossRef]
51. Al-Ghamdi, M.A.; Lanham-New, S.A.; Kahn, J.A. Differences in vitamin D status and calcium metabolism in Saudi Arabian boys and girls aged 6 to 18 years: Effects of age, gender, extent of veiling and physical activity with concomitant implications for bone health. *Public Health Nutr.* **2012**, *15*, 1845–1853. [CrossRef]

52. Al-Hazzaa, H.M. Pedometer-determined Physical Activity among Obese and Non-obese 8- to 12-year-old Saudi Schoolboys. *J. Physiol. Anthr.* **2007**, *26*, 459–465. [CrossRef]
53. Al-Hazzaa, H.M.; Abahussain, N.A.; Al-Sobayel, H.I.; Qahwaji, D.M.; Musaiger, A.O. Physical activity, sedentary behaviors and dietary habits among Saudi adolescents relative to age, gender and region. *Int. J. Behav. Nutr. Phys. Act.* **2011**, *8*, 140. [CrossRef]
54. Al-Hazzaa, H.M.; A Abahussain, N.; I Al-Sobayel, H.; Qahwaji, D.M.; O Musaiger, A. Lifestyle factors associated with overweight and obesity among Saudi adolescents. *BMC Public Health* **2012**, *12*, 354. [CrossRef]
55. Al-Hazzaa, H.M.; Alahmadi, M.A.; Al-Sobayel, H.I.; Abahussain, N.A.; Qahwaji, D.M.; Musaiger, A.O. Patterns and Determinants of Physical Activity Among Saudi Adolescents. *J. Phys. Act. Health* **2014**, *11*, 1202–1211. [CrossRef] [PubMed]
56. Al-Hazzaa, H.M.; Al-Hussain, M.H.; Alhowikan, A.M.; Obeid, O.A. Insufficient Sleep Duration and Its Association with Breakfast Intake, Overweight/Obesity, Socio-Demographics and Selected Lifestyle Behaviors Among Saudi School Children. *Nat. Sci. Sleep* **2019**, *11*, 253–263. [CrossRef]
57. Al-Hazzaa, H.M.; Al-Nakeeb, Y.; Duncan, M.J.; Al-Sobayel, H.I.; Abahussain, N.A.; Musaiger, A.O.; Lyons, M.; Collins, P.; Nevill, A. A Cross-Cultural Comparison of Health Behaviors between Saudi and British Adolescents Living in Urban Areas: Gender by Country Analyses. *Int. J. Environ. Res. Public Health* **2013**, *10*, 6701–6720. [CrossRef] [PubMed]
58. Al-Hazzaa, H.M.; Al-Rasheedi, A.A. Adiposity and physical activity levels among preschool children in Jeddah, Saudi Arabia. *Saudi Med. J.* **2007**, *28*, 766.
59. Al-Hazzaa, H.M.; Al-Sobayel, H.I.; Abahussain, N.A.; Qahwaji, D.M.; Alahmadi, M.A.; Musaiger, A.O. Association of dietary habits with levels of physical activity and screen time among adolescents living in Saudi Arabia. *J. Hum. Nutr. Diet.* **2013**, *27*, 204–213. [CrossRef]
60. Al-Hazzaa, H.M.; Al-Sobayel, H.I.; Musaiger, A.O. Convergent Validity of the Arab Teens Lifestyle Study (ATLS) Physical Activity Questionnaire. *Int. J. Environ. Res. Public Health* **2011**, *8*, 3810–3820. [CrossRef] [PubMed]
61. Al-Hazzaa, H.M.; Musaiger, A.O.; Abahussain, N.A.; Al-Sobayel, H.I.; Qahwaji, D.M. Lifestyle correlates of self-reported sleep duration among Saudi adolescents: A multicentre school-based cross-sectional study. *Child: Care Health Dev.* **2013**, *40*, 533–542. [CrossRef]
62. Alhusaini, A.A.; Al-Walah, M.A.; Melam, G.R.; Buragadda, S. Pedometer-determined physical activity levels of healthy children and children with Down's syndrome. *Somatosens. Mot. Res.* **2017**, *34*, 219–225. [CrossRef]
63. Alhusaini, A.A.; Buragadda, S.; Melam, G. Associations among Body Mass Index, sedentary behavior, physical activity, and academic performance in schoolchildren. *SSRN Electron. J.* **2020**, *60*, 1551–1557. [CrossRef]
64. Alhusaini, A.A.; Melam, G.R.; Buragadda, S. Cross-Cultural Variation in BMI, Sedentary Behavior, and Physical Activity in International School Girls Residing in Saudi Arabia. *Int. J. Environ. Res. Public Health* **2020**, *17*, 2057. [CrossRef]
65. Aliss, E.M.; Sutaih, R.H.; Kamfar, H.Z.; Alagha, A.E.; Marzouki, Z.M. Physical activity pattern and its relationship with overweight and obesity in Saudi children. *Int. J. Pediatr. Adolesc. Med.* **2020**, *7*, 181–185. [CrossRef] [PubMed]
66. Aljuhani, O.; Sandercock, G. Contribution of Physical Education to the Daily Physical Activity of Schoolchildren in Saudi Arabia. *Int. J. Environ. Res. Public Health* **2019**, *16*, 2397. [CrossRef] [PubMed]
67. Al-Kutbe, R.; Payne, A.; de Looy, A.; Rees, G.A. A comparison of nutritional intake and daily physical activity of girls aged 8–11 years old in Makkah, Saudi Arabia according to weight status. *BMC Public Health* **2017**, *17*, 592. [CrossRef]
68. Allafi, A.; Al-Haifi, A.R.; Al-Fayez, M.A.; Al-Athari, B.I.; Al-Ajmi, F.A.; Al-Hazzaa, H.M.; Musaiger, A.O.; Ahmed, F. Physical activity, sedentary behaviours and dietary habits among Kuwaiti adolescents: Gender differences. *Public Health Nutr.* **2013**, *17*, 2045–2052. [CrossRef]
69. Al-Nakeeb, Y.; Lyons, M.; Collins, P.; Al-Nuaim, A.; Al-Hazzaa, H.; Duncan, M.J.; Nevill, A. Obesity, Physical Activity and Sedentary Behavior Amongst British and Saudi Youth: A Cross-Cultural Study. *Int. J. Environ. Res. Public Health* **2012**, *9*, 1490–1506. [CrossRef]
70. Al-Nuaim, A.A.; Al-Nakeeb, Y.; Lyons, M.; Al-Hazzaa, H.M.; Nevill, A.; Collins, P.; Duncan, M.J. The Prevalence of Physical Activity and Sedentary Behaviours Relative to Obesity among Adolescents from Al-Ahsa, Saudi Arabia: Rural versus Urban Variations. *J. Nutr. Metab.* **2012**, *2012*, 1–9. [CrossRef] [PubMed]
71. Al-Sobayel, H.; Al-Hazzaa, H.M.; Abahussain, N.A.A.; Qahwaji, D.M.; Musaiger, A.O. Gender differences in leisure-time versus non-leisure-time physical activity among Saudi adolescents. *Ann. Agric. Environ. Med.* **2015**, *22*, 344–348. [CrossRef]
72. Altintaş, A.; Aşçi, F.H. Physical Self-Esteem of Adolescents with Regard to Physical Activity and Pubertal Status. *Pediatr. Exerc. Sci.* **2008**, *20*, 142–156. [CrossRef]
73. Altıntaş, A.; Aşçı, F.H.; Kin-İşler, A.; Güven-Karahan, B.; Kelecek, S.; Özkan, A.; Yılmaz, A.; Kara, F.M. The role of physical activity, body mass index and maturity status in body-related perceptions and self-esteem of adolescents. *Ann. Hum. Biol.* **2013**, *41*, 395–402. [CrossRef]
74. Amini, M.; Djazayery, A.; Majdzadeh, R.; Taghdisi, M.-H.; Sadrzadeh-Yeganeh, H.; Abdollahi, Z.; Hosseinpour-Niazi, N.; Chamari, M.; Nourmohammadi, M. A School-Based Intervention to Reduce Excess Weight in Overweight and Obese Primary School Students. *Biol. Res. Nurs.* **2016**, *18*, 531–540. [CrossRef] [PubMed]
75. Amiri, P.; Jalali-Farahani, S.; Zarkesh, M.; Barzin, M.; Kaviani, R.; Ahmadizad, S. Reliability and validity of the Iranian version of the QAPACE in adolescents. *Qual. Life Res.* **2014**, *23*, 1797–1802. [CrossRef]
76. Ardestani, M.; Niknami, S.; Hidarnia, A.; Hajizadeh, E. Predictors of Physical Activity among Adolescent Girl Students Based on the Social Cognitive Theory. *J. Res. Health Sci.* **2015**, *15*, 223–227. [PubMed]

77. Ardestani, M.; Niknami, S.; Hidarnia, A.; Hajizadeh, E. Psychometric properties of the Socail Cognitive Theory questionnaire for physical activity in a sample of Iranian adolescent girl students. *East. Mediterr. Health J.* **2016**, *22*, 318–326. [CrossRef] [PubMed]
78. Ardic, A.; Erdogan, S. The effectiveness of the COPE healthy lifestyles TEEN program: A school-based intervention in middle school adolescents with 12-month follow-up. *J. Adv. Nurs.* **2016**, *73*, 1377–1389. [CrossRef]
79. Aviram, R.; Harries, N.; Rabani, A.S.; Amro, A.; Nammourah, I.; Al-Jarrah, M.; Raanan, Y.; Hutzler, Y.; Bar-Haim, S. Comparison of Habitual Physical Activity and Sedentary Behavior in Adolescents and Young Adults with and Without Cerebral Palsy. *Pediatr. Exerc. Sci.* **2019**, *31*, 60–66. [CrossRef]
80. Azabdaftari, F.; Jafarpour, P.; Asghari-Jafarabadi, M.; Shokrvash, B.; Reyhani, P. Unrestricted prevalence of sedentary behaviors from early childhood. *BMC Public Health* **2020**, *20*, 255. [CrossRef] [PubMed]
81. Azadbakht, L.; Akbari, F.; Qorbani, M.; Motlagh, M.E.; Ardalan, G.; Heshmat, R.; Daneshzad, E.; Kelishadi, R. Dinner consumption and cardiovascular disease risk factors among a nationally representative sample of Iranian adolescents: The CASPIAN-III Study. *J. Cardiovasc. Thorac. Res.* **2019**, *11*, 138–146. [CrossRef]
82. Bagherniya, M.; Darani, F.M.; Sharma, M.; Maracy, M.R.; Birgani, R.A.; Ranjbar, G.; Taghipour, A.; Safraian, M.; Keshavarz, S.A. Assessment of the Efficacy of Physical Activity Level and Lifestyle Behavior Interventions Applying Social Cognitive Theory for Overweight and Obese Girl Adolescents. *J. Res. Health Sci.* **2018**, *18*, e00409.
83. Bagherniya, M.; Sharma, M.; Mostafavi, F.; Keshavarz, S.A. Application of Social Cognitive Theory in Predicting Childhood Obesity Prevention Behaviors in Overweight and Obese Iranian Adolescents. *Int. Q. Community Health Educ.* **2015**, *35*, 133–147. [CrossRef]
84. Baradaran Mahdavi, S.; Bolourinejad, P.; Heshmat, R.; Motlagh, M.E.; Ziaodini, H.; Taheri, M.; Ahadi, Z.; Qorbani, M.; Kelishadi, R. Association of Sedentary Leisure Time with School Performance in Children and Adolescents: The CASPI-AN-V Study. *Int. J. Pediatr.* **2019**. [CrossRef]
85. Mahdavi, S.B.; Mansourian, M.; Shams, E.; Qorbani, M.; Heshmat, R.; Motlagh, M.E.; Ziaodini, H.; Dashti, R.; Taheri, M.; Kelishadi, R. Association of Sunlight Exposure with Sleep Hours in Iranian Children and Adolescents: The CASPIAN-V Study. *J. Trop. Pediatr.* **2019**, *66*, 4–14. [CrossRef]
86. Bathrellou, E.; Lazarou, C.; Panagiotakos, D.B.; Sidossis, L.S. Physical Activity Patterns and Sedentary Behaviors of Children from Urban and Rural Areas of Cyprus. *Central Eur. J. Public Health* **2007**, *15*, 66–70. [CrossRef]
87. Baygi, F.; Dorosty, A.R.; Kelishadi, R.; Qorbani, M.; Asayesh, H.; Mansourian, M.; Mirkarimi, K. Determinants of Childhood Obesity in Representative Sample of Children in North East of Iran. *Cholesterol* **2012**, *2012*, 1–5. [CrossRef]
88. Baygi, F.; Heshmat, R.; Kelishadi, R.; Mohammadi, F.; Motlagh, M.E.; Ardalan, G.; Asayesh, H.; Larijani, B.; Qorbani, M. Regional Disparities in Sedentary Behaviors and Meal Frequency in Iranian Adolescents: The CASPIAN-III Study. *Iran. J. Pediatr.* **2015**, *25*, e182. [CrossRef]
89. Bicer, A.H.; Alsaffar, A.A. Dietary intake and physical activity levels of male adolescents with autism spectrum disorder (ASD) and normal to high body mass index (BMI)—A case series study. *Res. Autism Spectr. Disord.* **2016**, *31*, 1–10. [CrossRef]
90. Bucksch, J.; Sigmundova, D.; Hamrik, Z.; Troped, P.J.; Melkevik, O.; Ahluwalia, N.; Borraccino, A.; Tynjälä, J.; Kalman, M.; Inchley, J. International Trends in Adolescent Screen-Time Behaviors From 2002 to 2010. *J. Adolesc. Health* **2016**, *58*, 417–425. [CrossRef] [PubMed]
91. Camliguney, A.F.; Mengutay, S.; Pehlivan, A. Differences in Physical Activity Levels in 8-10 Year-old Girls Who Attend Physical Education Classes Only and Those Who Also Regularly Perform Extracurricular Sports Activities. *Procedia-Soc. Behav. Sci.* **2012**, *46*, 4708–4712. [CrossRef]
92. Cengiz, C.; Ince, M.L. Impact of Social-Ecologic Intervention on Physical Activity Knowledge and Behaviors of Rural Students. *J. Phys. Act. Health* **2014**, *11*, 1565–1572. [CrossRef] [PubMed]
93. Cermak, S.A.; Katz, N.; Weintraub, N.; Steinhart, S.; Raz-Silbiger, S.; Munoz, M.; Lifshitz, N. Participation in Physical Activity, Fitness, and Risk for Obesity in Children with Developmental Coordination Disorder: A Cross-cultural Study. *Occup. Ther. Int.* **2015**, *22*, 163–173. [CrossRef]
94. Chacar, H.R.; Salameh, P. Public schools adolescents' obesity and growth curves in Lebanon. *Leban. Med. J.* **2011**, *103*, 1–9.
95. Dagci, G.; Saygin, Ö. Investigation of Physical Activity Levels and Body Compositions of Adolescent Boys and Girls. *Stud. Ethno-Med.* **2015**, *9*, 385–390. [CrossRef]
96. Daşkapan, A.; Şanlı, C.; Aydoğan-Arslan, S.; Çiledağ-Özdemir, F.; Korkem, D.; Kara, U. Evaluation of the functional capacity, respiratory functions and musculoskeletal systems of the children with chest pain for non-cardiac reasons. *Turk. J. Pediatr.* **2017**, *59*, 295–303. [CrossRef] [PubMed]
97. Davidsson, L.; Al-Ghanim, J.; Al-Ati, T.; Al-Hamad, N.; Al-Mutairi, A.; Al-Olayan, L.; Preston, T. Total Energy Expenditure in Obese Kuwaiti Primary School Children Assessed by the Doubly-Labeled Water Technique. *Int. J. Environ. Res. Public Health* **2016**, *13*, 1007. [CrossRef] [PubMed]
98. De Bourdeaudhuij, I.; Verbestel, V.; De Henauw, S.; Maes, L.; Huybrechts, I.; Mårild, S.; Eiben, G.; Moreno, L.A.; Barba, G.; Kovács, É.; et al. Behavioural effects of a community-oriented setting-based intervention for prevention of childhood obesity in eight European countries. Main results from the IDEFICS study. *Obes. Rev.* **2015**, *16* (Suppl. S2), 30–40. [CrossRef]
99. Dianat, I.; Alipour, A.; Jafarabadi, M.A. Prevalence and risk factors of low back pain among school age children in Iran. *Health Promot. Perspect.* **2017**, *7*, 223–229. [CrossRef]

100. Didarloo, A.; Sharafkhani, N.; Shahnazi, H.; Sorkhabi, Z.; Sheikhi, S. Application of Theory of Planned Behavior to Improve Obesity-Preventive Lifestyle among Students: A School-based Interventional Study. *Int. J. Pediatr.* **2017**. [CrossRef]
101. Doaei, S.; Jarrahi, S.; Torki, S.; Haghshenas, R.; Jamshidi, Z.; Rezaei, S.; Moslem, A.; Ghorat, F.; Khodabakhshi, A.; Gholamalizadeh, M. Serum vitamin D level may be associated with body weight and body composition in male adolescents; a longitudinal study. *Pediatr. Endocrinol. Diabetes Metab.* **2020**, *26*, 125–131. [CrossRef] [PubMed]
102. Doğan, M.; Derman, O.; Kanbur, N.; Akgül, S.; Kutluk, T. The effects of nutrition and physical activity on bone development in male adolescents. *Turk. J. Pediatr.* **2010**, *51*, 545–550.
103. Duncan, M.J.; Al-Hazzaa, H.M.; Al-Nakeeb, Y.; Al-Sobayel, H.I.; Abahussain, N.A.; Musaiger, A.O.; Lyons, M.; Collins, P.; Nevill, A. Anthropometric and lifestyle characteristics of active and inactive Saudi and British adolescents. *Am. J. Hum. Biol.* **2014**, *26*, 635–642. [CrossRef]
104. Edalati, S.; Bagherzadeh, F.; Jafarabadi, M.A.; Ebrahimi-Mamaghani, M. Higher ultra-processed food intake is associated with higher DNA damage in healthy adolescents. *Br. J. Nutr.* **2020**, *125*, 568–576. [CrossRef]
105. Ejtahed, H.-S.; Mahmoodi, Z.; Qorbani, M.; Angoorani, P.; Motlagh, M.E.; Hasani-Ranjbar, S.; Ziaodini, H.; Taheri, M.; Heshmat, R.; Kelishadi, R. A comparison between body mass index and waist circumference for identifying continuous metabolic syndrome risk score components in Iranian school-aged children using a structural equation modeling approach: The CASPIAN-V study. *Eat. Weight. Disord.-Stud. Anorexia Bulim. Obes.* **2020**, *26*, 1609–1616. [CrossRef]
106. Eliacik, K.; Bolat, N.; Koçyiğit, C.; Kanik, A.; Selkie, E.; Yilmaz, H.; Catli, G.; Dundar, N.O.; Dundar, B.N. Internet addiction, sleep and health-related life quality among obese individuals: A comparison study of the growing problems in adolescent health. *Eat. Weight. Disord.-Stud. Anorexia, Bulim. Obes.* **2016**, *21*, 709–717. [CrossRef] [PubMed]
107. Elkholy, T.; Hassanen, N.H.M.; Rasha, M.H. Demographic, Socio-Economic Factors and Physical Activity Affecting the Nutritional Status of Young Children Under Five Years. *Life Sci.* **2012**, *9*, 3604–3614.
108. Erturan, G.; McBride, R.; Agbuga, B. Self-regulation and self-efficacy as mediators of achievement goals and leisure time physical activity: A proposed model. *Pedagog. Phys. Cult. Sports* **2019**, *24*, 12–20. [CrossRef]
109. Esatbeyoğlu, F.; İşler, A.K. Physical Activity Levels, BMI and Healthy Life Style Behaviors in Adolescents Living in a Rural District. *Turk. Klin. J. Sports Sci.* **2018**, *10*, 9–18. [CrossRef]
110. Esmaeilzadeh, S.; Ebadollahzadeh, K. Physical Fitness, Physical Activity and Sedentary Activities of 7 to 11 Year Old Boys with Different Body Mass Indexes. *Asian J. Sports Med.* **2012**, *3*, 105–112. [CrossRef]
111. Faridizad, R.; Ahadi, Z.; Heshmat, R.; Motlagh, M.E.; Sheidaei, A.; Ziaodini, H.; Taheri, M.; Qorbani, M.; Mahdavi, S.B.; Kelishadi, R. Association of screen time with subjective health complaints in Iranian school-aged children and adolescents: The CASPIAN-V study. *J. Public Health* **2019**, *28*, 31–40. [CrossRef]
112. Fazah, A.; Jacob, C.; Moussa, E.; El-Hage, R.; Youssef, H.; Delamarche, P. Activity, inactivity and quality of life among Lebanese adolescents. *Pediatr. Int.* **2009**, *52*, 573–578. [CrossRef]
113. Gencer-Atalay, K.; Karadag-Saygi, E.; Uzuncakmak, B.; Keskin, A.; Furtun, Y.; Guven, H.; Uzunoglu, I.; Kurtel, H. Daily Physical Activity in Children and Adolescents with Low Lumbar and Sacral Level Myelomeningocele. *Dev. Neurorehabilit.* **2020**, *24*, 145–149. [CrossRef]
114. Ghavamzadeh, S.; Khalkhali, H.R.; Alizadeh, M. TV Viewing, Independent of Physical Activity and Obesogenic Foods, Increases Overweight and Obesity in Adolescents. *J. Health Popul. Nutr.* **2013**, *31*, 334–342. [CrossRef] [PubMed]
115. Ghobadi, S.; Faghih, S. Eating breakfast and snacks while television viewing are associated with some cardio metabolic risk factors among Iranian children. *Diabetes Metab. Syndr. Clin. Res. Rev.* **2018**, *12*, 235–243. [CrossRef] [PubMed]
116. Faghih, S.; Ghobadi, S.; Rostami, Z.H.; Marzijarani, M.S. Association of vitamin D status and metabolic syndrome components in Iranian children. *Int. J. Prev. Med.* **2019**, *10*, 77. [CrossRef] [PubMed]
117. Ghobadi, S.; Zepetnek, J.O.T.d.; Hemmatdar, Z.; Bellissimo, N.; Barati, R.; Ahmadnia, H.; Salehi-Marzijarani, M.; Faghih, S. Association between overweight/obesity and eating habits while watching television among primary-school children in the city of Shiraz, Iran. *Public Health Nutr.* **2017**, *21*, 571–579. [CrossRef]
118. Güvenç, A.; Açikada, C.; Aslan, A.; Ozer, K. Daily Physical Activity and Physical Fitness in 11-to 15-year-old Trained and Untrained Turkish Boys. *J. Sports Sci. Med.* **2011**, *10*, 502–514.
119. Güvenç, A.; Aslan, A.; Açıkada, C. Objectively measured activity in 8–10-year-old Turkish children: Relationship to health-related fitness. *Pediatr. Int.* **2013**, *55*, 629–636. [CrossRef]
120. Hajian-Tilaki, K.; Heidari, B. Prevalences of overweight and obesity and their association with physical activity pattern among Iranian adolescents aged 12–17 years. *Public Health Nutr.* **2012**, *15*, 2246–2252. [CrossRef]
121. Hajian-Tilaki, K.; Heidari, B. Childhood Obesity, Overweight, Socio-Demographic and Life Style Determinants among Preschool Children in Babol, Northern Iran. *Iran. J. Public Health* **2013**, *42*, 1283–1291.
122. Hamaideh, S.H.; Al-Khateeb, R.Y.; Al-Rawashdeh, A.B. Overweight and Obesity and Their Correlates Among Jordanian Adolescents. *J. Nurs. Sch.* **2010**, *42*, 387–394. [CrossRef]
123. Hashem, R.; Rey-López, J.P.; Hamer, M.; McMunn, A.; Whincup, P.H.; Owen, C.G.; Rowlands, A.; Stamatakis, E. Physical Activity and Sedentary Behaviors Levels of Kuwaiti Adolescents: The Study of Health and Activity Among Adolescents in Kuwait. *J. Phys. Act. Health* **2018**, *15*, 255–262. [CrossRef]

124. Hashem, R.; Rey-López, J.P.; Hamer, M.; McMunn, A.; Rowlands, A.; Whincup, P.H.; Owen, C.G.; Ding, D.; Powell, L.; Stamatakis, E. Associations between objectively assessed and questionnaire-based sedentary behaviour with body mass index and systolic blood pressure in Kuwaiti adolescents. *BMC Res. Notes* **2019**, *12*, 588. [CrossRef] [PubMed]
125. Hassan, M.; Al-Kharusy, W. Physical fitness and fatness among Omani schoolboys: A pilot study. *J. Sci. Res.* **2000**, *2*, 37–41.
126. Hawi, N.S.; Rupert, M.S. Impact of e-Discipline on Children's Screen Time. *Cyberpsychol. Behav. Soc. Netw.* **2015**, *18*, 337–342. [CrossRef] [PubMed]
127. Henry, C.J.K.; Lightowler, H.J.; Al-Hourani, H.M. Physical activity and levels of inactivity in adolescent females ages 11–16 years in the United Arab Emirates. *Am. J. Hum. Biol.* **2004**, *16*, 346–353. [CrossRef] [PubMed]
128. Hovsepian, S.; Kelishadi, R.; Motlagh, M.E.; Kasaeian, A.; Shafiee, G.; Arefirad, T.; Najafi, F.; Khoramdad, M.; Asayesh, H.; Heshmat, R.; et al. Level of physical activity and screen time among Iranian children and adolescents at the national and provincial level: The CASPIAN-IV study. *Med. J. Islam. Repub. Iran* **2016**, *30*, 422.
129. Jalali-Farahani, S.; Amiri, P.; Chin, Y.S. Are physical activity, sedentary behaviors and sleep duration associated with body mass index-for-age and health-related quality of life among high school boys and girls? *Health Qual. Life Outcomes* **2016**, *14*, 1–9. [CrossRef]
130. Jalilpiran, Y.; Mozaffari, H.; Askari, M.; Jafari, A.; Azadbakht, L. The association between Healthy Beverage Index and anthropometric measures among children: A cross-sectional study. *Eat. Weight. Disord.-Stud. Anorexia, Bulim. Obes.* **2020**, *26*, 1437–1445. [CrossRef]
131. Kalantari, N.; Mohammadi, N.K.; Izadi, P.; Gholamalizadeh, M.; Doaei, S.; Eini-Zinab, H.; Salonurmi, T.; Rafieifar, S.; Janipoor, R.; Tabesh, G.A. A complete linkage disequilibrium in a haplotype of three SNPs in Fat Mass and Obesity associated (FTO) gene was strongly associated with anthropometric indices after controlling for calorie intake and physical activity. *BMC Med Genet.* **2018**, *19*, 146. [CrossRef]
132. Karaca, A.; Caglar, E.; Bilgili, N.; Ayaz, S. Screen time of adolescents in an economically developing country: The case of Turkey. *Ann. Hum. Biol.* **2010**, *38*, 28–33. [CrossRef]
133. Kelishadi, R. Association of physical activity and dietary behaviours in relation to the body mass index in a national sample of Iranian children and adolescents: CASPIAN Study. *Bull. World Health Organ.* **2007**, *85*, 19–26. [CrossRef]
134. Kelishadi, R.; Heidari, Z.; Kazemi, I.; Jafari-Koshki, T.; Mansourian, M.; Motlagh, M.-E.; Heshmat, R. A hierarchical Bayesian tri-variate analysis on factors associated with anthropometric measures in a large sample of children and adolescents: The CASPIAN-IV study. *J. Pediatr. Endocrinol. Metab.* **2018**, *31*, 443–449. [CrossRef]
135. Kelishadi, R.; Mirghaffari, N.; Poursafa, P.; Gidding, S.S. Lifestyle and environmental factors associated with inflammation, oxidative stress and insulin resistance in children. *Atherosclerosis* **2009**, *203*, 311–319. [CrossRef]
136. Kerkadi, A.; Sadig, A.H.; Bawadi, H.; Al Thani, A.A.M.; Al Chetachi, W.; Akram, H.; Al-Hazzaa, H.M.; Musaiger, A.O. The Relationship between Lifestyle Factors and Obesity Indices among Adolescents in Qatar. *Int. J. Environ. Res. Public Health* **2019**, *16*, 4428. [CrossRef]
137. Khader, Y.; Irshaidat, O.; Khasawneh, M.; Amarin, Z.; Alomari, M.; Batieha, A. Overweight and Obesity Among School Children in Jordan: Prevalence and Associated Factors. *Matern. Child Health J.* **2008**, *13*, 424–431. [CrossRef] [PubMed]
138. Khayyatzadeh, S.S.; Vatanparast, H.; Avan, A.; Bagherniya, M.; Bahrami, A.; Kiani, M.A.; Bahrami-Taghanaki, H.; Ferns, G.A.; Ghayour-Mobarhan, M. Serum Transaminase Concentrations and the Presence of Irritable Bowel Syndrome Are Associated with Serum 25-Hydroxy Vitamin D Concentrations in Adolescent Girls Who Are Overweight and Obese. *Ann. Nutr. Metab.* **2017**, *71*, 234–241. [CrossRef] [PubMed]
139. Khoo, S.; Al-Shamli, A.K. Leisure-Time Physical Activity and Physical Fitness of Male Adolescents in Oman. *Asia Pac. J. Public Health* **2010**, *24*, 128–135. [CrossRef]
140. Kilani, H.; Al-Hazzaa, H.; Waly, M.I.; Musaiger, A. Lifestyle Habits: Diet, Physical Activity and Sleep Duration among Omani Adolescents. *SQUMJ* **2013**, *13*, 510–519. [CrossRef] [PubMed]
141. Isler, A.K.; Asci, F.H.; Altintas, A.; Guven-Karahan, B. Physical activity levels and patterns of 11–4 year-old Turkish adolescents. *Adolescence* **2009**, *44*, 1005–1015.
142. Koçak, S.; Harris, M.B.; İşler, A.K.; Çiçek, Ş. Physical Activity Level, Sport Participation, and Parental Education Level in Turkish Junior High School Students. *Pediatr. Exerc. Sci.* **2002**, *14*, 147–154. [CrossRef]
143. Kocaoglu, B.; Manios, Y.; Dimitriou, M.; Kolotourou, M.; Keskin, Y.; Sur, H.; Hayran, O.; Manios, Y. Parental educational level and cardiovascular disease risk factors in schoolchildren in large urban areas of Turkey: Directions for public health policy. *BMC Public Health* **2005**, *5*, 13. [CrossRef]
144. Kondolot, M.; Poyrazoğlu, S.; Horoz, D.; Borlu, A.; Altunay, C.; Balcı, E.; Öztürk, A.; Mazıcıoğlu, M.M.; Kurtoğlu, S. Risk factors for overweight and obesity in children aged 2–6 years. *J. Pediatr. Endocrinol. Metab.* **2017**, *30*, 499–505. [CrossRef]
145. Kovács, E.; on behalf of the IDEFICS consortium; Siani, A.; Konstabel, K.; Hadjigeorgiou, C.; de Bourdeaudhuij, I.; Eiben, G.; Lissner, L.; Gwozdz, W.; Reisch, L.; et al. Adherence to the obesity-related lifestyle intervention targets in the IDEFICS study. *Int. J. Obes.* **2014**, *38*, S144–S151. [CrossRef]
146. Lazarou, C.; Matalas, A.-L. Breakfast intake is associated with nutritional status, Mediterranean diet adherence, serum iron and fasting glucose: The CYFamilies study. *Public Health Nutr.* **2014**, *18*, 1308–1316. [CrossRef] [PubMed]
147. Lazarou, C.; Panagiotakos, D.B.; Kouta, C.; Matalas, A.-L. Dietary and other lifestyle characteristics of Cypriot school children: Results from the nationwide CYKIDS study. *BMC Public Health* **2009**, *9*, 147. [CrossRef] [PubMed]

148. Loucaides, C.A. Seasonal differences in segmented-day physical activity and sedentary behaviour in primary school children. *Early Child Dev. Care* **2016**, *188*, 410–420. [CrossRef]
149. A Loucaides, C. Screen time behaviour in a sample of 11- to 12-year-old Greek-Cypriot children: A cross-sectional study of parental and child reports. *SAGE Open Med.* **2020**, *8*. [CrossRef]
150. Loucaides, C.A.; Chedzoy, S.M.; Bennett, N. Differences in physical activity levels between urban and rural school children in Cyprus. *Health Educ. Res.* **2004**, *19*, 138–147. [CrossRef] [PubMed]
151. Loucaides, C.A.; Jago, R. Correlates of Pedometer-Assessed Physical Activity in Cypriot Elementary School Children. *J. Phys. Act. Health* **2006**, *3*, 267–276. [CrossRef]
152. Loucaides, C.A.; Jago, R. Differences in physical activity by gender, weight status and travel mode to school in Cypriot children. *Prev. Med.* **2008**, *47*, 107–111. [CrossRef]
153. A Loucaides, C.; Jago, R.; Theophanous, M. Physical activity and sedentary behaviours in Greek-Cypriot children and adolescents: A cross-sectional study. *Int. J. Behav. Nutr. Phys. Act.* **2011**, *8*, 90. [CrossRef]
154. Manios, Y.; Dimitriou, M.; Moschonis, G.; Kocaoglu, B.; Sur, H.; Keskin, Y.; Hayran, O. Cardiovascular disease risk factors among children of different socioeconomic status in Istanbul, Turkey: Directions for public health and nutrition policy. *Lipids Health Dis.* **2004**, *3*, 11. [CrossRef] [PubMed]
155. Manios, Y.; Kolotourou, M.; Moschonis, G.; Sur, H.; Keskin, Y.; Kocaoglu, B.; Hayran, O. Macronutrient intake, physical activity, serum lipids and increased body weight in primary schoolchildren in Istanbul. *Pediatr. Int.* **2005**, *47*, 159–166. [CrossRef] [PubMed]
156. Marashi, T.; Safari-Moradabadi, A.; Ahmadi, F.; Alipour-Anbarani, M. The effect of education based on the theory of planned behavior on the promotion of physical activity and knowledge of students about diabetes prevention. *Int. J. Health Promot. Educ.* **2020**, *60*, 316–328. [CrossRef]
157. Mehranfar, S.; Jalilpiran, Y.; Surkan, P.J.; Azadbakht, L. Association between protein-rich dietary patterns and anthropometric measurements among children aged 6 years. *Nutr. Diet.* **2020**, *77*, 359–367. [CrossRef] [PubMed]
158. Miri, S.F.; Javadi, M.; Lin, C.-Y.; Griffiths, M.D.; Björk, M.; Pakpour, A.H. Effectiveness of cognitive-behavioral therapy on nutrition improvement and weight of overweight and obese adolescents: A randomized controlled trial. *Diabetes Metab. Syndr. Clin. Res. Rev.* **2019**, *13*, 2190–2197. [CrossRef]
159. Mohammadifard, N.; Mahdavi, A.; Khosravi, A.; Esmaillzadeh, A.; Feizi, A.; Sarrafzadegan, N. Salt intake and its sources in children, adolescents and adults in the Islamic Republic of Iran. *East. Mediterr. Health J.* **2021**, *27*, 279–286. [CrossRef]
160. Mohseni-Takalloo, S.; Mirmiran, P.; Hosseini-Esfahani, F.; Mehrabi, Y.; Azizi, F. Metabolic Syndrome and its Association with Healthy Eating Index-2005 in Adolescents: Tehran Lipid and Glucose Study. *J. Food Nutr. Res.* **2014**, *2*, 155–161. [CrossRef]
161. Moludi, J.; Ebrahimi, B.; Maleki, V.; Saiedi, S.; Tandoroost, A.; Jafari-Vayghyan, H.; Alizadeh, S.; Djafarian, K. Comparison of Dietary Macro and Micronutrient Intake with Physical Activity Levels among Children with and without Autism: A Case-Control Study. *Prog. Nutr.* **2020**, *21*, 49–55. [CrossRef]
162. Moradi, G.; Mostafavi, F.; Piroozi, B.; Zareie, B.; Mahboobi, M.; Rasouli, M.A. The prevalence of physical inactivity in Iranian adolescents and the impact of economic and social inequalities on it: Results of a National Study in 2018. *BMC Public Health* **2020**, *20*, 1499. [CrossRef]
163. Moradi-Lakeh, M.; El Bcheraoui, C.; Tuffaha, M.; Daoud, F.; Al Saeedi, M.; Basulaiman, M.; Memish, Z.A.; Al Mazroa, M.A.; Al Rabeeah, A.A.; Mokdad, A.H. The health of Saudi youths: Current challenges and future opportunities. *BMC Fam. Pr.* **2016**, *17*, 26. [CrossRef]
164. Motamed-Gorji, N.; Qorbani, M.; Nikkho, F.; Asadi, M.; Motlagh, M.E.; Safari, O.; Arefirad, T.; Asayesh, H.; Mohammadi, R.; Mansourian, M.; et al. Association of screen time and physical activity with health-related quality of life in Iranian children and adolescents. *Health Qual. Life Outcomes* **2019**, *17*, 1–11. [CrossRef] [PubMed]
165. Mozafarian, N.; Kelishadi, R.; Motlagh, M.E.; Maracy, M. Propensity Score Application in the Relationship of Screen Time and Metabolic Syndrome in Adolescents: The CASPIAN-III Study. *Int. J. Pediatr.* **2016**, *4*. [CrossRef]
166. Mozaffari, H.; Nabaei, B. Obesity and related risk factors. *Indian J. Pediatr.* **2007**, *74*, 265–267. [CrossRef] [PubMed]
167. Musaiger, A.O.; Al-Mufty, B.A.; Al-Hazzaa, H.M. Eating Habits, Inactivity, and Sedentary Behavior among Adolescents in Iraq: Sex Differences in the Hidden Risks of Noncommunicable Diseases. *Food Nutr. Bull.* **2014**, *35*, 12–19. [CrossRef] [PubMed]
168. Najafabadi, M.G.; Memari, A.-H.; Kordi, R.; Shayestehfar, M.; Eshghi, M.-A. Mental training can improve physical activity behavior in adolescent girls. *J. Sport Health Sci.* **2017**, *6*, 327–332. [CrossRef]
169. Naseri, P.; Amiri, P.; Momenyan, S.; Zayeri, F.; Karimi, M.; Azizi, F. Longitudinal association between body mass index and physical activity among adolescents with different parental risk: A parallel latent growth curve modeling approach. *Int. J. Behav. Nutr. Phys. Act.* **2020**, *17*, 1–13. [CrossRef]
170. Nasreddine, L.; Naja, F.; Akl, C.; Chamieh, M.C.; Karam, S.; Sibai, A.-M.; Hwalla, N. Dietary, Lifestyle and Socio-Economic Correlates of Overweight, Obesity and Central Adiposity in Lebanese Children and Adolescents. *Nutrients* **2014**, *6*, 1038–1062. [CrossRef]
171. Nejadsadeghi, E.; Sadeghi, R.; Shojaeizadeh, D.; Yekaninejad, M.S.; Djazayeri, A.; Majlesi, F. Influence of lifestyle factors on Body Mass Index in preschoolers in Behbahan city, southwest Iran, 2016. *Electron. Physician* **2018**, *10*, 6725–6732. [CrossRef]

172. Nemet, D.; Barkan, S.; Epstein, Y.; Friedland, O.; Kowen, G.; Eliakim, A. Short- and Long-Term Beneficial Effects of a Combined Dietary–Behavioral–Physical Activity Intervention for the Treatment of Childhood Obesity. *Pediatrics* **2005**, *115*, e443–e449. [CrossRef]
173. Nemet, D.; Levi, L.; Pantanowitz, M.; Eliakim, A. A combined nutritional-behavioral-physical activity intervention for the treatment of childhood obesity—A 7-year summary. *J. Pediatr. Endocrinol. Metab.* **2014**, *27*, 445–451. [CrossRef]
174. Tehrani, A.N.; Farhadnejad, H.; Salehpour, A.; Beyzai, B.; Hekmatdoost, A.; Rashidkhani, B. The association between nutrition knowledge and adherence to a Mediterranean dietary pattern in Iranian female adolescents. *Int. J. Adolesc. Med. Health* **2019**, *33*, 20180188. [CrossRef] [PubMed]
175. Ng, S.W.; Zaghloul, S.; Ali, H.; Harrison, G.; Yeatts, K.; El Sadig, M.; Popkin, B.M. Nutrition transition in the United Arab Emirates. *Eur. J. Clin. Nutr.* **2011**, *65*, 1328–1337. [CrossRef] [PubMed]
176. Kaluski, D.N.; Mazengia, G.D.; Shimony, T.; Goldsmith, R.; Berry, E.M. Prevalence and determinants of physical activity and lifestyle in relation to obesity among schoolchildren in Israel. *Public Health Nutr.* **2009**, *12*, 774–782. [CrossRef]
177. Nozari, R.A.; Farshbaf-Khalili, A.; Sattarzadeh, N.; Jafarabadi, M.A. The Effect of Counseling on Menstrual Hygiene, Physical Activity, and Nutritional Status of Female Adolescent Students: A Randomized Controlled Field Trial. *CJMB* **2019**, *6*, 393–402.
178. Okur, E.O.; Inal-Ince, D.; Saglam, M.; Vardar-Yagli, N.; Arikan, H. Physical activity patterns in children with cerebral palsy and typically developing peers. *Physiother. Theory Pr.* **2019**, *37*, 710–718. [CrossRef] [PubMed]
179. Olafsdottir, S.; Berg, C.; Eiben, G.; Lanfer, A.; Reisch, L.; Ahrens, W.; Kourides, Y.; Molnár, D.; A Moreno, L.; Siani, A.; et al. Young children's screen activities, sweet drink consumption and anthropometry: Results from a prospective European study. *Eur. J. Clin. Nutr.* **2013**, *68*, 223–228. [CrossRef]
180. Özmert, E.N.; Özdemir, R.; Pektaş, A.; Üçkardeş, Y.; Yurdakök, K. Effect of activity and television viewing on BMI z-score in early adolescents in Turkey. *World J. Pediatr.* **2010**, *7*, 37–40. [CrossRef] [PubMed]
181. Pinhas-Hamiel, O.; Bar-Zvi, E.; Boyko, V.; Reichman, B.; Lerner-Geva, L. Prevalence of overweight in kindergarten children in the centre of Israel - association with lifestyle habits. *Child: Care Health Dev.* **2009**, *35*, 147–152. [CrossRef]
182. Platat, C.; Jarrar, A. Reliability and validity of a physical activity questionnaire in children. *Int. J. Food Sci. Nutr.* **2011**, *63*, 637–644. [CrossRef]
183. Qahwaji, D. Physical activity and life style among Male Adolescents in Jeddah, Saudi Arabia. *Life Sci.* **2012**, *9*, 1163–1172.
184. Rahimi, H.; Yuzbashian, E.; Zareie, R.; Asghari, G.; Djazayery, A.; Movahedi, A.; Mirmiran, P. Dietary approaches to stop hypertension (DASH) score and obesity phenotypes in children and adolescents. *Nutr. J.* **2020**, *19*, 1–9. [CrossRef]
185. Raz-Silbiger, S.; Lifshitz, N.; Katz, N.; Steinhart, S.; Cermak, S.; Weintraub, N. Relationship between motor skills, participation in leisure activities and quality of life of children with Developmental Coordination Disorder: Temporal aspects. *Res. Dev. Disabil.* **2015**, *38*, 171–180. [CrossRef] [PubMed]
186. Kazemi, A.; Rostamian, M. Relationship between observational learning and health belief with physical activity among adolescents girl in Isfahan, Iran. *Iran. J. Nurs. Midwifery Res.* **2016**, *21*, 601–604. [CrossRef]
187. Rostami-Moez, M.; Hazavehei, S.M.M.; Karami, M.; Karimi-Shahanjarini, A.; Nazem, F.; Rezapur-Shahkolai, F. Decline in Physical Activity Among Iranian Girl Students Aged 10 to 16 and the Related Factors. *Health Scope* 2017, *in press*. [CrossRef]
188. Safiri, S.; Kelishadi, R.; Qorbani, M.; Abbasi-Ghah-Ramanloo, A.; Motlagh, M.E.; Ardalan, G.; Shafiee, G.; Ahadi, Z.; Sanaei, M.; Asayesh, H.; et al. Screen Time and its Relation to Cardiometabolic Risk among Children and Adolescents: The CASPIAN-III Study. *Iran. J. Public Health* **2015**, *44*, 35–44.
189. Saglam, D.; Samur, G.; Turan, S. Assessment of Vitamin D Status in Turkish Adolescents: Its Relation to Obesity, Car-diometabolic Risk Factors and Nutritional Status. *Progr. Nutr.* **2019**, *21*, 762–768. [CrossRef]
190. Salamoun, M.M.; Kizirian, A.S.; I Tannous, R.; Nabulsi, M.M.; Choucair, M.K.; E Deeb, M.; Fuleihan, G.A.E.-H. Low calcium and vitamin D intake in healthy children and adolescents and their correlates. *Eur. J. Clin. Nutr.* **2004**, *59*, 177–184. [CrossRef] [PubMed]
191. Sanaeinasab, H.; Saffari, M.; Nazeri, M.; Zarchi, A.K.; Cardinal, B.J. Descriptive analysis of Iranian adolescents' stages of change for physical activity behavior. *Nurs. Health Sci.* **2012**, *15*, 280–285. [CrossRef]
192. Sanaeinasab, H.; Tavakoli, R.; Karimizarchi, A.; Amini, Z.H.; Farokhian, A.; Najarkolaei, F.R. The Effectiveness of Education Using the Health Belief Model in Preventing Osteoporosis among Female Students. *EMHJ* **2014**, *19*, S38–S44. [CrossRef]
193. Sarsour, A.; Turban, M.; Al Wahaidi, A.; Abed, Y.; Alkahlout, H. Does gender influence food intake and physical activity pattern among Palestinian adolescents in the Gaza Strip? *East. Mediterr. Health J.* **2019**, *25*, 722–727. [CrossRef]
194. Saygin, O. Physical Activity Level and Obesity Prevalence of Primary and Secondary Students. *Anthropologist* **2014**, *18*, 371–377. [CrossRef]
195. Saygin, O.; Zorba, E.; Karacabey, K.; Mengutay, S. Gender and Maturation Differences in Health-Related Physical Fitness and Physical Activity in Turkish Children. *Pak. J. Biol. Sci.* **2007**, *10*, 1963–1969. [CrossRef]
196. Sedaghat, F.; Naja, F.; Darand, M.; Beyzai, B.; Rashidkhani, B. Adherence to a Mediterranean dietary pattern and overweight and obesity among female adolescents in Iran. *Int. J. Adolesc. Med. Health* **2017**, *31*. [CrossRef] [PubMed]
197. Sherman, G.; Nemet, D.; Moshe, V.; Consolaro, A.; Ravelli, A.; Ruperto, N.; Uziel, Y.; Paediatric Rheumatology International Trials Organisation (PRINTO). Disease activity, overweight, physical activity and screen time in a cohort of patients with juvenile idiopathic arthritis. *Clin. Exp. Rheumatol.* **2018**, *36*, 1110–1116.

198. Shokrvash, B.; Majlessi, F.; Montazeri, A.; Nedjat, S.; Rahimi, A.; Djazayeri, A.; Shojaeezadeh, D. Correlates of physical activity in adolescence: A study from a developing country. *Glob. Health Action* **2013**, *6*, 20327. [CrossRef] [PubMed]
199. Simsek, S.; Inal-Ince, D.; Cakmak, A.; Emiralioglu, N.; Calik-Kutukcu, E.; Saglam, M.; Vardar-Yagli, N.; Ozcelik, H.U.; Sonbahar-Ulu, H.; Bozdemir-Ozel, C.; et al. Reduced anaerobic and aerobic performance in children with primary ciliary dyskinesia. *Eur. J. Pediatr.* **2018**, *177*, 765–773. [CrossRef]
200. Smith, E.; Fazeli, F.; Wilkinson, K.; Clark, C.C.T. Physical behaviors and fundamental movement skills in British and Iranian children: An isotemporal substitution analysis. *Scand. J. Med. Sci. Sports* **2020**, *31*, 398–404. [CrossRef]
201. Soltanian, A.R.; Amiri, M.; Namazi, S.; Qaedi, H.; Kohan, G.R. Mental Health Changes and Its Predictors in Adolescents using the Path Analytic Model: A 7-Year Observational Study. *Iran. J. Psychiatry* **2014**, *9*, 1–7.
202. Sourtiji, H.; Hosseini, S.A.; Rassafiani, M.; Kohan, A.; Noroozi, M.; Motlagh, M.E. The Associations Between Screen Time, Sleep Duration, and Body Mass Index (BMI) in Under Five-Year-Old Children. *Arch. Neurosci.* **2018**, in press. [CrossRef]
203. Sur, H.; Kolotourou, M.; Dimitriou, M.; Kocaoglu, B.; Keskin, Y.; Hayran, O.; Manios, Y. Biochemical and behavioral indices related to BMI in schoolchildren in urban Turkey. *Prev. Med.* **2005**, *41*, 614–621. [CrossRef]
204. Tarakci, E.; Yeldan, I.; Mutlu, E.K.; Baydogan, S.N.; Kasapcopur, O. The relationship between physical activity level, anxiety, depression, and functional ability in children and adolescents with juvenile idiopathic arthritis. *Clin. Rheumatol.* **2011**, *30*, 1415–1420. [CrossRef]
205. Taymoori, P.; Berry, T.R.; Lubans, D.R. Tracking of physical activity during middle school transition in Iranian adolescents. *Health Educ. J.* **2011**, *71*, 631–641. [CrossRef]
206. Taymoori, P.; Lubans, D.R. Mediators of behavior change in two tailored physical activity interventions for adolescent girls. *Psychol. Sport Exerc.* **2008**, *9*, 605–619. [CrossRef]
207. Taymoori, P.; Niknami, S.; Berry, T.; Ghofranipour, F.; Kazemnejad, A. Application of the Health Promotion Model to Predict Stages of Exercise Behaviour in Iranian Adolescents. *EMHJ* **2009**, *15*, 1215–1225.
208. Taymoori, P.; Rhodes, R.E.; Berry, T.R. Application of a social cognitive model in explaining physical activity in Iranian female adolescents. *Health Educ. Res.* **2008**, *25*, 257–267. [CrossRef] [PubMed]
209. Tayyem, R.; Al-Hazzaa, H.; Abumweis, S.; Bawadi, H.; Musaiger, A.; Qatatsheh, A. Association of Lifestyle Factors with Obesity Indices among Adolescents Living in Amman. *MJN* **2014**, *20*, 51–62.
210. Tayyem, R.F.; Al-Hazzaa, H.M.; Abu-Mweis, S.S.; Bawadi, H.A.; Hammad, S.S.; Musaiger, A.O. Dietary Habits and Pysical Activity Levels in Jordanian Adolescents Attending Private versus Public Schools. *EMHJ* **2014**, *20*, 416–423. [PubMed]
211. Teber, S.; Saglam, M.; Ertugrul, I.; Vardar-Yagli, N.; Cakmak, A.; Calik-Kutukcu, E.; Inal-Ince, D.; Arikan, H.; Karagoz, T. Levels of Physical Activity and Physical Fitness in Pediatric Pacemaker Patients: A Cross-Sectional Study. *Pediatr. Cardiol.* **2020**, *41*, 1363–1369. [CrossRef]
212. Haghparast, A.; Rohani, C.; Vasli, P.; Salmani, F.; Marzaleh, M.A. the Effect of two educational methods of lecturing and peer group on physical activity among 12–15-year-old students in health promoting schools. *Iran. Red Crescent Med J.* **2020**, *22*. [CrossRef]
213. Yiallouros, P.K.; Economou, M.; Kolokotroni, O.; Savva, S.C.; Gavatha, M.; Ioannou, P.; Karpathios, T.; Middleton, N. Gender differences in objectively assessed physical activity in asthmatic and non-asthmatic children. *Pediatr. Pulmonol.* **2014**, *50*, 317–326. [CrossRef]
214. Yilmaz, G.; Caylan, N.D.; Karacan, C.D. An intervention to preschool children for reducing screen time: A randomized controlled trial. *Child: Care, Health Dev.* **2014**, *41*, 443–449. [CrossRef] [PubMed]
215. Yurdakul, H.; Baydemir, B. Comparison of physical activity and skinfold thickness of students living in rural and city center. *Pedagog. Phys. Cult. Sports* **2020**, *24*, 271–277. [CrossRef]
216. Sasaki, J.E.; John, D.; Freedson, P.S. Validation and comparison of ActiGraph activity monitors. *J. Sci. Med. Sport* **2011**, *14*, 411–416. [CrossRef] [PubMed]
217. Klippel, N.J.; Heil, D.P.F. Validation of energy expenditure prediction algorithms in adults using the actical electronic activity monitor. *Med. Sci. Sports Exerc.* **2003**, *35*, S284. [CrossRef]
218. Yegian, A.K.; Heymsfield, S.B.; Lieberman, D.E. Historical body temperature records as a population-level 'thermometer' of physical activity in the United States. *Curr. Biol.* **2021**, *31*, R1375–R1376. [CrossRef]
219. Epstein, L.H.; Paluch, R.A.; Kalakanis, L.E.; Goldfield, G.S.; Cerny, F.J.; Roemmich, J.N. How Much Activity Do Youth Get? A Quantitative Review of Heart-Rate Measured Activity. *Pediatrics* **2001**, *108*, e44. [CrossRef] [PubMed]
220. Brusseau, T.; Kulinna, P.; Tudor-Locke, C.; van der Mars, H.; Darst, P. Children's Step Counts on Weekend, Physical Education, and Non-Physical Education Days. *J. Hum. Kinet.* **2011**, *27*, 123–134. [CrossRef]
221. Telford, R.M.; Telford, R.D.; Olive, L.S.; Cochrane, T.; Davey, R. Why Are Girls Less Physically Active than Boys? Findings from the LOOK Longitudinal Study. *PLoS ONE* **2016**, *11*, e0150041. [CrossRef]
222. Colley, R.C.; Garriguet, D.; Janssen, I.; Craig, C.L.; Clarke, J.; Tremblay, M.S. Physical activity of Canadian children and youth: Accelerometer results from the 2007 to 2009 Canadian Health Measures Survey. *Health Rep.* **2011**, *22*, 15–23.
223. Duncan, M.J.; Al-Nakeeb, Y.; Woodfield, L.; Lyons, M. Pedometer determined physical activity levels in primary school children from central England. *Prev. Med.* **2007**, *44*, 416–420. [CrossRef] [PubMed]
224. Belton, S.; Brady, P.; Meegan, S.; Woods, C. Pedometer step count and BMI of Irish primary school children aged 6–9 years. *Prev. Med.* **2010**, *50*, 189–192. [CrossRef] [PubMed]

225. Mendonça, G.; Cheng, L.A.; Mélo, E.N.; de Farias Júnior, J.C. Physical activity and social support in adolescents: A systematic review. *Health Educ. Res.* **2014**, *29*, 822–839. [CrossRef] [PubMed]
226. Babic, M.J.; Morgan, P.J.; Plotnikoff, R.C.; Lonsdale, C.; White, R.L.; Lubans, D.R. Physical activity and physical self-concept in youth: Systematic review and meta-analysis. *Sports Med.* **2014**, *44*, 1589–1601. [CrossRef] [PubMed]
227. Bauman, A.; Bull, F.; Chey, T.; Craig, C.L.; Ainsworth, E.B.; Sallis, J.F.; Bowles, H.R.; Hagstromer, M.; Sjostrom, M.; Pratt, M.; et al. The International Prevalence Study on Physical Activity: Results from 20 countries. *Int. J. Behav. Nutr. Phys. Act.* **2009**, *6*, 21. [CrossRef] [PubMed]
228. Biddle, S.J.H.; Gorely, T.; Marshall, S.J. Is Television Viewing a Suitable Marker of Sedentary Behavior in Young People? *Ann. Behav. Med.* **2009**, *38*, 147–153. [CrossRef]
229. Clark, B.K.; Healy, G.N.; Winkler, E.A.H.; Gardiner, P.A.; Sugiyama, T.; Dunstan, D.W.; Matthews, C.E.; Owen, N. Relationship of Television Time with Accelerometer-Derived Sedentary Time. *Med. Sci. Sports Exerc.* **2011**, *43*, 822–828. [CrossRef]
230. Minton, H.A.M.; Thevenet-Morrison, K.; Fernandez, I.D. Using Television-Viewing Hours and Total Hours Sitting as Interchangeable Measures of Sedentary Behavior. *Am. J. Lifestyle Med.* **2016**, *13*, 98–105. [CrossRef]
231. Mullan, K. Technology and Children's Screen-Based Activities in the UK: The Story of the Millennium So Far. *Child Indic. Res.* **2017**, *11*, 1781–1800. [CrossRef]
232. Thomas, G.; Bennie, J.A.; De Cocker, K.; Castro, O.; Biddle, S.J.H. A Descriptive Epidemiology of Screen-Based Devices by Children and Adolescents: A Scoping Review of 130 Surveillance Studies Since 2000. *Child Indic. Res.* **2019**, *13*, 935–950. [CrossRef]
233. Sibai, A.M.; Semaan, A.; Tabbara, J.; Rizk, A. Ageing and health in the Arab region: Challenges, opportunities and the way forward. *Popul. Horizons* **2017**, *14*, 73–84. [CrossRef]
234. Sharara, E.; Akik, C.; Ghattas, H.; Obermeyer, C.M. Physical inactivity, gender and culture in Arab countries: A systematic assessment of the literature. *BMC Public Health* **2018**, *18*, 639. [CrossRef] [PubMed]

MDPI AG
Grosspeteranlage 5
4052 Basel
Switzerland
Tel.: +41 61 683 77 34

International Journal of Environmental Research and Public Health Editorial Office
E-mail: ijerph@mdpi.com
www.mdpi.com/journal/ijerph

www.ingramcontent.com/pod-product-compliance
Lightning Source LLC
Chambersburg PA
CBHW061605210926
51850CB00009B/2216
* 9 7 8 3 7 2 5 8 7 7 2 7 0 *